Arthritis Sourcebook

Basic Consumer Health Information about Specific Forms of Arthritis and Related Disorders, Including Rheumatoid Arthritis, Osteoarthritis, Gout, Polymyalgia Rheumatica, Psoriatic Arthritis, Spondyloarthropathies, Juvenile Rheumatoid Arthritis, and Juvenile Ankylosing Spondylitis; Along with Information about Medical, Surgical, and Alternative Treatment Options, and Including Strategies for Coping with Pain, Fatigue, and Stress

Edited by Allan R. Cook. 575 pages. 1998. 0-7808-0201-2. $78.

Back & Neck Disorders Sourcebook

Basic Information about Disorders and Injuries of the Spinal Cord and Vertebrae, Including Facts on Chiropractic Treatment, Surgical Interventions, Paralysis, and Rehabilitation, Along with Advice for Preventing Back Trouble

Edited by Karen Bellenir. 548 pages. 1997. 0-7808-0202-0. $78.

"The strength of this work is its basic, easy-to-read format. Recommended."
— *Reference and User Services Quarterly, Winter '97*

Blood & Circulatory Disorders Sourcebook

Basic Information about Blood and Its Components, Anemias, Leukemias, Bleeding Disorders, and Circulatory Disorders, Including Aplastic Anemia, Thalassemia, Sickle-Cell Disease, Hemochromatosis, Hemophilia, Von Willebrand Disease, and Vascular Diseases; Along with a Special Section on Blood Transfusions and Blood Supply Safety, a Glossary, and Source Listings for Further Help and Information

Edited by Karen Bellenir and Linda M. Shin. 575 pages. 1998. 0-7808-0203-9. $78.

Brain Disorders Sourcebook

Basic Consumer Health Information about Strokes, Epilepsy, Amyotrophic Lateral Sclerosis (ALS/Lou Gehrig's Disease), Parkinson's Disease, Brain Tumors, Cerebral Palsy, Headache, Tourette Syndrome, and More; Along with Statistical Data, Treatment and Rehabilitation Options, Coping Strategies, Reports on Current Research Initiatives, a Glossary, and Resource Listings for Additional Help and Information

Edited by Karen Bellenir. 600 pages. 1999. 0-7808-0229-2. $78.

Burns S

Basic Infor... Scalds, Inc... and Sun; ... ments, Ti... Prevention Suggestions, and First Aid

Edited by Allan R. Cook. 600 pages. 1999. 0-7808-0204-7. $78.

Cancer Sourcebook, 1st Edition

Basic Information on Cancer Types, Symptoms, Diagnostic Methods, and Treatments, Including Statistics on Cancer Occurrences Worldwide and the Risks Associated with Known Carcinogens and Activities

Edited by Frank E. Bair. 932 pages. 1990. 1-55888-888-8. $78.

"Written in nontechnical language. Useful for patients, their families, medical professionals, and librarians."
— *Guide to Reference Books, '96*

"Designed with the non-medical professional in mind. Libraries and medical facilities interested in patient education should certainly consider adding the *Cancer Sourcebook* to their holdings. This compact collection of reliable information . . . is an invaluable tool for helping patients and patients' families and friends to take the first steps in coping with the many difficulties of cancer."
— *Medical Reference Services Quarterly, Winter '91*

"Specifically created for the nontechnical reader . . . an important resource for the general reader trying to understand the complexities of cancer."
— *American Reference Books Annual, '91*

"This publication's nontechnical nature and very comprehensive format make it useful for both the general public and undergraduate students." — *Choice, Oct '90*

New Cancer Sourcebook, 2nd Edition

Basic Information about Major Forms and Stages of Cancer, Featuring Facts about Primary and Secondary Tumors of the Respiratory, Nervous, Lymphatic, Circulatory, Skeletal, and Gastrointestinal Systems, and Specific Organs; Statistical and Demographic Data; Treatment Options; and Strategies for Coping

Edited by Allan R. Cook. 1,313 pages. 1996. 0-7808-0041-9. $78.

"This book is an excellent resource for patients with newly diagnosed cancer and their families. The dialogue is simple, direct, and comprehensive. Highly recommended for patients and families to aid in their understanding of cancer and its treatment."
— *Booklist Health Sciences Supplement, Oct '97*

"The amount of factual and useful information is extensive. The writing is very clear, geared to general readers. Recommended for all levels." — *Choice, Jan '97*

Continues next page

Cancer Sourcebook, 3rd Edition

Basic Information about Major Forms and Stages of Cancer, Featuring Facts about Primary and Secondary Tumors of the Respiratory, Nervous, Lymphatic, Circulatory, Skeletal, and Gastrointestinal Systems, and Specific Organs, Statistical and Demographic Data, Treatment Options, and Strategies for Coping

Edited by Edward J. Prucha. 800 pages. 1999. 0-7808-0227-6. $78.

Cancer Sourcebook for Women

Basic Information about Specific Forms of Cancer That Affect Women, Featuring Facts about Breast Cancer, Cervical Cancer, Ovarian Cancer, Cancer of the Uterus and Uterine Sarcoma, Cancer of the Vagina, and Cancer of the Vulva; Statistical and Demographic Data; Treatments, Self-Help Management Suggestions, and Current Research Initiatives

Edited by Allan R. Cook and Peter D. Dresser. 524 pages. 1996. 0-7808-0076-1. $78.

"... written in easily understandable, non-technical language. Recommended for public libraries or hospital and academic libraries that collect patient education or consumer health materials."
— *Medical Reference Services Quarterly, Spring '97*

"Would be of value in a consumer health library. . . . written with the health care consumer in mind. Medical jargon is at a minimum, and medical terms are explained in clear, understandable sentences."
— *Bulletin of the MLA, Oct '96*

"The availability under one cover of all these pertinent publications, grouped under cohesive headings, makes this certainly a most useful sourcebook."
— *Choice, Jun '96*

"Presents a comprehensive knowledge base for general readers. Men and women both benefit from the gold mine of information nestled between the two covers of this book. Recommended."
— *Academic Library Book Review, Summer '96*

"This timely book is highly recommended for consumer health and patient education collections in all libraries."
— *Library Journal, Apr '96*

Cancer Sourcebook for Women, 2nd Edition

Basic Information about Specific Forms of Cancer That Affect Women, Featuring Facts about Breast Cancer, Cervical Cancer, Ovarian Cancer, Cancer of the Uterus and Uterine Sarcoma, Cancer of the Vagina, and Cancer of the Vulva, Statistical and Demographic Data, Treatments, Self-Help Management Suggestions, and Current Research Initiatives

Edited by Edward J. Prucha. 600 pages. 1999. 0-7808-0226-8. $78.

Cardiovascular Diseases & Disorders Sourcebook

Basic Information about Cardiovascular Diseases and Disorders, Featuring Facts about the Cardiovascular System, Demographic and Statistical Data, Descriptions of Pharmacological and Surgical Interventions, Lifestyle Modifications, and a Special Section Focusing on Heart Disorders in Children

Edited by Karen Bellenir and Peter D. Dresser. 683 pages. 1995. 0-7808-0032-X. $78.

". . . comprehensive format provides an extensive overview on this subject."
— *Choice, Jun '96*

". . . an easily understood, complete, up-to-date resource. This well executed public health tool will make valuable information available to those that need it most, patients and their families. The typeface, sturdy non-reflective paper, and library binding add a feel of quality found wanting in other publications. Highly recommended for academic and general libraries. "
— *Academic Library Book Review, Summer '96*

Communication Disorders Sourcebook

Basic Information about Deafness and Hearing Loss, Speech and Language Disorders, Voice Disorders, Balance and Vestibular Disorders, and Disorders of Smell, Taste, and Touch

Edited by Linda M. Ross. 533 pages. 1996. 0-7808-0077-X. $78.

"This is skillfully edited and is a welcome resource for the layperson. It should be found in every public and medical library."
— *Booklist Health Sciences Supplement, Oct '97*

Congenital Disorders Sourcebook

Basic Information about Disorders Acquired during Gestation, Including Spina Bifida, Hydrocephalus, Cerebral Palsy, Heart Defects, Craniofacial Abnormalities, Fetal Alcohol Syndrome, and More, Along with Current Treatment Options and Statistical Data

Edited by Karen Bellenir. 607 pages. 1997. 0-7808-0205-5. $78.

"Recommended reference source." — *Booklist, Oct '97*

Consumer Issues in Health Care Sourcebook

Basic Information about Health Care Fundamentals and Related Consumer Issues, Including Exams and Screening Tests, Physician Specialties, Choosing a Doctor, Using Prescription and Over-the-Counter Medications Safely, Avoiding Health Scams, Managing Common Health Risks in the Home, Care Options for Chronically or Terminally Ill Patients, and a List of Resources for Obtaining Help and Further Information

Edited by Karen Bellenir. 592 pages. 1998. 0-7808-0221-7. $78.

Continues in back end sheets

Alzheimer's Disease SOURCEBOOK

Second Edition

Health Reference Series

Second Edition

Alzheimer's Disease SOURCEBOOK

*Basic Consumer Health Information about
Alzheimer's Disease, Related Disorders, and
Other Dementias, Including Multi-Infarct
Dementia, AIDS-Related Dementia, Alcoholic
Dementia, Huntington's Disease, Delirium,
and Confusional States; Along with Reports
Detailing Current Research Efforts in
Prevention and Treatment, Long-Term
Care Issues, and Listings of Sources for
Additional Help and Information*

Edited by
Karen Bellenir

Omnigraphics, Inc.

Penobscot Building / Detroit, MI 48226

BIBLIOGRAPHIC NOTE

Because this page cannot legibly accommodate all the copyright notices, the Bibliographic Note portion of the Preface constitutes an extension of the copyright notice.

Beginning with books published in 1999, each volume of the *Health Reference Series* on a new topic will be individually titled and called a "First Edition." Subsequent updates will carry sequential edition numbers. To help avoid confusion and to provide maximum flexibility in our ability to respond to informational needs, the practice of consecutively numbering each volume will be discontinued.

Edited by Karen Bellenir
Peter D. Dresser, Managing Editor, *Health Reference Series*

Omnigraphics, Inc.
Tamekia Nichole Ashford, *Production Associate*
Matthew P. Barbour, *Manager, Production and Fulfillment*
Laurie Lanzen Harris, *Vice President, Editorial Director*
Joan Margeson, *Research Associate*
Margaret Mary Missar, *Research Coordinator*
Peter E. Ruffner, *Vice President, Administration*
James A. Sellgren, *Vice President, Operations and Finance*
Jane J. Steele, *Marketing Consultant*
Jenifer Swanson, *Research Associate*

Robert R. Tyler, Executive Vice President and Associate Publisher
Frederick G. Ruffner, Jr., Publisher

©1999, Omnigraphics, Inc.

Library of Congress Cataloging-in-Publication Data

Alzheimer's disease sourcebook / (edited by Karen Bellenir). -- 2nd ed.
    p. cm. -- (Health reference series ; v. 46) Includes bibliographical references and index.
    ISBN 0-7808-0223-3 (lib. bdg. ; alk. paper)
    1. Alzheimer's disease--Popular works.
    2. Dementia-- Popular works. I. Bellenir, Karen
II. Series.
RC523.2.A45 1999   98-51624
616.8'31--dc21   CIP

∞

This book is printed on acid-free paper meeting the ANSI Z39.48 Standard. The infinity symbol that appears above indicates that the paper in this book meets that standard.

Printed in the United States

Table of Contents

Preface

About This Book

Alzheimer's disease is not a normal part of aging; it is not something that inevitably happens in later life. Rather, it is a type of dementing disorder that affects a small but significant percentage of older Americans. Only five to six percent of older people are afflicted with Alzheimer's disease or a related dementia, but this means approximately three to four million Americans have one of these debilitating disorders. The annual economic toll of Alzheimer's disease in the United States in terms of health care expenses and lost wages of both patients and their caregivers is estimated at $80 to $100 billion.

Although much is still unknown about Alzheimer's disease, researchers have made significant progress in their efforts to identify some of its causes and risk factors. Many are working to find ways to slow its progression, delay its onset, or prevent it altogether. Investigators hope to unravel the mystery of what happens in the brain causing some nerve cells to lose their ability to communicate with each other. Other researchers seek to identify diagnostic markers of dementias and improve tests to determine the causes of mental declines. Scientists are also looking for better ways to treat the symptoms of Alzheimer's disease and improve the daily lives of patients with the disorder.

This *Sourcebook* will help readers recognize the warning signs of Alzheimer's disease and the symptoms of other dementias, including multi-infarct dementia, AIDS-related dementia, alcoholic dementia,

Huntington's disease, Binswanger's disease, metachromatic leukod-ystrophy, Pick's disease, corticobasal degeneration, delirium, and con-fusional states. It provides information to help patients and their families understand the differences between reversible and irrevers-ible causes of dementia, comprehend the results of current research initiatives, and know what to expect as Alzheimer's disease progresses. A glossary and resource listings provide additional sources of help and information.

How to Use This Book

This book is divided into parts and chapters. Parts focus on broad areas of interest. Chapters are devoted to single topics within a part.

Part I: Alzheimer's Disease provides general and statistical informa-tion about Alzheimer's disease and its warning signs. To help read-ers understand the disease process, it begins with an overview of normal brain functioning.

Part II: Other Dementias and Related Disorders describes types of non-Alzheimer's dementia and disorders that may be mistaken for Alzheimer's disease. These include multi-infarct dementia, cerebral atrophy, Huntington's disease, AIDS-related dementia, alcoholic de-mentia, and delirium.

Part III: Prevention and Treatment Research offers information about genetic, neurological, and pharmacological research initiatives focused on understanding, preventing, diagnosing, and treating Alzheimer's disease and its symptoms. Information about the Autopsy Assistance Network is included to assist families who may be considering an autopsy or the possibility of tissue donation for Alzheimer's disease research.

Part IV: Long-Term Care Issues gives caregivers and family members helpful information for coping with the day-to-day challenges of car-ing for someone with Alzheimer's disease.

Part V: Additional Help and Information provides a glossary of im-portant terms, a guide to federal programs for Alzheimer's disease, lists of state Agencies on Aging and long-term care ombudsman pro-grams, a directory of additional resources, and a list of reading ma-terials for Alzheimer's disease patients, family members, and caregivers.

Bibliographic Note

This volume contains documents and excerpts from publications issued by the following U.S. government agencies: Administration on Aging (AoA), Agency for Health Care Policy and Research (AHCPR), Alzheimer's Disease Education and Referral (ADEAR) Center, Health Care Financing Administration (HCFA), National Institute of Mental Health (NIMH), National Institute of Neurological Disorders and Stroke (NINDS), National Institute of Nursing Research (NINR), and the National Institute on Aging (NIA).

In addition, this volume contains copyrighted documents from the following organizations: Alzheimer's Association Autopsy Assistance Network, Alzheimer's Disease and Related Disorders Association, American Association of Homes and Services for the Aging, Dana Alliance, and Duke University Medical Center. Copyrighted articles from *AIDS Weekly Plus*; *American Family Physician; British Medical Journal; Journal of Neurology, Neurosurgery, and Psychiatry*; and *Patient Care* are also included. Full citation information is provided on the first page of each chapter. Every effort has been made to secure all necessary rights to reprint the copyrighted material. If any omissions have been made, please contact Omnigraphics to make corrections for future editions.

Acknowledgements

In addition to the many organizations listed above that provided the material presented in this volume, special thanks are due to researchers Margaret Mary Missar and Jenifer Swanson, permissions specialist Maria Franklin, verification assistant Dawn Matthews, indexer Edward J. Prucha, and document engineer Bruce Bellenir.

Note from the Editor

This book is part of Omnigraphics' *Health Reference Series*. The series provides basic consumer health information about a broad range of medical concerns. It is not intended to serve as a tool for diagnosing illness, in prescribing treatments, or as a substitute for the physician/patient relationship. All persons concerned about medical symptoms or the possibility of disease are encouraged to seek professional care from an appropriate health care provider.

Our Advisory Board

The *Health Reference Series* is reviewed by an Advisory Board comprised of librarians from public, academic, and medical libraries. We would like to thank the following board members for providing guidance to the development of this series:

Nancy Bulgarelli
William Beaumont Hospital Library, Royal Oak, MI

Karen Morgan
Mardigian Library, University of Michigan, Dearborn, MI

Rosemary Orlando
St. Clair Shores Public Library, St. Clair Shores, MI

Health Reference Series *Update Policy*

The inaugural book in the *Health Reference Series* was the first edition of *Cancer Sourcebook* published in 1992. Since then, the *Series* has been enthusiastically received by librarians and in the medical community. In order to maintain the standard of providing high-quality health information for the lay person, the editorial staff at Omnigraphics felt it was necessary to implement a policy of updating volumes when warranted.

Medical researchers have been making tremendous strides, and the challenge to stay current with the most recent advances is one our editors take seriously. Each decision to update a volume will be made on an individual basis. Some of the considerations will include how much new information is available and the feedback we receive from people who use the books. If there's a topic you would like to see added to the update list, or an area of medical concern you feel has not been adequately addressed, please write to:

Editor
Health Reference Series
Omnigraphics, Inc.
2500 Penobscot Bldg.
Detroit, MI 48226

The commitment to providing on-going coverage of important medical developments has also led to some technical changes in the *Health Reference Series*. Beginning with books published in 1999, each volume on a new topic will be individually titled and called a "First Edition." Subsequent updates will carry sequential edition numbers. To help avoid confusion and to provide maximum flexibility in our ability to respond to informational needs, the practice of consecutively numbering each volume will be discontinued.

Part One

Alzheimer's Disease

Chapter 1

Understanding How Your Brain Works

The brain is the most complex part of the human body. This three-pound organ is the seat of intelligence, the interpreter of the senses, the initiator of body movement, and the controller of behavior. Lying in its bony shell and washed by protective fluid, the brain is the source of all the qualities that define our humanity. The brain is the crown jewel of the human body.

For centuries, scientists and philosophers have been fascinated by the brain, but until recently they viewed the brain as nearly incomprehensible. Now, however, the brain is beginning to relinquish its secrets. Scientists have learned more about the brain in the last 10 years than in all the previous centuries of study due to the accelerating pace of neurological and behavioral science and the development of new research techniques. As a result, Congress has named the 1990s the Decade of the Brain. At the forefront of research on the brain and other elements of the nervous system is the National Institute of Neurological Disorders and Stroke (NINDS), which conducts and supports scientific studies in the United States and around the world.

This chapter is a basic introduction to the human brain. It may help you understand how the healthy brain works, how to keep it healthy, and what happens when the brain is diseased or dysfunctional.

"Know Your Brain," NIH Pub. No. 92-3440-2, 1992.

The Architecture of the Brain

The brain is like a committee of experts. All the parts of the brain work together, but each part has its own special properties. The brain can be divided into three basic units: the forebrain, the midbrain, and the hindbrain.

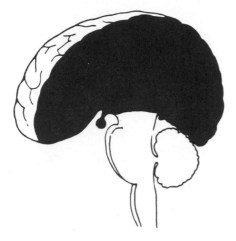

Figure 1.1. *The Forebrain.*

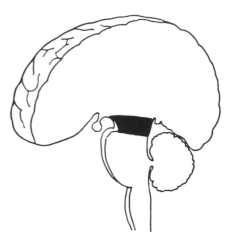
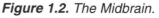

Figure 1.2. *The Midbrain.*

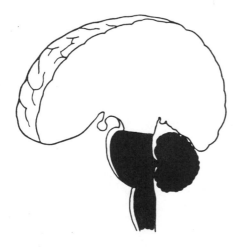

Figure 1.3. *The Hindbrain.*

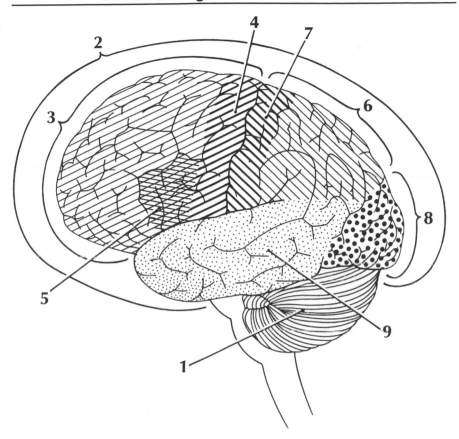

Figure 1.4. *The architecture of the brain.*

The hindbrain includes the upper part of the spinal cord, the brain stem, and a wrinkled ball of tissue called the **cerebellum** (1). The hindbrain controls the body's vital functions such as respiration and heart rate. The cerebellum is responsible for learned rote movements. When you play the piano or hit a tennis ball you are activating the cerebellum. Above the hindbrain lies the midbrain, which controls some reflex actions and is part of the circuit responsible for voluntary movements. The forebrain is the largest and most highly developed part of the human brain: it consists primarily of the **cerebrum** (2) and the structures hidden beneath it (see "The Inner Brain").

When people see pictures of the brain it is usually the cerebrum that they notice. The cerebrum sits at the topmost part of the brain and is the source of intellectual activities. It holds your memories, allows you to plan, enables you to imagine and think. It allows you to recognize friends, read books, and play games.

The cerebrum is split into two halves (hemispheres) by a deep fissure. Despite the split, the two cerebral hemispheres communicate with each other through a thick tract of nerve fibers that lies at the base of this fissure. Although the two hemispheres seem to be mirror images of each other, they are different. For instance, the ability to form words seems to lie primarily in the left hemisphere, while the right hemisphere seems to control many abstract reasoning skills.

For some as-yet-unknown reason, nearly all of the signals from the brain to the body and vice-versa cross over on their way to and from the brain. This means that the right cerebral hemisphere primarily controls the left side of the body and the left hemisphere primarily controls the right side. When one side of the brain is damaged, the opposite side of the body is affected. For example, a stroke in the right hemisphere of the brain can leave the left side of the body paralyzed.

The Geography of Thought

Each cerebral hemisphere can be divided into sections, or lobes, each of which specializes in different functions. To understand each lobe and its specialty we will take a tour of the cerebral hemispheres, starting with the two **frontal lobes** (3), which lie directly behind the forehead. When you plan a schedule, imagine the future, or use reasoned arguments, these two lobes are working. One of the ways the frontal lobes seem to do these things is by acting as short-term storage sites, allowing one idea to be kept in mind while other ideas are considered. In the rearmost portion of each frontal lobe is a **motor area** (4), which helps control voluntary movement. A nearby place on the left frontal lobe called **Broca's area** (5) allows thoughts to be transformed into words.

When you enjoy a good meal—the taste, aroma, and texture of the food—two sections behind the frontal lobes called the **parietal lobes** (6) are at work. The forward parts of these lobes, just behind the motor areas, are the primary **sensory areas** (7). These areas receive information about temperature, taste, touch, and movement from the rest of the body. Reading and arithmetic are also functions in the repertoire of each parietal lobe.

As you look at the words and pictures on this page, two areas at the back of the brain are at work. These lobes, called the **occipital lobes** (8), process images from the eyes and link that information with images stored in memory. Damage to the occipital lobes can cause blindness.

The last lobes on our tour of the cerebral hemispheres are the **temporal lobes** (9), which lie in front of the visual areas and nest under the parietal and frontal lobes. Whether you appreciate symphonies or rock music, your brain responds through the activity of these lobes. At the top of each temporal lobe is an area responsible for receiving information from the ears. The underside of each temporal lobe plays a crucial role in forming and retrieving memories, including those associated with music. Other parts of this lobe seem to integrate memories and sensations of taste, sound, sight, and touch.

The Cerebral Cortex

Coating the surface of the cerebrum and the cerebellum is a vital layer of tissue the thickness of a stack of two or three dimes. It is called the cortex, from the Latin word for bark. Most of the actual information processing in the brain takes place in the cerebral cortex. When people talk about "gray matter" in the brain they are talking about this thin rind. The cortex is gray because nerves in this area lack the insulation that makes most other parts of the brain appear to be white. The folds in the brain add to its surface area and therefore increase the amount of gray matter and the quantity of information that can be processed.

The Inner Brain

Deep within the brain, hidden from view, lie structures that are the gatekeepers between the spinal cord and the cerebral hemispheres. These structures not only determine our emotional state, they also modify our perceptions and responses depending on that state, and allow us to initiate movements that you make without thinking about them. Like the lobes in the cerebral hemispheres, the structures described below come in pairs: each is duplicated in the opposite half of the brain.

The **hypothalamus** (10), about the size of a pearl, directs a multitude of important functions. It wakes you up in the morning, and gets the adrenalin flowing during a test or job interview. The hypothalamus is also an important emotional center, controlling the molecules that make you feel exhilarated, angry, or unhappy. Near the hypothalamus lies the **thalamus** (11), a major clearinghouse for information going to and from the spinal cord and the cerebrum.

7

An arching tract of nerve cells leads from the hypothalamus and the thalamus to the **hippocampus** (12). This tiny nub acts as a memory indexer—sending memories out to the appropriate part of the cerebral hemisphere for long-term storage and retrieving them when necessary. The **basal ganglia** (not shown) are clusters of nerve cells surrounding the thalamus. They are responsible for initiating and integrating movements. Parkinson's disease, which results in tremors, rigidity, and a stiff, shuffling walk, is a disease of nerve cells that lead into the basal ganglia.

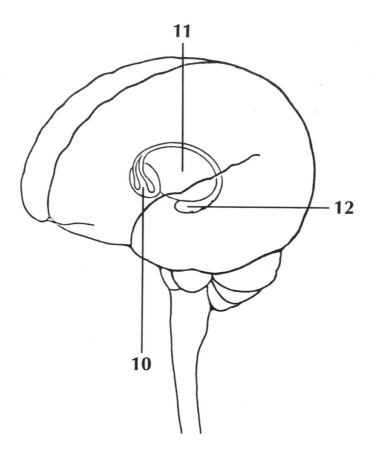

Figure 1.5. *The inner brain.*

Making Connections

The brain and the rest of the nervous system are composed of many different types of cells, but the primary functional unit is a cell called the neuron. All sensations, movements, thoughts, memories, and feelings are the result of signals that pass through neurons. Neurons consist of three parts. The **cell body** (13) contains the nucleus, where most of the molecules that the neuron needs to survive and function are manufactured. **Dendrites** (14) extend out from the cell body like

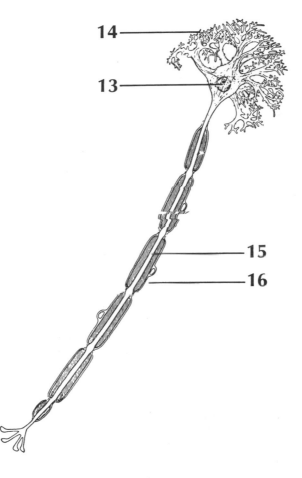

14

13

15

16

Figure 1.6. A neuron.

the branches of a tree and receive messages from other nerve cells. Signals then pass from the dendrites through the cell body and may travel away from the cell body down an **axon** (15) to another neuron, a muscle cell, or cells in some other organ. The neuron is usually surrounded by many support cells. Some types of cells wrap around the axon to form an insulating **sheath** (16). This sheath can include a fatty molecule called myelin, which provides insulation for the axon and helps nerve signals travel faster and farther. Axons may be very short, such as those that carry signals from one cell in the cortex to another cell less than a hair's width away. Or axons may be very long, such as those that carry messages from the brain all the way down the spinal cord.

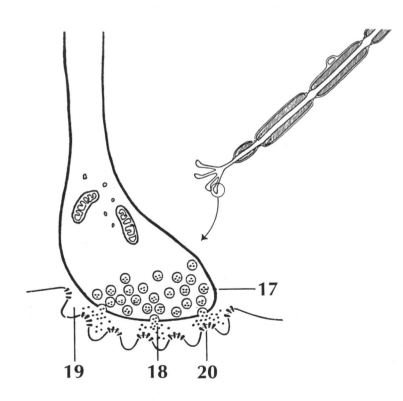

Figure 1.7. The synapse.

Scientists have learned a great deal about neurons by studying the synapse—the place where a signal passes from the neuron to another cell. When the signal reaches the end of the axon it stimulates tiny **sacs** (17). These sacs release chemicals known as **neurotransmitters** (18) into the **synapse** (19). The neurotransmitters cross the synapse and attach to **receptors** (20) on the neighboring cell. These receptors can change the properties of the receiving cell. If the receiving cell is also a neuron, the signal can continue the transmission to the next cell.

Some Key Neurotransmitters at Work

Acetylcholine is called an excitatory neurotransmitter because it generally makes cells more excitable. It governs muscle contractions and causes glands to secrete hormones. Alzheimer's disease, which initially affects memory formation, is associated with a shortage of acetylcholine.

GABA (gamma-aminobutyric acid) is called an inhibitory neurotransmitter because it tends to make cells less excitable. It helps control muscle activity and is an important part of the visual system. Drugs that increase GABA levels in the brain are used to treat epileptic seizures and tremors in patients with Huntington's disease.

Serotonin is an inhibitory neurotransmitter that constricts blood vessels and brings on sleep. It is also involved in temperature regulation. Dopamine is an inhibitory neurotransmitter involved in mood and the control of complex movements. The loss of dopamine activity in some portions of the brain leads to the muscular rigidity of Parkinson's disease. Many medications used to treat behavioral disorders work by modifying the action of dopamine in the brain.

Neurological Disorders

When the brain is healthy it functions quickly and automatically. But when problems occur, the results can be devastating. Some 50 million people in this country—one in five—suffer from damage to the nervous system. The NINDS supports research on more than 600 neurological diseases. Some of the major types of disorders include: neurogenetic diseases (such as Huntington's disease and muscular dystrophy), developmental disorders (such as cerebral palsy), degenerative diseases of adult life (such as Parkinson's disease and Alzheimer's disease), metabolic diseases (such as Gaucher's disease), cerebrovascular diseases (such as stroke and vascular dementia), trauma (such as spinal cord and head injury), convulsive disorders (such as epilepsy), infectious diseases (such as AIDS dementia), and brain tumors.

The National Institute of Neurological Disorders and Stroke

Since its creation by Congress in 1950, the NINDS has grown to become the leading supporter of neurological research in the United States. Most research funded by the NINDS is conducted by scientists in public and private institutions such as universities, medical schools, and hospitals. Government scientists also conduct a wide array of neurological research in the 21 laboratories and branches of the NINDS itself. This research ranges from studies on the structure and function of single brain cells to tests of new diagnostic tools and treatments for those with neurological disorders. For more information, write or call:

Neurological Institute
P.O. Box 5801
Bethesda, MD 20824
Phone: (301) 496-5751
Toll-free number: (800) 352-9424
Fax number: (301) 402-2186

Chapter 2

Is It Alzheimer's? Warning Signs You Should Know

Introduction

- Your wife always misplaces her keys. But last Tuesday, she couldn't remember what they were for.

- Your grandfather likes to take daily strolls around the neighborhood. But four times in the past month he's gotten lost and couldn't find his way home without help from a neighbor.

- Your favorite uncle can't remember your name or the names of your husband or children.

The memory loss, confusion, and disorientation described in these examples are symptoms of dementing illness. The most common dementing illness is Alzheimer's disease.

Unfortunately, many people fail to recognize that these symptoms indicate something is wrong. They may mistakenly assume that such behavior is a normal part of the aging process; it isn't. Or, symptoms may develop gradually and go unnoticed for a long time. Sometimes people refuse to act even when they know something's wrong.

It's important to see a physician when you recognize these symptoms. Only a physician can properly diagnose the person's condition, and sometimes symptoms are reversible. Even if the diagnosis is Alzheimer's disease, help is available to learn how to care for a person with dementia and where to find assistance for yourself, the caregiver.

Is It Alzheimer's? Ten Warning Signs

To help you know what warning signs to look for, the Alzheimer's Association has developed a checklist of common symptoms (some of them also may apply to other dementing illnesses). Review the list and check the symptoms that concern you. If you make several check marks, the individual with the symptoms should see a physician for a complete examination.

1. Recent Memory Loss That Affects Job Skills

It's normal to occasionally forget assignments, colleagues' names, or a business associate's telephone number and remember them later. Those with a dementia, such as Alzheimer's disease, may forget things more often, and not remember them later.

2. Difficulty Performing Familiar Tasks

Busy people can be so distracted from time to time that they may leave the carrots on the stove and only remember to serve them at the end of the meal. People with Alzheimer's disease could prepare a meal and not only forget to serve it, but also forget they made it.

3. Problems with Language

Everyone has trouble finding the right word sometimes, but a person with Alzheimer's disease may forget simple words or substitute inappropriate words, making his or her sentence incomprehensible.

4. Disorientation of Time and Place

It's normal to forget the day of the week or your destination for a moment. But people with Alzheimer's disease can become lost on their own street, not knowing where they are, how they got there or how to get back home.

5. Poor or Decreased Judgment

People can become so immersed in an activity that they temporarily forget the child they're watching. People with Alzheimer's disease could forget entirely the child under their care. They may also dress inappropriately, wearing several shirts or blouses.

6. Problems with Abstract Thinking

Balancing a checkbook may be disconcerting when the task is more complicated than usual. Someone with Alzheimer's disease could forget completely what the numbers are and what needs to be done with them.

7. Misplacing Things

Anyone can temporarily misplace a wallet or keys. A person with Alzheimer's disease may put things in inappropriate places: an iron in the freezer, or a wristwatch in the sugar bowl.

8. Changes in Mood or Behavior

Everyone becomes sad or moody from time to time. Someone with Alzheimer's disease can exhibit rapid mood swings—from calm to tears to anger—for no apparent reason.

9. Changes in Personality

People's personalities ordinarily change somewhat with age. But a person with Alzheimer's disease can change drastically, becoming extremely confused, suspicious, or fearful.

10. Loss of Initiative

It's normal to tire of housework, business activities, or social obligations, but most people regain their initiative. The person with Alzheimer's disease may become very passive and require cues and prompting to become involved.

Questions and Answers about Alzheimer's Disease

Q. What is Alzheimer's disease?

A. Alzheimer's disease is a progressive, degenerative disease of the brain in which brain cells die and are not replaced. It results in impaired memory, thinking, and behavior, and is the most common form of dementing illness.

Q. What are other causes of Alzheimer-like symptoms?

A. Depression, nutritional deficiencies, drug interaction or intoxication, and thyroid imbalances can cause symptoms similar to those related to Alzheimer's disease, and sometimes these symptoms are reversible with a physician's care. Symptoms are also found with dementias associated with stroke, Huntington's disease, Parkinson's disease, Pick's disease, and AIDS.

Q. How prevalent is the disease?

A. An estimated 4 million Americans are afflicted with Alzheimer's disease. It is the fourth leading cause of death among American adults. Because the population is aging, an estimated 14 million will have the disease by the year 2050.

Q. Who is afflicted with Alzheimer's disease?

A. Ten percent of those over 65, and almost half of those over age 85 have the disease. However, because of improved testing and greater public awareness, physicians are seeing an increase in diagnosed patients in their 40s and 50s. Alzheimer's disease strikes equally at men and women, all races, and all socioeconomic groups.

Q. What causes Alzheimer's disease?

A. The causes of Alzheimer's disease are still unknown, and there currently is no cure.

Q. What should I do if I have noticed these symptoms in a loved one?

A. Make an appointment with a physician for a complete examination. Discuss the symptoms you've noticed and your concerns. Your physician may refer you to a neurologist for additional testing.

Q. How is Alzheimer's disease diagnosed?

A. A definitive diagnosis of Alzheimer's disease is only possible with an autopsy. However, there has been enormous progress in diagnostic testing in recent years, leading to 80- to 90-percent accurate diagnoses of Alzheimer's by physicians. There is no single, or simple test to diagnose Alzheimer's disease. A detailed medical history and physical examination are done. Then a series of neurological tests may be conducted over a period of time. The process is intended to rule out any other possible cause of symptoms.

About the Alzheimer's Association

The Alzheimer's Association is the oldest and largest national voluntary organization dedicated to research for the causes, cure, and prevention of Alzheimer's disease and to providing education and support services to Alzheimer's patients, their families, and caregivers.

Founded in 1980 by dedicated family members, the Alzheimer's Association today works through a network of more than 220 local chapters, 2,000 support groups, and 35,000 volunteers. The group is officially known as the Alzheimer's Disease and Related Disorders Association.

The Alzheimer's Association is a major source of funding for Alzheimer's research. It is leading the way in defining and implementing quality of care guidelines for dementia patients. And it provides a wide range of programs and services to support patients and their families.

Information on Alzheimer's disease, current research, patient care, and assistance for family caregivers is available from the Alzheimer's Association. For information, or the location of the chapter nearest you, call: 1 (800) 272-3900.

Alzheimer's Association
919 North Michigan Avenue
Suite 1000
Chicago, IL 60611-1676

Chapter 3

Forgetfulness: It's Not Always What You Think

Many older people worry about becoming more forgetful. They think forgetfulness is the first sign of Alzheimer's disease. In the past, memory loss and confusion were considered a normal part of aging. However, scientists now know that most people remain both alert and able as they age, although it may take them longer to remember things.

A lot of people experience memory lapses. Some memory problems are serious, and others are not. People who have serious changes in their memory, personality, and behavior may suffer from a form of brain disease called dementia. Dementia seriously affects a person's ability to carry out daily activities. Alzheimer's disease is one of many types of dementia.

The term dementia describes a group of symptoms that are caused by changes in brain function. Dementia symptoms may include asking the same questions repeatedly; becoming lost in familiar places; being unable to follow directions; getting disoriented about time, people, and places; and neglecting personal safety, hygiene, and nutrition. People with dementia lose their abilities at different rates.

Dementia is caused by many conditions. Some conditions that cause dementia can be reversed, and others cannot. Further, many different medical conditions may cause symptoms that seem like Alzheimer's disease, but are not. Some of these medical conditions

National Institute on Aging (NIA) *Age Page*, 1996.

may be treatable. Reversible conditions can be caused by a high fever, dehydration, vitamin deficiency and poor nutrition, bad reactions to medicines, problems with the thyroid gland, or a minor head injury. Medical conditions like these can be serious and should be treated by a doctor as soon as possible.

Sometimes older people have emotional problems that can be mistaken for dementia. Feeling sad, lonely, worried, or bored may be more common for older people facing retirement or coping with the death of a spouse, relative, or friend. Adapting to these changes leaves some people feeling confused or forgetful. Emotional problems can be eased by supportive friends and family, or by professional help from a doctor or counselor.

The two most common forms of dementia in older people are Alzheimer's disease and multi-infarct dementia (sometimes called vascular dementia). These types of dementia are irreversible, which means they cannot be cured. In Alzheimer's disease, nerve cell changes in certain parts of the brain result in the death of a large number of cells. Symptoms of Alzheimer's disease begin slowly and become steadily worse. As the disease progresses, symptoms range from mild forgetfulness to serious impairments in thinking, judgment, and the ability to perform daily activities. Eventually, patients may need total care.

In multi-infarct dementia, a series of small strokes or changes in the brain's blood supply may result in the death of brain tissue. The location in the brain where the small strokes occur determines the seriousness of the problem and the symptoms that arise. Symptoms that begin suddenly may be a sign of this kind of dementia. People with multi-infarct dementia are likely to show signs of improvement or remain stable for long periods of time, then quickly develop new symptoms if more strokes occur. In many people with multi-infarct dementia, high blood pressure is to blame. One of the most important reasons for controlling high blood pressure is to prevent strokes.

Diagnosis

People who are worried about memory problems should see their doctor. If the doctor believes that the problem is serious, then a thorough physical, neurological, and psychiatric evaluation may be recommended. A complete medical examination for memory loss may include gathering information about the person's medical history, including use of prescription and over-the-counter medicines, diet, past medical problems, and general health. Because a correct diagnosis depends on recalling these details accurately, the doctor also may ask a family member for information about the person.

Tests of blood and urine may be done to help the doctor find any problems. There are also tests of mental abilities (tests of memory, problem solving, counting, and language). A brain CT scan may assist the doctor in ruling out a curable disorder. A scan also may show signs of normal age-related changes in the brain. It may be necessary to have another scan at a later date to see if there have been further changes in the brain.

Alzheimer's disease and multi-infarct dementia can exist together, making it hard for the doctor to diagnose either one specifically. Scientists once thought that multi-infarct dementia and other types of vascular dementia caused most cases of irreversible mental impairment. They now believe that most older people with irreversible dementia have Alzheimer's disease.

Treatment

Even if the doctor diagnoses an irreversible form of dementia, much still can be done to treat the patient and help the family cope. A person with dementia should be under a doctor's care, and may see a neurologist, psychiatrist, family doctor, internist, or geriatrician. The doctor can treat the patient's physical and behavioral problems and answer the many questions that the person or family may have.

For some people in the early and middle stages of Alzheimer's disease, the drug tacrine (also known as Cognex or THA) is prescribed to possibly delay the worsening of some of the disease's symptoms. Doctors believe it is very important for people with multi-infarct dementia to try to prevent further strokes by controlling high blood pressure, monitoring and treating high blood cholesterol and diabetes, and not smoking.

Many people with dementia need no medication for behavioral problems. But for some people, doctors may prescribe medications to reduce agitation, anxiety, depression, or sleeping problems. These troublesome behaviors are common in people with dementia. Careful use of doctor-prescribed drugs may make some people with dementia more comfortable and make caring for them easier.

A healthy diet is important. Although no special diets or nutritional supplements have been found to prevent or reverse Alzheimer's disease or multi-infarct dementia, a balanced diet helps maintain overall good health. In cases of multi-infarct dementia, improving the diet may play a role in preventing more strokes.

Family members and friends can assist people with dementia in continuing their daily routines, physical activities, and social contacts. People with dementia should be kept up to date about the details of their lives, such as the time of day, where they live, and what is happening at home or in the world. Memory aids may help in the day-to-day living of patients in the earlier stages of dementia. Some families find that a big calendar, a list of daily plans, notes about simple safety measures, and written directions describing how to use common household items are very useful aids.

Advice for Today

Scientists are working to develop new drugs that someday may slow, reverse, or prevent the damage caused by Alzheimer's disease and multi-infarct dementia. In the meantime, people who have no dementia symptoms can try to keep their memory sharp.

Some suggestions include developing interests or hobbies and staying involved in activities that stimulate both the mind and body. Giving careful attention to physical fitness and exercise also may go a long way toward keeping a healthy state of mind. Limiting the use of alcoholic beverages is important, because heavy drinking over time can cause permanent brain damage.

Many people find it useful to plan tasks; make "things-to-do" lists; and use notes, calendars, and other memory aids. They also may remember things better by mentally connecting them to other meaningful things, such as a familiar name, song, or lines from a poem.

Stress, anxiety, or depression can make a person more forgetful. Forgetfulness caused by these emotions usually is temporary and goes away when the feelings fade. However, if these feelings last for a long period of time, getting help from a professional is important. Treatment may include counseling or medication, or a combination of both.

Some physical and mental changes occur with age in healthy people. However, much pain and suffering can be avoided if older people, their families, and their doctors recognize dementia as a disease, not part of normal aging.

Resources

Having accurate, current information about dementia also is important. The Alzheimer's Disease Education and Referral (ADEAR)

Center is a clearinghouse supported by the National Institute on Aging. For more information about Alzheimer's disease and multi-infarct dementia, contact:

ADEAR Center
PO Box 8250
Silver Spring, MD 20907-8250
toll-free 800-438-4380
e-mail: adear@alzheimers.org
Internet Web site: http://www.alzheimers.org/adear

Families often need information about community resources, such as home care, adult day care, respite programs, and nursing homes. This information usually is available from State or Area Agencies on Aging. For help in finding the appropriate agency in your area, call the Eldercare Locator, toll-free at 800-677-1116.

Chapter 4

Alzheimer's Disease

What Is Alzheimer's?

"Alzheimer's disease" is the term used to describe a dementing disorder marked by certain brain changes, regardless of the age of onset. Alzheimer's disease is not a normal part of aging—it is not something that inevitably happens in later life. Rather, it is one of the dementing disorders, a group of brain diseases that lead to the loss of mental and physical functions. The disorder, whose cause is unknown, affects a small but significant percentage of older Americans. A very small minority of Alzheimer's patients are under 50 years of age. Most are over 65.

Alzheimer's disease is the exception, rather than the rule, in old age. Only 5 to 6 percent of older people are afflicted by Alzheimer's disease or a related dementia—but this means approximately 3 to 4 million Americans have one of these debilitating disorders. Research indicates that 1 percent of the population aged 65-74 has severe dementia, increasing to 7 percent of those aged 75-84 and to 25 percent of those 85 or older. At least half the people in U.S. nursing homes have Alzheimer's disease or a related disorder; in 1991, the annual cost of caring for individuals with Alzheimer's disease and related dementias in institutional and community settings was estimated between $24 billion and $48 billion for direct costs alone and is probably higher today. As our population ages and the number of Alzheimer's patients increases, costs of care will rise as well.

National Institute of Mental Health (NIMH), NIH Pub. No. 94-3676, 1994.

Although Alzheimer's disease is not curable or reversible, there are ways to alleviate symptoms and suffering and to assist families. Not every person with this illness must necessarily move to a nursing home. Many thousands of patients—especially those in the early stages of the disease—are cared for by their families in the community. Indeed, one of the most important aspects of medical management is family education and family support services. When, or whether, to transfer a patient to a nursing home is a decision to be carefully considered by the family.

Who Gets Alzheimer's Disease?

The main risk factor for Alzheimer's disease is increased age. The rates of the disease increase markedly with advancing age, with 25 percent of people over 85 suffering from Alzheimer's or other severe dementia.

Some investigators, describing a family pattern of Alzheimer's disease, suggest that in some cases heredity may influence its development. A genetic basis has been identified through the discovery of several genetic markers on chromosomes 21 and 14 for a small subgroup of families in which the disease has frequently occurred at relatively early ages (beginning before age 50). Some evidence points to chromosome 19 as implicated in certain other families that have frequently had the disease develop at later ages.

At the same time, data indicate that the likelihood that a close relative (sibling, child, or parent) of an afflicted individual will develop Alzheimer's disease is low. In most cases, such an individual's risk is only slightly higher than that of someone in the general population, where the lifetime risk is below 1 percent. And, of course, many disorders have a genetic potential that is never expressed—that is, despite being at risk for a certain illness, one might go through life without ever developing any symptom of the disease.

What to Expect When Someone Has Alzheimer's Disease

Mary Ellen's friends thought she was the perfect mother, wife, friend, and hostess. Her husband George, a prolific author, counted on her to edit his work and manage his schedule. He was the first to notice that she was no longer able to remember her good friends' names, her children's birthdays, or the details of her busy life. During social occasions, she could be seen sitting on the sidelines, answering politely but vaguely if spoken to, but never engaged in meaningful conversation. She was no longer able to go shopping or pay the household bills as she had done for the past 30 years. George was bewildered and could not understand what had happened to his close companion of so many years.

The onset of Alzheimer's disease is usually very slow and gradual, seldom occurring before age 65. Over time, however, it follows a progressively more serious course. Among the symptoms that typically develop, none is unique to Alzheimer's disease at its various stages. It is therefore essential for suspicious changes to be thoroughly evaluated before they become inappropriately or negligently labeled Alzheimer's disease.

Problems of memory, particularly recent or short-term memory, are common early in the course of the disease. For example, the individual may, on repeated occasions, forget to turn off the iron or may not recall which of the morning's medicines were taken. Mild personality changes, such as less spontaneity or a sense of apathy and a tendency to withdraw from social interactions, may occur early in the illness. As the disease progresses, problems in abstract thinking or in intellectual functioning develop. The individual may begin to have trouble with figures when working on bills, with understanding what is being read, or with organizing the day's work. Further disturbances in behavior and appearance may also be seen at this point, such as agitation, irritability, quarrelsomeness, and diminishing ability to dress appropriately.

Later in the course of the disorder, the affected individuals may become confused or disoriented about what month or year it is and be unable to describe accurately where they live or to name correctly a place being visited. Eventually they may wander, be unable to engage in conversation, seem inattentive and erratic in mood, appear uncooperative, lose bladder and bowel control, and, in extreme cases, become totally incapable of caring for themselves if the final stage is reached. Death then follows, perhaps from pneumonia or some other problem that occurs in severely deteriorated states of health. The average course of the disease from the time it is recognized to death is about 6 to 8 years, but it may range from under 2 to over 20 years. Those who develop the disorder later in life may die from other illnesses (such as heart disease) before Alzheimer's disease reaches its final and most serious stage.

27

Though the changes just described represent the general range of symptoms for Alzheimer's disease, the specific problems, along with the rate and severity of decline, can vary considerably with different individuals. Indeed, most persons with Alzheimer's disease can function at a reasonable level and remain at home far into the course of the disorder. Moreover, throughout much of the course of the illness individuals maintain the capacity for giving and receiving love, for sharing warm interpersonal relationships, and for participating in a variety of meaningful activities with family and friends.

A person with Alzheimer's disease may no longer be able to do math, but still be able to read a magazine with pleasure for months or years to come. Playing the piano might become too stressful in the face of increasing mistakes, but singing along with others may still be satisfying. The chess board may have to be put away, but one may still be able to play tennis. Thus, despite the many exasperating moments in the lives of Alzheimer patients and their families, many opportunities remain for positive interactions. Challenge, frustration, closeness, anger, warmth, sadness, and satisfaction may all be experienced by those who work to help the person with Alzheimer's disease cope as well as possible with the disease.

The reaction of an individual to the illness—his or her capacity to cope with it—also varies and may depend on such factors as lifelong personality patterns and the nature and severity of stress in the immediate environment. Depression, severe uneasiness, and paranoia or delusions may accompany or result from the disease, but they can often be alleviated by appropriate treatments. Although there is no cure for Alzheimer's disease, treatments are available to alleviate many of the symptoms that cause suffering.

The Diagnosis of Alzheimer's Disease

Abnormal Brain Tissue Findings

1. Plaques and Tangles

Microscopic brain tissue changes have been described in Alzheimer's disease since Alois Alzheimer first reported them in 1906. The two principal changes are senile or neuritic plaques (chemical deposits consisting of degenerating nerve cells combined with a form of protein called beta amyloid) and neurofibrillary tangles (malformations within nerve cells). The brains of Alzheimer's disease patients of all ages reveal these findings on autopsy examination.

The plaques found in the brains of people with Alzheimer's disease appear to be made, in part, from protein molecules—amyloid precursor protein (APP)—that normally are essential components of the brain. Plaques are made when an enzyme snips APP apart at a specific place and then leaves the fragments—beta amyloid—in brain tissue where they come together in abnormal deposits. It has not as yet been definitely determined how neurofibrillary tangles are formed.

As research on Alzheimer's disease progresses, scientists are describing other abnormal anatomical and chemical changes associated with the disease. These include nerve cell degeneration in the brain's nucleus basalis of Meynert and reduced levels of the neurotransmitter acetylcholine in the brains of Alzheimer's disease victims. But from a practical standpoint, the "classical" plaque and tangle changes seen in the brain at autopsy typically suffice for a diagnosis of Alzheimer's disease. In fact, it is still only through the study of brain tissue from a person who was thought to have Alzheimer's disease that a definitive diagnosis of the disorder can be made.

2. Brain Scans

Computer-Assisted Tomography (CAT scan) changes become more evident as the disease progresses—not necessarily early on. Thus a CAT scan performed in the first stages of the disease cannot in itself be used to make a definitive diagnosis of Alzheimer's disease; its value is in helping to establish whether certain disorders (some reversible) that mimic Alzheimer's disease are present. Later on, CAT scans often reveal changes characteristic of Alzheimer's disease, namely an atrophied (shrunken) brain with widened sulci (tissue indentations) and enlarged cerebral ventricles (fluid-filled chambers).

Several new types of instrumentation are enabling researchers to learn even more about the brain. Both positron emission tomography (PET scan) and SPECT (single photon emission computerized tomography) can map regional cerebral blood flow, metabolic activity, and distribution of specific receptors, as well as integrity of the blood-brain barrier. These procedures may reveal abnormalities characteristic of Alzheimer's disease. Another method, magnetic-resonance imaging (MRI), probes the brain by examining the interaction of the magnetic properties of atoms with an external magnetic field. MRI provides both structural and chemical information and distinguishes moving blood from static brain tissue (Taylor, 1990).

Clinical Features of Alzheimer's Disease

The "clinical" features of Alzheimer's disease, as opposed to the "tissue" changes, are threefold:

1. Dementia—significant loss of intellectual abilities such as memory capacity, severe enough to interfere with social or occupational functioning;

2. Insidious onset of symptoms—subtly progressive and irreversible course with documented deterioration over time;

3. Exclusion of all other specific causes of dementia by history, physical examination, laboratory tests, psychometric, and other studies.

Diagnosis by Exclusion

Based on these criteria, the clinical diagnosis of Alzheimer's disease has been referred to as "a diagnosis by exclusion," and one that can only be made in the face of clinical deterioration over time. There is no specific clinical test or finding that is unique to Alzheimer's disease. Hence, all disorders that can bring on similar symptoms must be systematically excluded or "ruled out." This explains why diagnostic workups of individuals where the question of Alzheimer's disease has been raised can be so frustrating to patient and family alike; they are not told that Alzheimer's disease has been specifically diagnosed, but that other possible diagnoses have been dismissed, leaving Alzheimer's disease as the likely diagnosis by the process of elimination.

Some scientists think that the results from biochemical research may lead to a diagnostic "marker" for certain persons evaluated for Alzheimer's disease. For example, research has discovered a protein, called Alzheimer's Disease Associated Protein (ADAP), in the autopsied brains of Alzheimer's patients. The protein, which seems to appear only in people with Alzheimer's, is mainly concentrated in the cortex covering the front and side sections of the brain, regions involved in memory function. Researchers have found ADAP not only in brain tissue but also in spinal fluid. If they can perfect a test to detect the protein in the cerebrospinal fluid, or potentially even circulating in the blood, it may be possible to use this method of diagnosis on living patients.

Many scientists are working at developing other tests or procedures that may someday identify living persons with the disorder, perhaps even early in its course before behavioral changes become evident. Still, a reliable, specific diagnostic marker for Alzheimer's disease is not yet available.

Meanwhile, Alzheimer's disease is the most overdiagnosed and misdiagnosed disorder of mental functioning in older adults. Part of the problem, already alluded to, is that many other disorders show symptoms that resemble those of Alzheimer's disease. The crucial difference, though, is that many of these disorders—unlike Alzheimer's disease—may be stopped, reversed, or cured with appropriate treatment. But first they must be identified and not dismissed as Alzheimer's disease or senility.

Conditions that affect the brain and result in intellectual, behavioral, and psychological dysfunction are referred to as "organic mental disorders." These disorders represent a broad grouping of diseases and include Alzheimer's disease. Organic mental disorders that can cause clinical problems like those of Alzheimer's disease, but which might be reversible or controlled with proper diagnosis and treatment, include the following:

- **Side Effects of Medications:** Unusual reactions to medications, too much or too little of prescribed medications, combinations of medications which, when taken together, cause adverse side effects.

- **Substance Abuse:** Abuse of legal and/or illegal drugs, alcohol abuse.

- **Metabolic Disorders:** Thyroid problems, nutritional deficiencies, anemias, etc.

- **Circulatory Disorders:** Heart problems, strokes, etc.

- **Neurological Disorders:** Normal-pressure hydrocephalus, multiple sclerosis, etc.

- **Infections:** Especially viral or fungal infections of the brain.

- **Trauma:** Injuries to the head.

- **Toxic Factors:** Carbon monoxide, methyl alcohol, etc.

- **Tumors:** Any type within the skull—whether originating or metastasizing there.

In addition to organic mental disorders resulting from these diverse causes, other forms of mental dysfunction or mental health problems can also be confused with Alzheimer's disease. For example, severe forms of depression can cause problems with memory and concentration that initially may be indistinguishable from early symptoms of Alzheimer's disease. Sometimes these conditions, referred to as "pseudodementia," can be reversed. Other psychiatric problems can similarly masquerade as Alzheimer's disease, and, like depression, respond to treatment.

Of course, not all memory changes or complaints in later life signal Alzheimer's disease or mental disorder. Many memory changes are only temporary, such as those that occur with bereavement or any stressful situation that makes it difficult to concentrate. In fact, older people are often accused or accuse themselves of memory changes which are not really taking place. If a person in his thirties misplaces keys or a wallet, forgets the name of a neighbor, or calls one sibling by another's name, nobody gives it a second thought. But the same normal forgetfulness for people in their seventies may raise unjustifiable concern. On the other hand, serious memory difficulties should not be dismissed as an unavoidable part of normal aging. Since rigorous studies on intelligence in later life show that healthy people who stay intellectually active maintain a sharp mind throughout the life cycle, noticeable decline in older adults that interferes with functioning should be clinically explored for an underlying problem.

The Importance of a Comprehensive Clinical Evaluation

Because of the many other disorders that can be confused with Alzheimer's disease, a comprehensive clinical evaluation is essential to arrive at a correct diagnosis of symptoms that look like those of Alzheimer's disease. Such an assessment should include at least three major components—(1) a thorough general medical workup, (2) a neurological examination, and (3) a psychiatric evaluation that may include psychological or psychometric testing. The family physician can be consulted about the best way to get the necessary examinations.

George tried to get Mary Ellen to see their family physician but she refused. Finally, he suggested that they both go in to have their blood pressure checked. The doctor was shocked at the deterioration in Mary Ellen's personality and scheduled a complete physical examination for her. He also made an appointment with a neurologist for further neurological examination, including a

CAT scan. A psychiatrist working in the same office conducted a psychiatric evaluation. George helped by giving them many details of Mary Ellen's history. A tentative diagnosis of Alzheimer's disease was made, and George was instructed to bring Mary Ellen back in 6 months for further evaluation. George still hoped that Mary Ellen's condition was temporary and told no one of his distress. When their two daughters called, he always made excuses as to why their mother did not answer the telephone. He neglected his writing as more of his time was taken up with household tasks that Mary Ellen no longer even tried to do.

The Search for the Cause of Alzheimer's Disease

Alzheimer's disease has emerged as one of the great mysteries in modern day medicine, with a growing number of clues but still no answers as to its cause. The quest to uncover its cause has the air of a veritable whodunit saga. Though none of the leading theories about the genesis of Alzheimer's disease has resolved the mystery, each has led to certain intriguing findings that suggest further investigation is needed. It is important to examine these theories, not only to understand current thinking on Alzheimer's disease, but also to learn what popular ideas have proved to be incorrect. There have been at least five prominent theories about the cause of Alzheimer's disease:

1. Chemical Theories (Deficiencies and Toxic Excesses)

A. Biochemical Changes in Growth (Trophic) Factors: Much research is taking place in the examination of naturally occurring substances that may affect the nervous system and that may contribute to the dysfunction or death of brain cells in Alzheimer's. It is possible that one reason for nerve cell death in Alzheimer's patients is a decline in growth-promoting factors that maintain the functioning of brain cells, or, conversely, a spontaneous increase in factors that are toxic to brain cells.

A naturally occurring substance of interest is nerve growth factor (NGF). Experiments in aged rats indicate that specific nerve growth factors can stimulate the growth of new synaptic connections in the hippocampus and, as a result, restore some memory loss. Although there could be neurotoxic as well as growth-enhancing effects in the use of NGF, scientists are investigating methods of safely introducing NGF into the brain, possibly through the transplant of genetically engineered cells.

Other research is exploring whether changes or an imbalance in the metabolism of certain elements like calcium in brain cells may be part of the process by which the cells degenerate and die in Alzheimer's disease.

B. Chemical Deficiencies: One of the ways in which brain cells communicate with one another is through chemicals called neurotransmitters. Studies of Alzheimer's disease brains have uncovered diminished levels of various neurotransmitters that are thought to influence intellectual functioning and behavior. For example, reduced levels of the neurotransmitter acetylcholine (ACh) have been found in Alzheimer's disease. This finding has been coupled with observations that drugs whose side effects lower ACh levels in the brain can cause reversible memory problems. These findings have led to a number of drug studies employing pharmacologic agents to elevate ACh in patients. The treatments have included lecithin, choline, physostigmine, deprenyl, tacrine hydrochloride (THA), and others, used

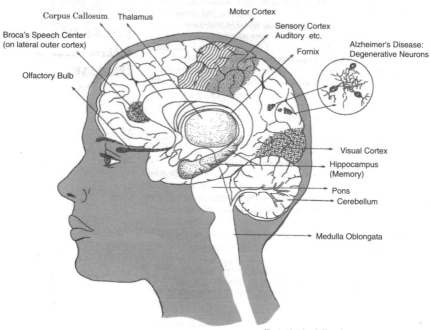

Illustration by Jeffrey Aarons

Figure 4.1. The brain.

alone or in different combinations with one another. The results of these experiments are difficult to interpret. In some of these studies, a few Alzheimer's disease patients seem to show minor improvement over a brief but not sustained period of time. Typically, any improvement may be on certain narrow test measures—and not usually on significant activities of daily living which would be more important to the person's family and physician. Nonetheless, the researchers' enthusiasm is understandable, for they are dealing with the potential modifiability of underlying physiological phenomena that influence the Alzheimer's disease symptoms. The drugs they are studying now may not be the right ones, but they may point the way to the discovery of more effective pharmacologic agents.

One drug in particular, THA or tacrine (trade name, Cognex), has been studied extensively. Early studies indicated that THA appeared to have a slightly positive effect on patient functioning, but assessment by a skilled observer showed no overall improvement. More recent studies conducted on patients with mild or moderate Alzheimer's, using a higher dosage of tacrine than the earlier studies, showed a statistically significant improvement, both in clinical and caregiver evaluations and in quality of life measurements. These results caused the Food and Drug Administration in the fall of 1993 to approve the drug. Tacrine can, however, have side effects, including elevation of liver functioning tests. The family of the patient should be aware that the patient must take the medication 4 times a day, that blood must be drawn weekly during the dose adjustment phase, and that a third of patients experience significant adverse effects. As is always the case, but particularly while better drugs are being developed, caregivers and patients will have to weigh the possible benefits of the available drug against the cost and the potential problems incurred.

C. Toxic Chemical Excesses: Although some researchers have found increased levels of aluminum, mercury, or other metals in the brains of Alzheimer's disease victims, others have not. And while some investigators have hypothesized that aluminum may play a role in the genesis of Alzheimer's disease, most have regarded aluminum as an effect of the disorder rather than its cause. In other words, instead of aluminum's acting to induce brain tissue changes in Alzheimer's disease, it more likely accumulates in response to such changes. Research continues in an effort to better understand this phenomenon and to determine whether the aluminum deposits are a cause or a consequence of the disease, and, if the latter, whether they contribute further to the impairment already experienced.

2. The Genetic Theory

Genetic aspects of many diseases are confusing. For example, a disorder can occur more frequently in certain families than in others, but still not be genetic. Since family members living together are exposed to the same environment, they would all be at increased risk if an environmental toxin or infectious agent were the causative factor in a particular disease. Furthermore, a disorder can be congenital and not hereditary—that is, prenatal problems can cause developmental defects not brought on by heredity. And an illness can be hereditary but remain in a latent state if some other disease factor does not occur to trigger its onset.

Several connections between Alzheimer's disease and Down's syndrome led researchers initially to look for genetic factors in Alzheimer's disease on chromosome 21—the chromosome that is affected in Down's syndrome. At the present time, several genetic markers have been identified on chromosomes 21 and 14 in that small number of families where Alzheimer's disease has occurred with unusual frequency at relatively early ages. In families where the disease has tended to develop at later ages, other studies suggest that Alzheimer's disease is unusually frequent in persons who have a particular form of the apolipoprotein E (ApoE) gene found on chromosome 19. Only a minority of the general population show this version (ApoE4) of the gene, out of several variants that occur.

Despite these findings, the extent of genetic and hereditary involvement in Alzheimer's disease remains unclear. There are a vast number of people affected with this disorder who are not part of a strong family pattern. Furthermore, the genetic factors associated with the disease clearly vary for different families. This has led some investigators to postulate that there may be a number of subtypes of Alzheimer's disease, with differing risk factors and causes.

The National Institute of Mental Health (NIMH) is supporting research to locate the genes that cause Alzheimer's disease, schizophrenia, and manic depression. Ten diagnostic centers, three of which study Alzheimer's, provide genetic material to a central gene bank. Scientists at the centers use identical diagnostic tests, chosen for their sensitivity and reliability, to select members of families whose blood is sent to the gene bank for processing, storage, and distribution. Participating families must have several members affected by one of the diseases. The centers studying Alzheimer's are: The Johns Hopkins University, Baltimore, Maryland; Massachusetts General Hospital, Boston, Massachusetts; and University of Alabama, Birmingham, Alabama.

3. The Autoimmune Theory

The body's immune system, which protects against potentially harmful foreign invaders, may erroneously begin to attack its own tissues, producing antibodies to its own essential cells. This is called an autoimmune response, and it may take place in the brain. Some scientists speculate that certain late life changes in aging neurons (the major nerve cells of the brain) might be triggering an autoimmune response that evokes symptoms of Alzheimer's disease in vulnerable individuals. Curiously, some antibrain antibodies have been identified in the brains of those with Alzheimer's disease. Their significance, though, is not known, especially since some antibrain antibodies have also been identified in aging brains without Alzheimer's disease. Moreover, even if changes are occurring in brain neurons to trigger an autoimmune response, what originally induces these brain cell changes is not known.

4. The Slow Virus Theory

Because a slow-acting virus has been identified as a cause of some brain disorders that closely resemble Alzheimer's disease (for example, Creutzfeldt-Jakob disease), a slow virus has been postulated in Alzheimer's disease. Various researchers have suggested that suspicious brain tissue changes in Alzheimer's disease victims may be caused by a virus. However, to date a virus has not been isolated from the brains of those with Alzheimer's disease, and no immune reaction has been found in the brains of Alzheimer's patients, comparable to that found in patients with other viral dementias. At present, the possibility of a viral cause of Alzheimer's cannot be either decisively eliminated or confirmed.

5. The Blood Vessel Theory

Defects in blood vessels supplying blood to the brain have been studied as a possible cause of Alzheimer's disease. Hardening of the brain's arteries, also known as cerebroarteriosclerosis, proved not to be a cause of Alzheimer's disease. Thus, the hyperbaric oxygen chamber treatment proved ineffective as a therapy for Alzheimer's.

Stroke, another blood vessel problem that most often occurs later in life, can cause symptoms like those of Alzheimer's disease. But this condition, called multi-infarct dementia, differs from Alzheimer's disease. More recently, the blood vessel theory has been expanded to hypothesize potential defects in the blood-brain barrier, a protective membrane-like mechanism that guards the brain from foreign bodies or toxic agents circulating in the blood stream outside the brain.

There have been several reports of a possible association between serious head injuries involving a loss of consciousness and later onset of Alzheimer's disease. One theory as to why this connection might occur has to do with possible breaks in the blood-brain barrier as a result of these injuries to the brain.

The Treatment of Alzheimer's Disease

Two critical crossroads reached in the approach to treatment for Alzheimer's disease were (1) the recognition of Alzheimer's disease as a disorder distinct from the normal aging process; and (2) the realization that, in developing therapeutic and social interventions for a major illness or disability, the concept of care can be as important as that of cure. Moreover, in addition to the symptoms of Alzheimer's disease mentioned earlier, other symptoms and aggravating factors may compound the problem. Patient, environmental, and family stresses can converge to exaggerate patient dysfunction and family burden during the clinical course of Alzheimer's disease. Identifying these stresses and making appropriate changes can provide the foundation for more effective treatment and fewer everyday problems.

In the Alzheimer's disease patient, depression or delusions can aggravate dysfunction. These problems, which emerge during the course of the disorder in some individuals with Alzheimer's disease, compound memory impairment; they make the affected individual do worse than would be expected from the dementia alone—causing clinical conditions referred to as "excess disability" states. Depression by itself can mimic dementia—a condition that is sometimes termed pseudodementia. When combined with dementia, depression exacts yet greater incapacity and suffering in the Alzheimer's disease patient. Depression in Alzheimer's disease can be treated. Indeed this highlights one of the truly extraordinary phenomena that can be observed in Alzheimer's disease: By alleviating an excess disability state, actual clinical improvement can result—even though the underlying disease process is advancing. In other words, at a given point in time, the patient's symptoms can be reduced, suffering lowered, capacity to cope buttressed, with family burden eased as a further result. These are traditional goals of treatment for all illnesses.

Researchers in the NIMH Intramural program have developed and are testing a Dementia Mood Assessment Scale, designed to rate mood in Alzheimer's patients. This scale tracks the mood states of the patients over the course of their illness and thus may be helpful in testing various antidepressant treatments.

The patient's immediate environment can also interfere with coping, adding to the level of impairment. Modifying the surroundings can reduce stresses imposed by environmental factors. There is the matter of safety, as in the need to protect the person from wandering toward a stairway and subsequently falling. There is the matter of lowering the individual's frustration level, such as by placing different cues in the immediate environment to combat memory loss and to reduce resulting stress and disorganization. There is the matter of finding the most protective but least restrictive setting for care which at some point may involve a move away from home to a nursing home or other care facility well equipped to deal with those who have Alzheimer's disease.

Stress on the family can take a toll on patient and caregiver alike. Caregivers are usually family members—either spouses or children— and are preponderantly wives and daughters. As time passes and the burden mounts, it not only places the mental health of family caregivers at risk, it also diminishes their ability to provide care to the Alzheimer's disease patient. Hence, assistance to the family as a whole must be considered.

As the disease progresses, families experience increasing anxiety and pain at seeing unsettling changes in a loved one, and they commonly feel guilt over not being able to do enough. The prevalence of reactive depression among family members in this situation is disturbingly high—caregivers are chronically stressed and are much more likely to suffer from depression than the average person. If caregivers have been forced to retire from positions outside the home, they feel progressively more isolated and no longer productive members of society.

An NIMH-funded study shows that caregivers not only have increased rates of infectious illness and depression, but often have suppressed immune systems. Another study of caregivers found depressed mood in 54 percent of caregivers and anger in 67 percent. Researchers hypothesize that the caregivers who hold in their anger may be at greater risk of cardiovascular disease.

The likelihood, intensity, and duration of depression among caregivers can all be lowered through available interventions. For example, to the extent that family members can offer emotional support to each other and perhaps seek professional consultation, they will be better prepared to help their loved one manage the illness and to recognize the limits of what they themselves can reasonably do.

George and Mary Ellen's neighbors had become increasingly concerned as it was obvious something was very wrong. When they noticed that the newspaper had not been taken in one morning, two neighbors came over. When no one answered the door, they tried it, found it unlocked, and entered. George was lying on the floor near the telephone, and Mary Ellen was sitting at the piano trying to pick out a tune. The neighbors called an ambulance for George and then placed a long-distance call to one of his daughters. George, in the hospital suffering from a heart attack, for the first time shared with his children the events of the past months and realized that he must make plans for the future. One of his daughters stayed with him and Mary Ellen for 2 months after he left the hospital. She arranged for someone to come in once a week to clean the house. She also contacted Meals-on-Wheels to ensure nourishing meals for her parents. Through her parents' church, she enrolled Mary Ellen in a 5-day-a-week daycare program for the elderly. Each morning Mary Ellen was picked up by the daycare van and was brought back late in the afternoon. George, relieved of constant anxiety, recovered rapidly and began to catch up on his writing projects. Though he missed the social life they had once enjoyed with their friends, there were times when he and Mary Ellen still felt a close relationship. George now accepted the fact that someday Mary Ellen might have to enter a nursing home, but with the support of his family, friends, church, and community he would be able to deal with whatever came.

Since the components of the problem vary, so too should the focus, nature, and sources of interventions. Interventions should focus on the patient's symptoms, the affected individual's everyday environment, and the family support system. Specific interventions can involve support from the family, the help of a homemaker or other aide in the home, employment of behavioral therapies, and the use of medication. The sources for interventions can range from family support groups such as those available through the Alzheimer's Association (AA), to professional consultations for the patient and family with a mental health specialist, to a variety of community programs such as day or respite care. Information on what assistance is available in a given community can be gained by contacting the local Office on Aging, a Community Mental Health Center or local Medical Society, or a local chapter of the AA. In addition, every State has an agency on aging that provides information on services and programs.

See Part V "Additional Help and Information" in this book for sources of help.

Though Alzheimer's disease cannot at present be cured, reversed, or stopped in its progression, much can be done to help both the patient and the family live through the course of the illness with greater dignity and less discomfort. Toward this goal, appropriate clinical interventions and community services should be vigorously sought.

Hope for the Future Through Research

While Alzheimer's disease remains a mystery, with its cause and cure not yet found, there is considerable excitement and hope about new findings that are unfolding in numerous research settings. The connecting pieces to the puzzle called Alzheimer's disease continue to be found. At the same time, there are more and more partners involved in the effort, with growing national and international interest. Government, industry, academia, and the volunteer sector are all becoming more and more active; Federal, State, community, corporate, and foundation support for new studies and better services are all on the rise.

The U.S. Department of Health and Human Services established a Departmental Task Force on Alzheimer's Disease, which first met in April 1983. This Task Force, later legislatively mandated as the Council on Alzheimer's Disease, is composed of representatives from the following agencies that have programs related to Alzheimer's disease: the National Institute of Mental Health, the National Institute on Aging, the National Institute of Neurological Disorders and Stroke, the National Institute of Allergy and Infectious Diseases, the National Institute for Nursing Research, the Administration on Aging, the Agency for Health Care Policy and Research, the Health Care Financing Administration, the Health Resources and Services Administration, the National Center for Health Statistics, and the Department of Veterans Affairs. The Council, which also includes both the Surgeon General and the Assistant Secretary for Planning and Evaluation as members, is chaired by the Assistant Secretary for Health. The Council's recommendations are sent in an annual report to Congress.

In addition, a non-Federal Advisory Panel on Alzheimer's Disease was established by congressional action. The Panel, which works closely with the Council, consists of 15 national authorities on Alzheimer's disease selected for their depth and breadth of expertise in this area. The Panel has issued four reports, for 1988-89, 1990,

1991, and 1992. The activities of both the Council and the Panel reflect the scope of concern and interest that is being focused by the Federal Government on Alzheimer's disease.

Chapter 5

Prevalence and Costs of Alzheimer's Disease

Alzheimer's Disease

Alzheimer's disease (AD) is a progressive brain disorder that occurs gradually and results in memory loss, unusual behavior, personality changes, and a decline in thinking abilities that cannot be reversed. These mental losses are related to the death of brain cells and the breakdown of the connections between them. The course of this disease varies from person to person, as does the rate of decline. On average, AD patients live from 4 to 8 years after they are diagnosed; however, the disease can continue for up to 20 years.

AD advances by stages, from early, mild forgetfulness to severe dementia. Dementia is a specific case of loss of healthy mental function. In most people with AD, symptoms appear after age 60. First symptoms often include loss of recent memory, faulty judgment, and changes in personality. Often, people with AD think less clearly and forget the names of familiar people and common objects. Later in the disease, they may forget how to do simple tasks like washing their hands. Eventually, people with AD lose all reasoning abilities and come to depend on other people for their everyday care. Finally, the disease becomes so debilitating that patients are bedridden and likely to develop coexisting illnesses. Most commonly, people with AD die from pneumonia.

Excerpted from *Progress Report on Alzheimer's Disease, 1997,* National Institute on Aging (NIA), NIH Pub. No. 97-4014, 1997.

The risk of developing AD increases with age, but AD and dementia symptoms are not a part of normal aging. AD and other dementing disorders in old age are caused by diseases. In the absence of a disease, the human brain often can function well into the tenth decade of life and beyond.

Prevalence and Costs of Alzheimer's Disease

AD is the most common cause of dementia among people age 65 and older. AD affects approximately 4 million Americans; slightly more than half of these people receive care at home, while the others are in many different health care institutions. Before long, ongoing population studies may give estimates of the number of people at different stages of the disease.

The prevalence of AD and other dementias doubles every 5 years beyond age 65. Prevalence is the number of people in a population with a disease at a given time. In fact, some studies indicate that nearly half of all people age 85 and older have symptoms of AD.

Life expectancy has increased dramatically since the turn of the century. About 33 million people—13 percent of the total population of the United States—are age 65 and older. According to the Bureau of the Census, this percentage will climb to 20 percent by the year 2025. In addition, the proportion of very old people (those aged 85 and older)—who often are most in need of care—will increase considerably. In most industrialized countries, the 85 and older age group is the fastest growing segment of the population over age 65. Now 3.5 million, the number of American aged 85 and older will total nearly 9 million by the year 2030.

A great many spouses, relatives, and friends take care of people with AD. These caregivers are the backbone of the Nation's informal system of long-term care for AD patients; their numbers also can be expected to grow significantly as the population ages.

During years of caregiving, families experience emotional, physical, and financial stresses. They watch their loved ones become more and more forgetful, frustrated, and confused. Many caregivers—most of them women—juggle child care and jobs with caring at home for relatives with AD who cannot function on their own. As the disease runs its course and the abilities of people with AD steadily decline, family members face painful decisions about the long-term care of their loved ones.

AD puts a heavy economic burden on society as well. A recent study estimated that the cost of caring for one AD patient with severe cognitive impairments at home or in a nursing home, excluding indirect losses in productivity or wages, is more than $47,000 a year. For a disease that can span from 2 to 20 years, the overall cost of AD to families and to society is staggering. The annual economic toll of AD in the United States in terms of health care expenses and lost wages of both patients and their caregivers is estimated at $80 to $100 billion.

AD is a major health problem and expense for the United States. Until researchers find a way to cure or prevent AD, a large and growing number of people, especially those who live to be very old (85+), will be at risk for AD. Providing and financing the care of this growing older population will increase the strain on our already burdened health care system.

Chapter 6

Ethnic and Cultural Issues in Alzheimer's Disease and Related Dementias

Report on Ethnic and Cultural Issues in Alzheimer's Disease and Related Dementias

Alzheimer's disease and related dementias (ADRD) affect millions of Americans, without regard to their social class, racial or ethnic group, or country of origin. Ethnicity, race, and economic status exert a complex set of influences upon the manner in which ADRD, and many other diseases, present themselves and how families respond to these disorders. Thus, dementia must be understood by researchers and treated by clinicians within its cultural as well as biophysiological and psychological contexts. Such clarification will benefit the mainstream population as well as ethnic subpopulations, since significant cultural variations exist within the general population as well.

Today, discussion of cultural diversity—ethnicity—most often identifies four major U.S. ethnic subgroups: African Americans (Blacks), Asian Americans and Pacific Islanders (or Pan-Asian populations), American Indians and Alaska Natives, and Hispanics (or Latinos). These four classifications, albeit a shorthand for a widely diverse set of populations within each subgroup, have been found useful for sociopolitical purposes. (Indeed, the term "Asian Americans" represents more than 50 distinct linguistic groups. African Americans

Excerpted from *"Fourth Report of the Advisory Panel on Alzheimer's Disease,"* National Institute of Mental Health (NIMH), NIH Pub. No. 93-3520, February 1993.

include persons who can trace their roots to Africa, who were born in Africa, or who were born in the Caribbean Islands. Hispanics count more than 25 different countries of national origin. American Indians and Alaska Natives encompass over 500 federally recognized tribes and groups, with at least 30 different languages.) Thus, they will be used in this report as reflecting current usage and operational convention. The combined phrase "ethnic minority" is used occasionally in this report as a reminder that the subject populations are characterized and differentiated from others by both ethnocultural factors and status as a minority population.

Race is a cultural or folk concept of relatively recent historical origin, used primarily in the United States and a few other cultures. Practically speaking, race, as a scientific variable, refers to the phenotype or physical appearance of a group, with the main racial designations identified broadly as caucasoid, negroid, and mongoloid. As a dominant factor in American life, race may be an appropriate variable in research evaluating access to service systems and the distribution of resources, particularly in situations in which political power and influence are, or historically have been, involved. Thus, as in the case of other health and human service realms, racial discrimination may be a factor in access to and resource allocation regarding ADRD services. However, this issue, like those of culture and ethnicity, must be approached, not as a tacit assumption, but as an empirical question. Furthermore, research should be undertaken to examine whether social class factors—rather than either ethnic/cultural or racial considerations—may be the principal influences impeding access to, and utilization of, services.

Issues of cultural diversity have not been a major focus of those engaged either in the conduct of research or the development of service systems related to ADRD. From the scientific perspective, the diversity among ADRD patients of differing ethnic backgrounds and cultural settings may help us elucidate the common biophysiological core of the Alzheimer's disease process itself. Moreover, if greater equity in the treatment of ADRD patients and their families within our Nation's health care and social services systems is to be achieved, programs must be designed that take account of cultural diversity among ADRD victims.

In past reports, the Advisory Panel on Alzheimer's Disease has noted the special needs of what traditionally have been medically underserved populations; it has identified how issues of diagnosis, access to care, and the course of treatment may differ across our heterogeneous aging population. This supplemental report of the Panel focuses more closely upon the effects that ethnic and cultural differences in ADRD can have in the conduct of scientific inquiry into the dementias and the effects these differences already are having in the treatment of patients with ADRD. It discusses not only the research needs in the field, but also the current problems faced by ethnic elders in seeking and accepting ADRD related services. The Panel's recommendations, by necessity, are not specific to any single ethnic or cultural population. What is presented is a framework within which research and health care service delivery may function in a culturally sensitive manner.

Demographic Trends

The overall population of ethnic elders—African Americans, Asian Americans and Pacific Islanders, American Indians and Alaska Natives, and Hispanics—is growing rapidly; their needs for health care are growing concomitantly. While the proportion of elderly within most ethnic groups in the United States is lower than is found in our general population, the ethnically and racially diverse elderly population is growing at more than twice the rate of the overall elderly population. The number of U.S. ethnic elderly has doubled with each census since 1960, a pattern expected to continue well into the next century. Among Asian Americans, for example, the Chinese and Japanese populations are aging particularly rapidly as children bring older parents to the United States in increasing numbers. By the year 2030, ethnic elderly minority groups combined may well constitute a majority of the elderly population, particularly in some regions and urban areas.

Notwithstanding the growing numbers of ethnic elderly, many local communities lack the vital information, education, and resources necessary to aid ethnic elders and families who are confronting ADRD. Ethnic populations may have differing expectations and understanding of the normal aging process; indeed, variations may be found not just across ethnic populations, but within them as well. Thus, ADRD may not be recognized until late in the disease process, at which point some caregiving options may be foreclosed. Moreover, long-term care programs, oriented predominantly toward the majority U.S. population, may lack the organized capacity to work with and appropriately serve some ethnic group ADRD victims and their caregivers. With the tremendous increase in the population of ethnic elders, greater attention to these concerns is both timely and imperative. Alzheimer's disease research and health services delivery

49

agendas should be broadened to reflect the wide cultural diversity encountered in our society.

Dimensions Often Confused with Ethnic Status

To gain a clear understanding of the "ethnic experience," it is necessary to identify systemic, social class, and ethnocultural variables that may impinge on patterns of behavior. The four sociopolitical groupings described above, by necessity, intermix such critical dimensions as culture or ethnicity, language, degree of acculturation to the mainstream culture, education and literacy, religion, socioeconomic status, race, and genetic or other biophysical differences. Systemic variation also exists in social environments and resources available to the individual, sometimes reflecting institutional racism or other types of discrimination, sometimes reflecting individual choice.

For example, older Asians who have recently immigrated to the United States to be with their children face multiple jeopardies of culture shock, linguistic difficulty, decreased value in the new environment for their cultural knowledge or experience, and greater social alienation. Their situation may be substantially different from that confronting older Asian Americans who have resided in the United States for an extended period of time. So-called "culture-bound syndromes"—disorders occurring solely within a particular culture or ethnic group—have been described for Asian Americans, some American Indians and Alaska Natives, and some recently immigrated Hispanics. The disorders are not recognized in the majority culture and are often difficult to translate in terms comprehensible to Western medicine. Moreover, the language used by many ethnic elders to describe affective concerns and philosophies is often difficult to translate.

Among Hispanic elders and in a number of other ethnic subcultures, the pattern of not seeking services and treatment beyond the informal caregiving network is believed to be based, in part, on having available a wide scope of kinship relationships. Whether such kinship bonds in fact obtain for most of the ethnic elders (or have been overly idealized by policymakers), and whether these account for the elders' service utilization decisions, are questions that have not been well researched. In contrast, there is a widespread perception that African American elders may avoid using formal services because they have experienced relative inequalities in the health care and educational systems, leaving them with inadequate knowledge of and minimal trust in such systems. More research is needed to determine the accuracy of these perceptions and beliefs.

Thus, while the fact of minority subgroup membership is held in common by the ethnic elderly, and many basic issues are similar, each ethnic group has had a unique experience. Moreover, within each ethnic group, different constellations of problems arise based on such factors as socioeconomic status, sociopolitical history, and duration of U.S. residency, among others. If we fail to distinguish among, and control or account for these factors, they will confuse our interpretation of any observed differences among groups, whether we are concerned with sociopolitical issues in service delivery or with basic questions about ADRD as diseases.

Incidence and Prevalence of AD in Ethnic Populations

Insufficient data have been amassed regarding the relative prevalence of AD among our Nation's various ethnic groups. For example, a recent study in China that found the prevalence of AD in Shanghai to be similar to that encountered in the mainland U.S. population is interesting, but its findings cannot be extrapolated into conclusions about the prevalence of AD in Asian Americans. Research to clarify the relative prevalence of AD among U.S. ethnic groups has become all the more important in light of increased prevalence estimates for the Nation's general population, based on a recent study.

Several tentative leads have emerged. The Epidemiological Catchment Area studies conducted by NIMH and another small clinical study suggest that African Americans (and, perhaps, also Asian Americans) appear to show relatively higher prevalence rates for multi-infarct dementia than the general population. This finding may corroborate a hypothesis of long standing that such a pattern would hold true due to elevated levels of hypertension and other cardiovascular risk factors in these groups.

Only a few studies have examined ADRD in ethnic populations. While some larger studies have included certain ethnic subgroups in their samples, the absolute numbers of these subjects are often too limited to provide data adequate to generate reliable estimates. Moreover, data are not gathered with sufficient precision to control for the heterogeneity of the ethnic subgroups themselves. For example, in addition to the problem that few of the available databases have separated Hispanics from non-Hispanic whites, in most studies in which they have been separated, the population remains pooled, not taking into account the heterogeneous subgroups that comprise the Hispanic population.

Alternately, those few studies that have documented heterogeneity tend to have subgroups that are too small or unrepresentative to address

ADRD concerns. The three Hispanic subgroups in the Hispanic Health and Nutrition Examination Survey, for example, included only a few hundred older persons, and no subjects age 75 or older. Further inquiry is needed to determine whether overall differences found between the major ethnic classifications can be substantiated across the various subgroups within these classifications and, if so, whether they are due to a genetic factor, differences in lifestyle (e.g., diet), or social class factors. At this point, no controlled studies permit such determinations.

Quite simply, insufficient epidemiologic data have been collected to provide precise delineation of the incidence and prevalence of AD among each of the four major ethnic groupings—African Americans, Hispanics, Asian Americans and Pacific Islanders, and American Indians and Alaska Natives. The closest proxy information has come from studies that have classified their subjects not by diagnostic categories (such as AD or multi-infarct dementia) but by degree of cognitive impairment.

Data from a number of these studies have suggested that cognitive impairment, a possible early manifestation of dementing disease, is more frequent in ethnic populations. The Epidemiological Catchment Area studies that administered a version of the Mini-Mental State Examination reported relatively high levels of cognitive impairment among adult African American and Hispanic populations, almost double the levels of cognitive impairment found in the general population. The work of W. Lopes-Aqueres et al. ("Health Needs of the Hispanic Elderly"; *Journal of the American Geriatrics Society*, 32:191-98, 1984.) with a community sample of Hispanics also found higher than average levels of cognitive impairment.

The explanatory factors for these differences remain open to question. Some research has suggested that the purported differences in cognitive impairment among ethnic U.S. populations may be an artifact linked to the instruments chosen to measure that impairment. Measures such as the Mini-Mental State Examination may be insufficiently attuned to cultural differences exhibited by ethnic populations in the United States to reflect accurately the level of cognitive impairment both within and across the populations. If this is the case, the data on cognitive impairment may severely misrepresent the actual incidence and prevalence of ADRD in U.S. ethnic populations. Alternatively, other research suggests that the cognitive impairment data are not artifactual, but indeed reflect, or are paralleled by, higher rates of functional impairment and/or associated brain pathology in some ethnic minority groups. For example, according to data from the

Household Survey component of the 1987 National Medical Expenditure Survey, compared with Caucasians, African Americans also show a higher prevalence of deficits in activities of daily living, the conventional measure of everyday functional (as opposed to purely cognitive) limitations.

Efforts to respond to the foregoing problems require attention if we are to gain a more focused picture of the incidence and prevalence of ADRD across our multiethnic society. The challenge for clinical and epidemiological researchers is to develop a dementia research technology that transcends ethnic and cross-cultural differences and appropriately distinguishes between the person actually suffering from a dementing disease and the individual who tests in the impaired range because of a cultural heritage that is incongruent with the instruments or procedures used to evaluate ADRD or cognitive impairment. Until this impasse is resolved, both clinical and epidemiological studies of ADRD will be suspected of embodying cultural biases in their cognitive testing, diagnostic, and/or other research procedures, and we will not be able to determine with accuracy the incidence and prevalence of ADRD in our multicultural society.

Ethnic Populations and ADRD Care and Services

Similarities and Differences In Understanding ADRD

Ethnic populations exhibit both similarities to, and differences from, the majority population in their recognition and understanding of the symptoms and facts about ADRD. In part, the special approach of any ethnic group to ADRD can be traced both to culture-bound understanding of the diseases and disorders that produce cognitive impairment or dementia in late life and to long-held beliefs, attitudes, and practices about the best ways to identify and care for persons evidencing such changes.

Because of an "acculturation dynamic", members of any individual ethnic group, to a greater or lesser degree, may come to share concepts and attitudes about ADRD held by the larger society. Some members may adopt fully the ADRD knowledge base and diagnostic/treatment conventions that have been developed by the research community, the Alzheimer's Association, and other organizations. In contrast, other members of the particular ethnic group may rely on culture-specific constructs in which the disease may be viewed as a normal part of aging, to be expected in people's later years, or an abnormality or punishment brought about by prior behavior deemed

53

culturally inappropriate. However, attitudes will vary along the acculturation continuum, depending in large part upon the degree to which assimilation has been achieved or, indeed, even desired.

A number of investigators of various ethnic populations have observed that early signs and symptoms of elders' loss of memory or other cognitive function may evoke relatively little concern; the elder and other family members may not perceive the cognitive decline or may not feel disturbed about it even though family members may have recognized the subtle and insidious cognitive changes found in ADRD in their elders many years prior to seeking assistance. At present, data are not available that allow conclusions as to whether lack of concern regarding cognitive changes is actually more frequent in ethnic minority groups than in the majority population. As indicated by a broad survey of service providers, one reason for this lack of concern may be that ethnic minority populations have very little knowledge about dementia as a disorder and often attribute the changes involved to normal aging. Likewise, in the traditional U.S. Black southern culture, which often emphasizes affective aspects of relationships, symptoms of dementia are frequently attributed to various folk illnesses, such as "worration" (worry) or "spells." Common terms used to describe such mental illness include "going off," "having trouble," "not clothed in the right mind," or "not right in the head."

Significantly, these conditions often do not prompt movement toward the formal health care system. However, disintegration of personality function—a later symptom of ADRD—generally is approached more seriously and often precipitates a search for health care and social support services. Although it has not been established to what extent these ethnic minority patterns differ from those characteristic of the majority population and whether the differences relate to ethnicity, social class, or other factors, what is clear is that many affected ethnic elders come to clinical attention only when they have reached quite advanced stages of the disease.

Thus, our understanding of how Alzheimer's disease is viewed must include a comparison of the knowledge, attitudes, and practices of the overall ethnic group or of individual group members with the viewpoints of the majority society on the dementias. In this way, we can better plan and develop mechanisms to provide education and services that will be useful for that population. Though complex, this perspective is facilitated in research by gathering information about (a) the ethnic group's knowledge, beliefs, attitudes, and practices about aging and dementia and (b) the elder's and significant others' understanding of the disease. These cultural differences in viewpoints must be approached in a value-neutral fashion. Because of lack of research on these particular issues and on the general outcomes of providing formal or informal care to ADRD patients, few empirical data are available to clarify what repercussions either the majority-culture viewpoint or the ethnic minority approach have on the quality of life experienced by individuals with ADRD and their families.

While the need for community education about ADRD in ethnic populations is great, if that information is to be meaningful, it must be couched in appropriate ways, using the language and nuances of that particular culture. Experience in support group contexts has shown that complex technical information about ADRD can be both understood and integrated by non-English-speaking members of traditional ethnocultural groups when presented in a manner attuned to the ethnic group's core body of knowledge, attitudes, and practices and built upon this base.

Help-Seeking and Help-Accepting Behavior

Whether or not AD is a uniform biophysical process across cultures, responses to the illness vary, particularly with regard to help-seeking and help-accepting behaviors. Differences in the help-seeking and help-accepting behaviors typically shown by cognitively impaired elders and family caregivers in the various U.S. ethnic groups may well be related to the health maintenance behaviors characteristic of their cultures of origin as well as to characteristics of the U.S. health care delivery system. The response to illness must be distinguished from the disease entity itself.

Little or no literature has been produced bearing on the use of traditional, culture-specific forms of health care for ADRD treatment by ethnic populations, such as reliance on medicine men and women by American Indians and Alaska Natives, herbalists by Chinese Americans, spiritual healers or root doctors by African Americans, or curanderos by Mexican Americans. There is, however, considerable need for empirical data to validate the knowledge, attitudes, and practices regarding traditional treatments that characterize various minority groups, relative to those attributed to them in the emergent literature on this topic.

Information about the help-seeking and help-accepting patterns of ethnic groups with respect to ADRD, unfortunately, has not been widely reported in the research literature. An emerging area of study that centers around caregiver response to the disease process, however, appears to suggest certain salient features in care-seeking and accepting behavior among the four core ethnic populations. For example, African American caregivers appear to emphasize religiosity as a coping mechanism; they report higher use of internalizing or cognitive coping strategies. Furthermore, African Americans tend to maintain large caregiver households and to use a wide range of informal social supports.

Hispanic populations report greater utilization of informal support systems than traditional health care providers. Caregivers in some American Indian groups appear to manage stress by passive forbearance, with relatively little reference to control as a concept. An analysis of caregiving networks based on data from the 1982 National Long-Term Care Survey and associated Informal Caregivers Survey indicated that, in comparison to the majority population, ethnic frail elderly are more likely to have non-kin primary caregivers.

Whether or not relatives seek formal care for the demented elderly also depends upon such factors as acculturation, level of education, and literacy. Some studies have suggested that ethnic elders suffering from dementia and significant numbers of their family caregivers tend to have low levels of formal education and minimal operational or working knowledge of services and how best to link themselves to services and formal caregiving systems. Where others might seek services, they generally turn inward for assistance—to themselves and their network of significant others. Their informal caregiving networks seem to involve a greater number of individuals than found in the networks of comparable elders in the majority population; the tasks of assisting elders with their activities of daily living are distributed differently within these ethnic networks.

Unfortunately, study of caregiver response in ADRD is limited, not only with respect to the ethnic elderly population but also with respect to any large, representative population bases. Exploration of both the formal and informal networks of care used by ethnic elders suffering from ADRD is critical if we are to better understand how formal services may be structured to meet their individual needs optimally, in a culturally sensitive, empathetic manner. However, rather than either assuming the benefits of formal services or idealizing the informal care patterns observed among ethnic elders with ADRD, we need research comparing the empirical outcomes on such dimensions as the ethnic elder's health, daily functional level, socialization, and quality of life and also on the family's level of stress and burden. If reliance on informal caring networks is associated with detrimental outcomes, such research can also help clarify barriers that impede access to services. Alternatively, should the research show that some informal care outcomes are not altogether negative, the majority culture may have much to learn from the ways in which individuals with dementia are viewed and managed within ethnic subcultures.

Ethnic Group Access to Formal Services

Access to ADRD care by culturally diverse ethnic populations lags behind that of the majority population. Although exceptions may be cited (such as Casa Central in Chicago or On Lok in San Francisco), overall, long-term care services and clinical health care delivery programs are not designed with accessibility for ethnic populations in mind. Much of the overall health care system, and the long-term care system in particular, lacks culturally and linguistically accessible information and referral capacities. Social and health care services for ADRD elders are not always able to incorporate or make use of the informal caregiving networks of culturally diverse ethnic elders. The reliance for caregiving by many ethnic elders not only on the immediate family but also on friends, extended family, and the church is a positive asset but may present a challenge to service delivery organizations when attempting to include such caregivers in planning, patient management, and decisionmaking. Moreover, case management services frequently lack sensitivity to these sorts of cultural issues, whether because personnel lack the ability to communicate with non-English-speaking elderly or because the personnel are not attuned to traditional cultural values held by ethnic elderly clients. Financing mechanisms that address the special service eligibility concerns of immigrant and refugee ADRD victims, who are generally not eligible for Medicare or many other programs of assistance, are also lacking.

Thus, it is important to train ADRD service personnel to meet the culturally disparate needs of the ethnic elderly population. With increasing numbers of ethnic elderly, culturally capable long-term care staff should be increasingly available to work with both patients and families. Most studies in this area reveal the importance of barriers between patient and provider created by differences in language, cultural relevance, needs, and ethnicity. Bilingual ethnic professionals and paraprofessionals will be helpful in working with both newly immigrated elderly and those who have not yet learned fluent English. Use of translators may limit communication between patients and professional personnel, and perhaps limit treatment options as well. (Studies have found that family translators either may impart their own affect into the statements of their non-English-speaking relatives or may be embarrassed to translate candidly. Patients may hesitate to disclose important information when a family translator is used. Professional translators who are not of the patient's native culture may translate too literally to convey the culture-based message behind the words themselves.) Bilingual, ethnic health care and social services professionals may share with a patient a common understanding of attitudes and nonverbal communication. While acculturation differs from ethnic elder to ethnic elder, the ability to provide care in an environment sensitive to traditions and the ethos of the native culture is critical, particularly as the numbers of ethnic elders increase.

African Americans and Hispanics use long-term care facilities less than would be expected from their numbers within the population. To a large degree, the underrepresentation of ethnic populations within the long-term care system, particularly within nursing homes, may be due to socioeconomic and systemic factors such as poverty, absence of insurance, maldistribution of services, lack of educational opportunity, and behavior patterns reactive to the longstanding experience of having been underserved by the existing social and medical service system. Cultural factors obviously also influence the participation of ethnic elders in such facilities. Differences in language, attitudes, expectations, or tolerance for particular ADRD symptoms may make it more difficult for certain ethnic populations to adjust to nursing home or other formal care settings. Outreach and followup with such individuals by culturally sensitive social workers, home health nurses, and others involved in the health care and social services systems could begin to remove many obstacles that may be keeping formal care from being accessible for ethnic elders.

The absence of substantial numbers of ethnic group members within nursing homes and related long-term care services is also associated with the tendency for family members and others who provide informal support to maintain the caregiving function for a longer period, though the direction of causality in this association is unclear. Since this dynamic has been reported in the caregiver literature with respect to many ethnic groups, more comparative cross-cultural research may help to elucidate the factors involved, in particular, whether socioeconomic or cultural factors more strongly govern this pattern.

One of the most significant barriers to formal care for the ethnic elderly lies in the screening instruments used to detect both ADRD and the cognitive impairments found in these disorders. Variations in culture, education, and literacy profoundly affect these assessments; formidable problems have arisen in efforts to control for these influences in research protocols. Before ADRD treatment and research can move forward on behalf of ethnic minorities, it is necessary to validate the efficacy of existing screening instruments and, as necessary, to develop improved instruments or alternative techniques to detect dementia across ethnically and educationally different subpopulations.

Because few evaluative instruments have been validated directly with ethnic populations, both research and clinical work have relied on instruments and techniques that have been normed only on the Nation's majority population. Such methodology is inadequate both for resolving scientific questions regarding the incidence and prevalence of the cognitive deficits associated with ADRD in these populations and for undertaking individual clinical evaluations of the ethnic elderly. For example, test items based on orientation to time may be less relevant to certain ethnic subpopulations. Rather, what may be more salient is an understanding of kinship terms or power relationships (as in the Chinese and African American populations) or seasons (as in some Mexican and Mexican American groups) or knowledge of clans (as in some American Indian groups). By failing to determine the relevant, culturally based expressions of cognition, findings regarding functional capacity and cognitive ability may be distorted.

L.H. Rogler ("The Meaning of Culturally Sensitive Research in Mental Health," *American Journal of Psychiatry* 146:296-303, 1989.) has suggested that research and clinical work in ADRD and in other areas of mental illness must be made "culturally sensitive." The process through which this occurs extends far beyond translating a screening instrument into another language or applying nomenclature of one society to another. Rather, it requires extensive immersion in the culture of the study or treatment group, evaluating whether the concepts underlying the proposed test instruments fit the constructs of the study group itself. Only after such a fit is achieved should the translation of specific items begin. During the process of translation, care and attention must be given to ensuring that the instrument reflects the ways in which the population expresses itself. Only with this information in hand should final development of instruments begin. The process is complex, time-consuming, and expensive, but is necessary to ensure the requisite mesh between cultural components of the population and either the research intent or the clinical process.

Several factors in combination are likely to facilitate access to services by ethnic populations in need of long-term care assistance. First, the program (whether providing only patient care or combining care with research) ideally should be located within the target ethnic community.

Second, professional and technically competent personnel who are ethnically and culturally compatible with (or specially sensitive to) the patients to be served should be employed at all levels of the system. Thus, culturally capable geriatricians, internists, neurologists, neuropsychologists, psychiatrists, nurses, social workers, and other professionals and paraprofessionals should be working as part of the ADRD clinical intervention or research team. Since, as noted above, inadequate numbers of culturally capable specialists are now available, special training in cultural sensitivity must be emphasized in professional and paraprofessional education.

Third, the provision of social and health care services and the conduct of research on ADRD in ethnic minority populations should be accompanied by sustained, culturally relevant outreach and community-wide education. Specialized personnel, again, should be located and trained to facilitate this effort.

Fourth, screening instruments used to establish cognitive impairment as the first steps in the ADRD diagnostic process should be "culture-fair," that is, responsive to the particular culture-based belief systems, acculturation level, education, and ethos of the individuals being assessed.

Fifth, research data gathering must increase and must focus on documenting the ethnic group dynamics surrounding the disease, and the clinical and family outcomes experienced as a result of the forms of care rendered, as well as on probing the disease process itself. When formal services have been structured to fit the target ethnic group's knowledge, attitudes, and expectations regarding help-seeking and help-accepting behaviors, ethnic group members generally have shown a greater willingness to make use of these services.

A recent initiative by the Administration on Aging (AOA) to fund special projects on minority access to ADRD services generated a large number of applications and demonstrated that service providers in many localities are concerned about and attempting to address this issue. Three grants to develop new materials and methods for informing ethnic elders with dementia and their caregivers about available services, and for helping connect them to needed services, were awarded by AOA during 1990 to the Executive Office on Aging in

Honolulu, Hawaii; the Morehouse School of Medicine in Atlanta, Georgia; and the Institute for Community Research in Hartford, Connecticut. (In addition, a demonstration project recently funded by HCFA is allowing the State of Arizona to provide long-term care services, through community contracts, to Arizona residents, including American Indians.)

The context in which health care is provided to elderly American Indians and Alaska Natives living on reservations differs from that of other ethnic elders. Virtually all health care services for reservation-based American Indian elders are coordinated by the Indian Health Service (IHS), either directly or through contracts with tribes. While historically little attention has been paid to specifically geriatric issues for these elders, the recent establishment of an advisory IHS Workgroup on Aging concerned with the delivery of services to elders on reservations may lead to changes in the quality and availability of community care, home care, and other ADRD-relevant services for this subpopulation. Stronger linkages between the services provided and outside research investigators, if facilitated as a part of these changes, would also be a positive development.

Biomedical Science and Cross-Cultural Research in ADRD

Cross-cultural and cross-ethnic research has the unique potential to clarify the effects of cultural diversity on the presentation and diagnosis of Alzheimer's disease. The scientific value of multicultural research as well as its importance for sociopolitical purposes must not be overlooked.

Cognitive Screening Procedures

As noted earlier, the efficacy of existing cognitive screening instruments in accurately detecting cognitive impairment in the ethnic elderly of various origins has been questioned. For example, the high level of cognitive impairment found among African Americans and Hispanics may be valid or may be an erroneous finding based on an instrument lacking cultural sensitivity or plagued by other problems, such as the influence of respondents' educational status, interviewer characteristics, or poorly understood difficulties of administering the instrument in the field.

Research is already under way in New York, San Diego, Los Angeles, and San Antonio to validate screening instruments for Hispanic and African American populations. Preliminary findings from the work in New York comparing African American, Hispanic, and non-Hispanic white populations on five cognitive screening procedures suggests that a different procedure was most sensitive for each ethnic group. A task force of the multicenter Consortium to Establish a Registry for Alzheimer's Disease (CERAD) has been working to validate a brief neuropsychological battery for use with Hispanics and African Americans. In international research, the Blessed Dementia Rating Scale and the Mini-Mental State Examination have been tested with a Chinese population, as have components of a neuropsychological battery. Norms for these various populations have not yet been established, since many of the data are still being collected and analyzed.

The screening procedures that emerge from this ongoing research will have been validated for cultural fairness relative to the specific ethnocultural populations studied, meeting the culture-fair challenge inherent in earlier reports. Various studies are also attempting to resolve the effects that education and literacy appear to have on screening instruments and other assessments of cognitive function. A number of studies suggest that the current cognitive screening procedures (particularly the Mini-Mental State Examination) require a certain degree of educational attainment; even when the norms are scaled downward, existing items on such instruments may not be sufficient to measure cognitive impairment accurately or yield accurate diagnoses among those of lower educational attainment (e.g., less than ninth-grade education). Rather, additional items may be necessary to tap into various dimensions of cognitive impairment among those with very limited or no formal education. This idea is evident from a diagnostic study of AD in Shanghai in which the study population contained a large percentage of persons without any formal education. Twenty-six percent of the sample classified as illiterate also demonstrated exceptionally high levels of cognitive impairment on the Mini-Mental State Examination.

Researchers presently have great difficulty adequately screening nonliterate and semiliterate people for dementia, regardless of their culture, and can do so only by adding on extensive and expensive clinical diagnostic protocols. Several efforts are currently underway in the United States to disentangle the effects of education and low literacy from cultural artifacts in screening procedures. The already mentioned San Diego project with Hispanics is seeking to distinguish educational from cultural artifacts in three cognitive screening procedures—the Mental Status Questionnaire, Information-Memory-Concentration Test and the Mini-Mental State Examination. Research on alternate testing and diagnostic approaches that are less language-based and potentially more culturally fair, such as reaction time procedures, also is worth pursuing. Until cognitive screening procedures have been calibrated for nonliterate and semiliterate individuals, not only within linguistically and culturally diverse groups but also in the general population, prevalence studies will continue to report questionable rates of cognitive impairment in community populations, particularly in ethnic groups.

Yet, even the best testing instruments are only as good as the individuals administering them. The research community is in need of professionals who speak the language of the subgroups and who can explain things in terms familiar to the particular ethnic population. People who must communicate in a second language or through translators often appear to be curt and brusque simply because their vocabulary is limited and their knowledge of idiom absent. As noted earlier, translators create problems as well. Family translators restrict the test subject's freedom to speak; professional translators may over- or under-interpret in communications both from and to the interviewer.

Obviously, no resolution has yet been reached about the best testing instruments or about the most clearly efficacious approach to the study of ethnic populations. However, these issues require priority attention. Whether or not the biophysiology of AD may vary across racial and ethnic groups, patient and family recognition of and response to the disease may range widely. The challenge for clinical and epidemiological researchers at this point is to develop a dementia screening technology that transcends educational, ethnic, and cross-cultural differences. Until this impasse is resolved, both clinical and epidemiological studies of ADRD will suffer from cultural and educational biases inherent in their cognitive testing, diagnostic, and/or other research procedures.

Clinical Intervention Studies

Many of the same barriers that limit access by ethnic populations to long-term care services also affect their participation in basic, epidemiological, and clinical ADRD research. It has proven quite difficult for researchers to recruit ethnic population subjects in major clinical trials of psychopharmacological treatments for ADRD and other mental disorders. However, differences in drug metabolism of psychoactive agents are well documented and may extend to drugs being developed for ADRD. Some indications from other areas of psychopharmacological research suggest that physiologic systems vary, and appropriate medication dosage levels may differ among ethnic groups. A recently established Center on the Psychobiology of Ethnicity at the Harbor-University of California, Los Angeles, Medical Center has as its goal the study of the ways in which different ethnic groups physiologically process and respond to psychotropic medications. Findings from this NIMH-supported center's studies may help delineate physiological and sociocultural differences that may influence the appropriate use and dosages for psychotropic medications used in the treatment of disorders collateral to ADRD.

It is particularly important to test the safety and efficacy of drugs in a broad spectrum of patients as early as possible in clinical trials. However, the imperative to develop such drugs should not allow the difficulty in recruiting ethnic ADRD patients into clinical trials to slow the drug development process. Rather, this problem should encourage detailed study of ethnic populations in the later phases of the drug approval process or even postapproval surveillance studies.

Epidemiological and Population Studies

By identifying and subsequently testing variables of potential etiological significance, population studies and epidemiological research have great potential for uncovering causes of ADRD. However, no major etiologically oriented research on ADRD across ethnically diverse populations has been reported in the United States. One recently funded study, however, is beginning to evaluate, for cognitive deficits, a tri-ethnic population in New York City's North Manhattan, including a large group of now-elderly migrants from the Dominican Republic who may be at high risk for neurodegenerative changes because of earlier exposure to pesticides as field workers. Greater attention needs to be paid to including such ethnic comparisons in ongoing ADRD biomedical research, including autopsy efforts. In an effort to include more ethnic population elders in ongoing ADRD research, NIA has initiated a program of developing additional diagnostic and treatment centers as satellites to its Alzheimer's Disease Research Centers. These satellites expand the ADRC clinical operations to other geographic sites to facilitate the entry of minority, rural, and other underserved populations into AD research and drug trials.

While research has demonstrated convincingly that at least some cases of AD are genetically linked, scientific inquiry has not yet conclusively identified other robust risk factors aside from advancing age. Our ability to search more aggressively and broadly for modifiable risk factors in ADRD demands that the conduct of research extend across cultural boundaries. Comparative research on population groups in various cultures with different environmental exposures and habits may offer clues to the etiology of the disease that are not available from research undertaken within a single culture. These clues may emerge from differences in age-specific incidence and prevalence rates between distinct subpopulations or by acquired characteristics and may lead to new etiological research hypotheses.

With the exception of the epidemiological project conducted in Shanghai, the available literature provides little guidance relative to cross-cultural ADRD population studies. Although research on these important issues has not been adequately supported to date, several recently begun projects reflect growing interest in cross-cultural studies. Ongoing efforts include a World Health Organization multisite study involving Canada, Chile, Malta, Nigeria, and Spain as well as the United States that is developing culturally fair screening instruments and other tests needed as tools for conducting epidemiological comparisons. Another international collaboration is supporting a normative study in the elderly population of Italy of computerized technology developed in the United States for assessing cognitive impairment. Studies of ADRD in Japanese Americans are beginning in Seattle and Honolulu and will include parallel studies in Japan, thereby yielding an opportunity for migration studies. Other likely parallel study sites include Taiwan and, possibly, South Korea. U.S. investment in such ADRD studies, though increasing, has been minimal and needs to be expanded. The scientific value of such research needs to be more broadly recognized and receive greater emphasis. Though costly, the dividends from these studies are potentially great.

Chapter 7

Early Alzheimer's Disease: A Guide for Patients and Families

Purpose of This Chapter

This chapter is about Alzheimer's disease and other types of dementia. It presents information for patients, family members, and other caregivers. It talks about the effects Alzheimer's disease can have on you, your family members, and your friends.

The text describes the early signs and symptoms of Alzheimer's disease. Sources of medical, social, and financial support are listed at the end of the chapter. This chapter is not about treating Alzheimer's disease.

What Is Alzheimer's Disease?

In Alzheimer's disease and other dementias, problems with memory, judgment, and thought processes make it hard for a person to work and take part in day-to-day family and social life. Changes in mood and personality also may occur. These changes can result in loss of self-control and other problems.

Some 2 to 4 million persons have dementia associated with aging. Of these individuals, as many as two-thirds have Alzheimer's disease.

Although there is no cure for Alzheimer's disease at this time, it may be possible to relieve some of the symptoms, such as wandering and incontinence.

Consumer Version, Clinical Practice Guideline, Number 19, Agency for Health Care Policy and Research (AHCPR) Pub. No. 96-0704, September 1996.

The earlier the diagnosis, the more likely your symptoms will respond to treatment. Talk to your doctor as soon as possible if you think you or a family member may have signs of Alzheimer's disease.

Research is under way to find better ways to treat Alzheimer's disease. Ask your doctor if there are any new developments that might help you.

What Are Risk Factors for Alzheimer's Disease?

The chances of getting Alzheimer's disease increase with age. It usually occurs after age 65. Most people are not affected even at advanced ages. There are only two definite factors that increase the risk for Alzheimer's disease: a family history of dementia and Down syndrome.

Family History of Dementia

Some forms of Alzheimer's disease are inherited. If Alzheimer's disease has occurred in your family members, other members are more likely to develop it. Discuss any family history of dementia with your family doctor.

Down Syndrome

Persons with Down syndrome have a higher chance of getting Alzheimer's disease. Close relatives of persons with Down syndrome also may be at risk.

What Are the Signs of Alzheimer's Disease?

The classic sign of early Alzheimer's disease is gradual loss of short-term memory. Other signs include:

- Problems finding or speaking the right word.

- Inability to recognize objects.

- Forgetting how to use simple, ordinary things, such as a pencil.

- Forgetting to turn off the stove, close windows, or lock doors.

Mood and personality changes also may occur. Agitation, problems with memory, and poor judgment may cause unusual behavior. These symptoms vary from one person to the next.

Symptoms appear gradually in persons with Alzheimer's disease but may progress more slowly in some persons than in others. In other forms of dementia, symptoms may appear suddenly or may come and go.

If you have some of these signs, this does not mean you have Alzheimer's disease. Anyone can have a lapse of memory or show poor judgment now and then. When such lapses become frequent or dangerous, however, you should tell your doctor about them immediately.

Possible Signs of Alzheimer's Disease

Do you have problems with any of these activities?

- **Learning and remembering new information.** Do you repeat things that you say or do? Forget conversations or appointments? Forget where you put things?

- **Handling complex tasks.** Do you have trouble performing tasks that require many steps such as balancing a checkbook or cooking a meal?

- **Reasoning ability.** Do you have trouble solving everyday problems at work or home, such as knowing what to do if the bathroom is flooded?

- **Spatial ability and orientation.** Do you have trouble driving or finding your way around familiar places?

- **Language.** Do you have trouble finding the words to express what you want to say?

- **Behavior.** Do you have trouble paying attention? Are you more irritable or less trusting than usual?

Remember, everyone has occasional memory lapses. Just because you can't recall where you put the car keys doesn't mean you have Alzheimer's disease.

Consulting the Doctor

Identifying mild cases of Alzheimer's disease can be very difficult. Your doctor will review your health and mental status, both past and present. Changes from your previous, usual mental and physical functioning are especially important.

Persons with Alzheimer's disease may not realize the severity of their condition. Your doctor will probably want to talk with family members or a close friend about their impressions of your condition.

The doctor's first assessment for Alzheimer's disease should include a focused history, a physical examination, a functional status assessment, and a mental status assessment.

Medical and Family History

Questions the doctor may ask in taking your history include: How and when did problems begin? Have the symptoms progressed in steps or worsened steadily? Do they vary from day to day? How long have they lasted?

Your doctor will ask about past and current medical problems and whether other family members have had Alzheimer's disease or another form of dementia.

Education and other cultural factors can make a difference in how you will do on mental ability tests. Language problems (for example, difficulty speaking English) can cause misunderstanding. Be sure to tell the doctor about any language problems that could affect your test results.

It is important to tell the doctor about all the drugs you take and how long you have been taking them. Drug reactions can cause dementia. Bring all medication bottles and pills to the appointment with your doctor.

Do you take any medications? Even over-the-counter drugs, eye drops, and alcohol can cause a decline in mental ability. Tell your doctor about all the drugs you take. Ask if the drugs are safe when taken together.

Physical Examination

A physical examination can determine whether medical problems may be causing symptoms of dementia. This is important because prompt treatment may relieve some symptoms.

Functional Status Assessment

The doctor may ask you questions about your ability to live alone. Sometimes, a family member or close friend may be asked how well you can do activities like these:

• Write checks, pay bills, or balance a checkbook.

- Shop alone for clothing, food, and household needs.

- Play a game of skill or work on a hobby.

- Heat water, make coffee, and turn off stove.

- Pay attention to, understand, and discuss a TV show, book, or magazine.

- Remember appointments, family occasions, holidays, and medications.

- Travel out of the neighborhood, drive, or use public transportation.

Sometimes a family member or friend is not available to answer such questions. Then, the doctor may ask you to perform a series of tasks ("performance testing").

Mental Status Assessment

Several other tests may be used to assess your mental status. These tests usually have only a few simple questions. They test mental functioning, including orientation, attention, memory, and language skills. Age, educational level, and cultural influences may affect how you perform on mental status tests. Your doctor will consider these factors in interpreting test results.

Alzheimer's disease affects two major types of abilities

1. The ability to carry out everyday activities such as bathing, dressing, using the toilet, eating, and walking.

2. The ability to perform more complex tasks such as using the telephone, managing finances, driving a car, planning meals, and working in a job.

When a person has Alzheimer's disease, problems with complex tasks appear first and over time progress to more simple activities.

Treatable Causes of Dementia

Sometimes the physical examination reveals a condition that can be treated. Symptoms may respond to early treatment when they are caused by:

- Medication (including over-the-counter drugs).
- Alcohol.
- Delirium.
- Depression.
- Tumors.
- Problems with the heart, lungs, or blood vessels.
- Metabolic disorders (such as thyroid problems).
- Head injury.
- Infection.
- Vision or hearing problems.

Drug reactions. Drug reactions are the most common cause of treatable symptoms. Older persons may have reactions when they take certain medications. Some medications should not be taken together. Sometimes, adjusting the dose can improve symptoms.

Delirium and depression. Delirium and depression may be mistaken for or occur with Alzheimer's disease. These conditions require prompt treatment. See "Terms You Need to Know" below for more information on delirium and depression.

Special Tests

Gathering as much information as possible will help your doctor diagnose early Alzheimer's disease while the condition is mild. You may be referred to other specialists for further testing.

Some special tests can show a person's mental strengths and weaknesses and detect differences between mild, moderate, and severe impairment. Tests also can tell the difference between changes due to normal aging and those caused by Alzheimer's disease.

If you go to a special doctor for these tests, he or she should return all test results to your regular family doctor. The results will help your doctor track the progress of your condition, prescribe treatment, and monitor treatment effects.

Getting the Right Care

When the diagnosis is Alzheimer's disease, you and your family members have serious issues to consider. Talk with your doctor about what to expect in the near future and later on, as your condition progresses. Getting help early will help ensure that you get the care that is best for you.

When tests do not indicate Alzheimer's disease, but your symptoms continue or worsen, check back with your doctor. More tests may be needed. If you still have concerns, even though your doctor says you do not have Alzheimer's disease, you may want to get a second opinion. Whatever the diagnosis, followup is important.

Report any changes in your symptoms. Ask the doctor what followup is right for you. Your doctor should keep the results of the first round of tests for later use. After treatment of other health problems, new tests may show a change in your condition.

Recognizing Alzheimer's disease in its early stages, when treatment may relieve mild symptoms, gives you time to adjust. During this time, you and your family can make financial, legal, and medical plans for the future.

Coordinating Care

Your health care team may include your family doctor and medical specialists such as psychiatrists or neurologists, psychologists, therapists, nurses, social workers, and counselors. They can work together to help you understand your condition, suggest memory aids, and tell you and your family about ways you can stay independent as long as possible.

Talk with your doctors about activities that could be dangerous for you or others, such as driving or cooking. Explore different ways to do things.

Telling Family and Friends

Ask your doctor for help in telling people who need to know that you have Alzheimer's disease—members of your family, friends, and coworkers, for example.

Alzheimer's disease is stressful for you and your family. You and your caregiver will need support from others. Working together eases the stress on everyone.

Where to Get Help?

Learning that you have Alzheimer's disease can be very hard to deal with. It is important to share your feelings with family and friends.

Many kinds of help are available for persons with Alzheimer's disease, their families, and caregivers. Turn to the back of this chapter for a list of resources for patients and families. These resources include:

- **Support groups.** Sometimes it helps to talk things over with other people and families who are coping with Alzheimer's disease. Families and friends of people with Alzheimer's disease have formed support groups. The Alzheimer's Association has active groups across the country. Many hospitals also sponsor education programs and support groups to help patients and families.

- **Financial and medical planning.** Time to plan can be a major benefit of identifying Alzheimer's disease early. You and your family will need to decide where you will live and who will provide help and care when you need them.

- **Legal matters.** It is also important to think about certain legal matters. An attorney can give you legal advice and help you and your family make plans for the future. A special document called an advance directive lets others know what you would like them to do if you become unable to think clearly or speak for yourself.

Terms You Need to Know

Dementia. Dementia is a medical condition that interferes with the way the brain works. Symptoms include anxiety, paranoia, personality changes, lack of initiative, and difficulty acquiring new skills. Besides Alzheimer's disease, some other types or causes of dementia include: alcoholic dementia, depression, delirium, HIV/AIDS-related dementia, Huntington's disease (a disorder of the nervous system), inflammatory disease (for example, syphilis), vascular dementia (blood vessel disease in the brain), tumors, and Parkinson's disease.

Alzheimer's disease. Alzheimer's disease is the most common form of dementia. It proceeds in stages over months or years and gradually destroys memory, reason, judgment, language, and eventually the ability to carry out even simple tasks.

Delirium. Delirium is a state of temporary but acute mental confusion that comes on suddenly. Symptoms may include anxiety, disorientation, tremors, hallucinations, delusions, and incoherence. Delirium can occur in older persons who have short-term illnesses, heart or lung disease, long-term infections, poor nutrition, or hormone disorders. Alcohol or drugs (including medications) also may cause confusion.

Delirium may be life-threatening and requires immediate medical attention.

Depression. Depression can occur in older persons, especially those with physical problems. Symptoms include sadness, inactivity, difficulty thinking and concentrating, and feelings of despair. Depressed persons often have trouble sleeping, changes in appetite, fatigue, and agitation. Depression usually can be treated successfully.

Other Booklets Are Available

The information in this chapter is based on *Recognition and Initial Assessment of Alzheimer's Disease and Related Dementias: Clinical Practice Guideline No. 19.* A multidisciplinary panel of physicians, psychiatrists, psychologists, neurologists, nurses, a geriatrician, a social worker, and two consumer representatives developed the guideline. The Agency for Health Care Policy and Research (AHCPR), an agency of the U.S. Department of Health and Human Services, supported its development. Other AHCPR guidelines may be helpful to families affected by Alzheimer's disease. They include:

- *Depression Is a Treatable Illness: Patient Guide* discusses major depressive disorder, which usually can be treated successfully with the help of a health professional. (AHCPR Publication No. 93-0053)

- *Recovering After a Stroke: Patient and Family Guide* tells how to help a person who has had a stroke achieve the best possible recovery. (AHCPR Publication No. 95-0664)

- *Understanding Urinary Incontinence in Adults: Patient Guide* describes why people lose urine when they don't want to and what can be done about it. (AHCPR Publication No. 96-0684)

- *Preventing Pressure Ulcers: Patient Guide* discusses symptoms and causes of bed sores and ways to prevent them. (AHCPR Publication No. 92-0048)

- *Treating Pressure Sores: Consumer Guide* describes basic steps of care for bed sores. (AHCPR Publication No. 95-0654)

For more information on these or other guidelines, or to receive more copies of this text, call toll-free: 800-358-9295. Or write to:

Agency for Health Care Policy and Research
Publications Clearinghouse
P.O. Box 8547
Silver Spring, MD 20907

Resources for Patients and Families

Many kinds of help are available for patients with Alzheimer's disease, their families and caregivers. The list below gives information for contacting national organizations. They can refer you to local chapters and other resources where you live.

Alzheimer's Association
Chicago, IL
(312) 335-8700; 800-272-3900

Alzheimer's Disease Education and Referral (ADEAR) Center
Silver Spring, MD
800-438-4380

Administration on Aging
Washington, DC
(202)619-1006

Eldercare Locator
Washington, DC
800-677-1116

American Association of Retired Persons (AARP)
Washington, DC
(202)434-2277; 800-424-3410

Children of Aging Parents
Levittown, PA
(215) 945-6900

National Association For Continence (formerly Help for Incontinent People)
Spartanburg, SC
(800) 252-3337; 800-BLADDER

76

Insurance Consumer Helpline
Washington, DC
800-942-4242

Medicare Hotline
Baltimore, MD
800-638-6833

National Hospice Organization
Arlington, VA
(703)243-5900; 800-658-8898

Social Security Information
800-772-1213
(open 7 am–7 pm in all time zones)

Chapter 8

How Doctors Diagnose Alzheimer's Disease and Related Dementias

Purpose and Scope

Dementia is a syndrome of progressive decline that relentlessly erodes intellectual abilities, causing cognitive and functional deterioration leading to impairment of social and occupational functioning. Because Alzheimer's disease is the most common dementing illness in the United States, it is used as a prototype for dementia in this chapter unless otherwise stated.

An estimated 5 to 10 percent of the U.S. adult population ages 65 and older is affected by a dementing disorder, and incidence doubles every 5 years after age 65. Despite its prevalence, dementia is often unrecognized or misdiagnosed in its early stages. Failure to identify early-stage dementia can result in inappropriate treatment, hazardous situations, and needless distress. Early recognition of dementia, however, not only can prevent problems but also can allow the patient and family to plan for the future and consider participation in trials of promising new therapies as they are developed.

A number of characteristics distinguish early-stage dementia from normal aging and from other syndromes that involve cognitive problems, including depression. This chapter provides information to help

Costa PT Jr, Williams TF, Somerfield M, et al. *Early Identification of Alzheimer's Disease and Related Dementias. Clinical Practice Guideline, Quick Reference Guide for Clinicians, No. 19.* Rockville, MD: U.S. Department of Health and Human Services, Public Health Service, Agency for Health Care Policy and Research. AHCPR Publication No. 97-0703, November 1996.

clinicians recognize those characteristics as symptoms suggestive of a dementing disorder and to conduct an initial assessment of mental and functional status. The recommendations are intended for use by primary care clinicians, including but not limited to family physicians, internists, geriatricians, psychologists, psychiatrists, nurses, and nurse practitioners. They are not intended to replace existing recommendations for a differential diagnosis once dementia has been identified.

Recognizing Symptoms

Certain "triggers" (clues, symptoms) should prompt a clinician to conduct an initial assessment for dementia rather than attribute apparent signs of decline to aging. Examples of such triggers appear in Table 8.1. Although the patient, family members, or others often bring their concerns about symptoms to the clinician's attention, clinicians also should be alert to such signs during office visits.

Table 8.1 is a clinical guide, not a validated test instrument. In asymptomatic persons who have possible risk factors, the clinician's judgment and knowledge of the patient's current condition, history, and social situation (living arrangements, support services, isolation) must guide the decision to initiate an assessment for dementia.

For Alzheimer's disease, the only well-established risk factors are family history of dementia and the presence of Down syndrome. Genetic studies show that autosomal-dominant forms of Alzheimer's disease are associated with early onset and early death. Recent research also suggests an association of certain apolipoprotein E (apoE) genotypes and late-onset Alzheimer's disease; however, apoE genotyping is not a definitive diagnostic tool.

Evidence also suggests the possibility of a modest but significant association with earlier head trauma involving loss of consciousness.

Initiating and Assessment

To help determine whether a patient's symptoms meet current criteria for dementia, an initial assessment should combine information from several sources. The basic components of this assessment are a focused history, a physical examination, a functional status assessment, and a mental status assessment. The recommended assessment process is presented in Figure 8.2.

According to current criteria, a diagnosis of dementia requires evidence of decline from previous levels of functioning and impairment

Table 8.1. Symptoms that may indicate dementia.

Does the person have increased difficulty with any of the activities listed below?[a]

- ❑ *Learning and retaining new information.* Is more repetitive; has trouble remembering recent conversations, events, appointments; frequently misplaces objects.

- ❑ *Handling complex tasks.* Has trouble following a complex train of thought or performing tasks that require many steps such as balancing a checkbook or cooking a meal.

- ❑ *Reasoning ability.* Is unable to respond with a reasonable plan to problems at work or home, such as knowing what to do if the bathroom is flooded; shows uncharacteristic disregard for rules of social conduct.

- ❑ *Spatial ability and orientation.* Has trouble driving, organizing objects around the house, finding his or her way around familiar places.

- ❑ *Language.* Has increasing difficulty with finding the words to express what he or she wants to say and with following conversations.

- ❑ *Behavior.* Appears more passive and less responsive; is more irritable than usual; is more suspicious than usual; misinterprets visual or auditory stimuli.

  In addition to failure to arrive at the right time for appointments, the clinician can look for difficulty discussing current events in an area of interest, and changes in behavior or dress. It also may be helpful to follow up on areas of concern by asking the patient or family members relevant questions.

[a] Positive findings in any of these areas generally indicate the need for further assessment for the presence of dementia. Source: Guideline panel.

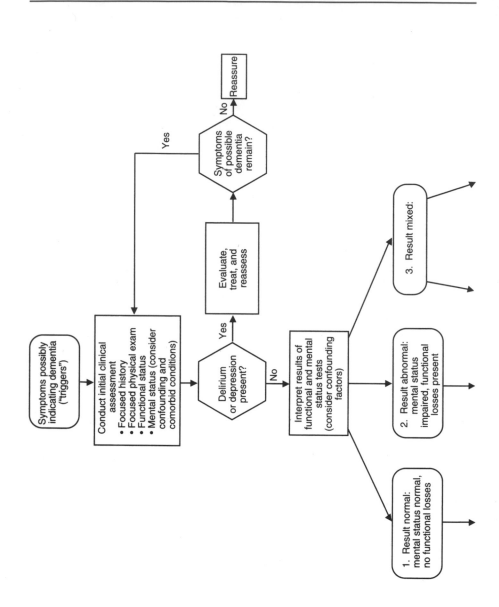

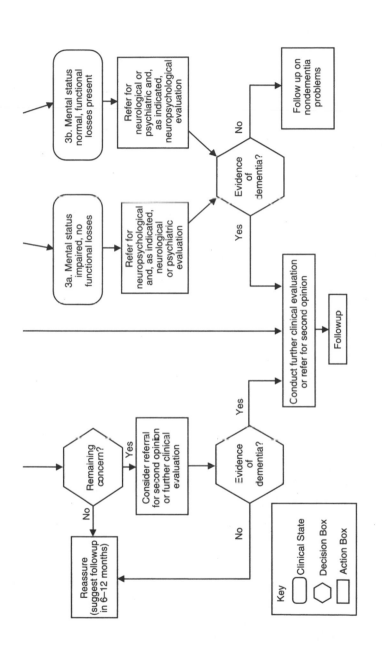

Figure 8.2. Flow chart for recognition and initial assessment of Alzheimer's disease and related dementias.

in multiple cognitive domains (see *Diagnostic and Statistical Manual of Mental Disorders, Fourth Edition* [DSM-IV], American Psychiatric Association, 1994).

Focused History

A focused history is critical in the assessment for dementia. It must identify signs and symptoms such as those listed in Table 8.1 and document the chronology of problems. Particularly important are

- Mode of onset (abrupt versus gradual).

- Progression (stepwise versus continuous decline; worsening versus fluctuating versus improving).

- Duration of symptoms.

In addition to containing a detailed description of the chief complaint, a focused history should include relevant medical, family, social and cultural, and medication history (including alcohol use).

Medical history. Ask about relevant systemic diseases; psychiatric disorders; known neurological disorders, including history of head trauma; alcohol or substance abuse; and exposure to environmental toxins. Because many medical conditions may cause or contribute to cognitive impairment, review information about any intercurrent, infectious, or metabolic illness, such as pneumonia, urinary tract infection, diabetes, or acute or chronic renal failure.

Family history. Inquire about a family history of early-onset Alzheimer's disease or other rare genetic conditions that lead to dementia, such as Huntington's disease.

Social and cultural history. Include information about recent life events and social support networks, education, literacy, and socioeconomic, ethnic, and cultural background. These factors may affect performance on mental status tests; some studies have found that they may affect the risk for dementia as well.

Medication history. This is a critical component of the initial evaluation, because drug toxicity is the most common cause of dementias that can be resolved or significantly ameliorated. A wide range of drugs have been associated with cognitive changes (see Table 8.3). Consider any drug, including over-the-counter medications and

Table 8.3. Some medications that may cause cognitive impairment

Type of medication and generic name [a]

Antiarrhythmic agents: disopyramide, quinidine, tocainide

Antibiotics: cephalexin, cephalothin, metronidazole, ciprofloxacin, ofloxacin

Anticholinergic agents: benztropine, homatropine, scopolamine, trihexyphenidyl

Antidepressants: amitryptyline, imipramine, desipramine, fluoxetine

Anticonvulsants: phenytoin, valproic acid, carbamazepine

Antiemetics: promethazine, hydroxyzine, metoclopramide, prochlorperazine

Antihypertensive agents: propranolol, metoprolol, atenolol, verapamil, methyldopa, prazosin, nifedipine

Antineoplastic agents: chlorambucil, cytarabine, interleukin-2

Antimanic agents: lithium

Anti-Parkinsonian agents: levodopa, pergolide, bromocryptine

Antihistamines/decongestants: phenylpropanolamin, diphenhydramine, chlorpheniramine, brompheniramine, pseudoephedrine

Cardiotonic agents: digoxin

Corticosteroids: hydrocortisone, prednisone

H2 receptor antagonists: cimetidine, ranitidine

Immunosuppressive agents: cyclosporine, interferon

Narcotic analgesics: codeine, hydrocodone, oxycodone, meperidine, propoxyphene

Muscle relaxants: baclofen, cyclobenzaprine, methocarbimol

Nonsteroidal anti-inflammatory agents: aspirin, ibuprofen, indomethacin, naproxen, sulindac

Radiocontrast agents: metrizamide, iothalamate, iohexol

Sedatives: alprazolam, diazepam, lorazepam, phenobarbital, butabarbital, chloral hydrate

[a] *These are examples only; new medications appear regularly. Many compounds contain other active ingredients. Source: Guideline panel.*

alcohol, as potentially suspect. Encourage patients to bring all medication bottles and pills to the appointment.

Informant reports. Whenever possible, obtain the history from both the patient and reliable informants, such as family members or close friends. Informant reports can supplement information from patients who have experienced memory loss and may lack insight into the severity of their decline.

Reports from relatives, however, may be influenced by the nature of the relationship to the patient. For this reason, more than one family informant or a family consensus approach can increase the accuracy of conclusions about the presence and range of cognitive impairments in persons suspected of having dementia.

When an informant is available:

- Interview the patient alone first, to respect the patient's dignity.

- Tell the patient that others will be interviewed.

- Interview informants separately from the patient to increase the likelihood of candor.

- Consider the possibility of questionable motives in informant reports. For example, symptoms may be minimized if the family is concerned about the patient's being denied admission to a nursing home; conversely, symptoms may be exaggerated or fabricated if an informant is motivated by financial or other considerations.

Focused Physical Examination

Use standard medical principles to guide a focused physical examination conducted as part of an initial assessment for dementia: life-threatening or rapidly progressing conditions must be identified first. Life-threatening conditions include mass lesions, vascular lesions, and infections. Assess carefully for conditions that cause delirium, which is a medical emergency requiring immediate attention (see Assessing for Delirium section). Also be alert to signs of abuse and neglect of patients by caregivers, and report suspected abuse to the proper authorities.

Functional Status Assessment

Use a standardized test to evaluate functional status. For evaluating complex or difficult cases, informant-based scales are particularly important.

Among standardized tests, the Functional Activities Questionnaire (FAQ) is currently the best discriminator for early-stage dementia (see Clinical Practice Guideline for details of meta-analyses). The FAQ is an informant-based measure. Every effort should be made to find a reliable informant.

Mental Status Assessment

A quantitative mental status examination should be part of an initial assessment for dementia. Although a comprehensive mental status examination that provides a detailed cognitive profile of the patient is desirable, it is impractical for most clinicians. Several brief, quantitative tests can provide useful information about mental status. They feature systematic, structured questions or tasks that can be scored easily.

Brief mental status tests are not diagnostic. They are used to:

- Develop a multidimensional clinical picture in conjunction with functional performance and the patient's signs and symptoms.

- Provide a baseline for monitoring the course of cognitive impairment over time.

- Reassess mental status in persons who have treatable delirium or depression on initial evaluation.

- Document multiple cognitive impairments, as required for a diagnosis of dementia.

No single mental status test is clearly superior (see *Clinical Practice Guideline* for details of meta-analyses). The following four brief mental status tests are largely equivalent in their discriminative ability:

- Mini-Mental State Examination (MMSE).
- The Blessed Information-Memory-Concentration Test (BIMC).
- The Blessed Orientation-Memory-Concentration Test (BOMC).
- Short Test of Mental Status (STMS).

Any of the tests is acceptable, if its utility is not limited by a patient's confounding or comorbid conditions (see below).

The MMSE is the most widely used brief mental status test in the United States and the most comprehensive of the brief tests; however, several studies have shown that it has differential sensitivity for various cognitive domains. On the basis of these studies, an MMSE finding of impairments in memory and at least one other cognitive area suggests dementia, but a finding of impairment only in memory does not necessarily exclude the possibility of dementia.

In diagnosing mild dementia, reliable informants' accounts of minor cognitive changes in a person suspected of dementia may be as important as—or more important than—quantitative assessments, which can be insensitive to mild impairment.

Confounding and comorbid conditions. Visual and auditory impairments and physical disabilities may affect performance on both mental status and neuropsychological tests. Assess the patient for such conditions and consider them in the selection of tests. For example, the MMSE's praxis and drawing portions make it unsuitable for a patient who has impaired motor control. In such cases, use other tests (e.g., the BIMC).

When possible, correct visual and auditory deficits before testing. When this is not possible or when a physical disability is present, consider referral for neuropsychological evaluation that uses the patient's unimpaired faculties and capacities. For testing any older adult, make sure that the following conditions are adequate: lighting, contrast of visual stimuli, and volume and distinctiveness of auditory stimuli.

Assessing for Delirium and Depression

During the focused history and physical examination, look for evidence of an acute confusional state or delirium, and for dysphoric mood suggesting depression. These conditions can be mistaken for, or coexist with, dementia; they also can occur together.

Delirium and depression need to be addressed promptly and explicitly. If symptoms suggesting dementia remain after the patient has been treated for delirium or depression, continue the assessment for dementia.

Delirium

Although delirium is common in older persons with acute or chronic illnesses, it is underrecognized in clinical settings. This underrecognition can have serious consequences, because delirium is a medical emergency requiring immediate further evaluation and treatment. Some of the underlying causes (e.g., bacterial meningitis or hypoglycemia) can be fatal. If delirium is recognized early, it may be possible to prevent disability and irreversible deterioration.

A person who displays the following symptoms is likely to have delirium rather than uncomplicated dementia:

- Sudden onset of cognitive impairment.
- Disorientation.
- Disturbances in attention.
- Decline in level of consciousness.
- Perceptual disturbances (e.g., hallucinations).

In addition to common medical conditions, adverse effects of the following types of medications are also common causes of delirium:

- Anticholinergic agents.
- Antipsychotic agents.
- Antidepressants.
- Digoxin.
- H_2-blocking agents.
- Antihypertensive agents.

To improve recognition of delirium, use mental status tests to identify patients with cognitive impairment, and establish the symptoms' history of onset and degree of fluctuations. Several systematic methods of assessing for delirium have been found effective (see Selected Bibliography below).

Depression

Although depression is the most common psychiatric illness in older persons, it is often underdiagnosed, especially when physical illness is present. Diagnosis is complicated because (a) depression is often mistaken for dementia and vice versa, (b) each may present as the other, and (c) they may coexist (e.g., DSM-IV categories of dementia with depressed mood). Changes in memory, attention, and executive function suggest depression; marked visuospatial or language impairment suggests a dementing process.

Problems are associated with misdiagnosing dementia as depression. In addition to the unnecessary expense, inappropriate treatment for nonexistent depression in a person with progressive dementia may exacerbate the condition because antidepressants that have anticholinergic properties may worsen confusion or memory impairment. In persons with coexisting depression and Alzheimer's disease, failure to diagnose and treat the depression may cause unnecessary emotional, physical, and social discomfort for both patient and family.

For these reasons, assessing for depression is an important part of the initial evaluation of any older adult suspected of cognitive impairment, especially for persons who complain of memory difficulty.

When taking the history, look for symptoms consistent with the DSM-IV definition of depression. If depression is suspected, (a) evaluate further, (b) treat appropriately (depression in older adults often responds to treatment with antidepressants, psychotherapy, electroconvulsive therapy, or all of the above), and then (c) reassess the patient for dementia.

Clinical interview. The clinical interview is the mainstay for evaluating and diagnosing depression in older adults. The DSM-IV provides some guidance on obtaining relevant information and observations. In applying DSM-IV criteria, however, be aware that physical conditions or behavioral changes common among older persons may account for many DSM-IV symptoms of major depression, such as:

- Changes in sleep pattern or appetite.
- Fatigue.
- Behavioral slowing or agitation.
- Complaints of diminished ability to think or concentrate.

Drug interactions that result from polypharmacy also can produce depression or depression-related symptoms and contribute to cognitive impairment.

Depression assessment instruments. Brief self-report questionnaires can facilitate initial screening for depression. The following two self-report instruments have established reliability and validity:

- *The Geriatric Depression Scale (GDS)*, developed specifically for use with older adults, is a 30-item questionnaire that has a simple yes/no format and takes only 8 to 10 minutes to administer. A 15-item form of the GDS is also available.

- The *Center for Epidemiological Studies Depression Scale (CES-D)* is a 20-item questionnaire that can be administered in 5 to 8 minutes.

Self-report instruments have shown lower frequencies of depression-related symptoms in patients with Alzheimer's disease compared with informant sources or trained clinical observers. They should be used with caution for persons suspected of having dementia. Depression screening in patients suspected of dementia should include informa-tion from both a patient self-report and a caregiver (or informant) report, as well as direct clinician observation of the patient's behav-ior. A good time to ask about other symptoms is right after the func-tional assessment.

Memory difficulty, agitation, disrupted sleep-wake cycle, and per-sonality changes (e.g., apathy, increased dependence) are classic symp-toms of Alzheimer's disease that may be mistaken for depressive signs of poor concentration, decreased interest, changes in psychomotor activity, sleep disturbance, and fatigue.

Interpreting Findings

The combination of findings from the assessments of mental and functional status can yield three possible results: (a) normal, (b) ab-normal, and (c) mixed. The following recommendations, geared to each of these results, provide a framework for clinical decisions and should be used in conjunction with patient-specific circumstances.

Normal Results

If findings from both the mental and the functional assessment are normal, reassure the patient and concerned family members or friends and suggest reassessment in 6 to 12 months (or whenever further concerns develop). If concerns remain, consider referral for a second opinion or for further clinical evaluation:

- For concern about the adequacy of the mental status test, refer for further neuropsychological testing.

- For concern about possible depression or other emotional prob-lems, refer for further psychiatric or psychological evaluation.

- For concern about possible loss of social and instrumental func-tioning caused by a neurological disorder not detected in the functional assessment, refer to a neurologist.

Abnormal Results

If findings from both the mental and the functional assessment are abnormal, the patient is likely to have a dementing illness and should have further clinical evaluation. This evaluation should include dif-ferential diagnosis, treatment, and continuing care as indicated. The Selected Bibliography lists guidelines for further clinical evaluation.

Laboratory tests may be appropriate when specific medical conditions are suspected. However, a laboratory test should not be used as a screening procedure solely to identify probable early-stage dementia or as a routine part of an initial assessment for dementia.

Mixed Results

Mixed results—abnormal findings on the mental status test with no abnormalities in functional assessment or vice versa—call for further evaluation. For example:

- Patients who have abnormal results on only the mental status test require more complete neuropsychological testing. If results indicate possible neuropsychiatric or systemic neurological problems as well, refer to an appropriate specialist.

- Patients who have declining function but normal mental status test results require either (a) further neurological evaluation for systemic neurological diseases or (b) psychiatric or psychological evaluation, if evidence suggests depression or other emotional problems.

Clinical presentations that could produce mixed results include:

- A person with lifelong borderline or retarded intellectual functioning who has learned to perform routine activities of daily living (ADLs) adequately.

- A person with a dementing illness who lives in an environment where functional supports mask evidence of significant functional impairment.

- A person with high intelligence and education who scores within the normal range on a mental status test but shows clear functional decline, especially on demanding tasks (e.g., instrumental activities of daily living [IADLs]).

Importance of Cognitive Baselines

Because cognitive performance can vary from day to day, an initial assessment of cognitive impairment needs to be verified by reassessment. A cognitive baseline is an important benchmark for confirming cognitive decline and evaluating its nature and magnitude. A baseline measure is especially useful for:

- Persons of initially high cognitive ability whose early decline may be difficult to find on initial testing.

- Persons found to have only mild impairment who require several examinations conducted weeks or months apart to document stable or progressing cognitive problems.

- Persons who minimize or deny problems because of lack of insight.

Confounding Factors

Assess confounding factors such as age, educational level, and cultural influences and consider them in the interpretation of mental status test scores.

Age and educational influences. Both age and education can affect performance on most mental status and neuropsychological tests. On the MMSE, for example, significant correlations have been found between MMSE scores and both age and years of schooling. Evidence suggests that:

- Low education increases the likelihood that an unimpaired person will test as cognitively impaired (false-positive error), especially for those who have fewer than 9 years of education.

- A high educational level increases the likelihood that a cognitively impaired person will test as unimpaired (false-negative error).

Age- and education-stratified data are available only for the MMSE. If the MMSE is the mental status test used, refer to these stratified data in interpreting test results. For other brief mental status tests, take these factors into account in setting the threshold for dementia for test results. As always, the clinician's knowledge of each patient should guide consideration of these confounding factors.

Cultural influences. Primary language, race, ethnicity, and cultural bias also can affect performance on mental status tests and some neuropsychological tests.

Research suggests that several neuropsychological tests (e.g., some Wechsler Adult Intelligence Scale Revised [WAIS-R] subtests, the FAS Controlled Oral Word Association Test) may place Hispanic persons and possibly members of other racial or ethnic groups at a disadvantage, particularly in the use of culturally inappropriate norms or cutpoints. The Consortium to Establish a Registry for Alzheimer's Disease (CERAD) has developed Spanish-language versions of its clinical and neuropsychological assessments. Copies are available from CERAD (see Resources section).

Use the focused history and physical examination to evaluate English language ability. Then determine whether it is appropriate to administer an English-language version of a mental status test or make a referral to someone who is competent in the patient's primary language.

Role of Neuropsychological Testing

Neuropsychological assessment can make an important contribution to identification of mild dementia, particularly when delayed recall is measured. It can

- Give information about the specific nature of strengths and deficits in cognitive functions.

- Assist in diagnosis, particularly in cases of mild impairment, high premorbid intellectual ability, or an unusual combination of cognitive impairments.

- Contribute to recommendations for treatment and management of behavior problems.

- Provide a baseline measurement for judging the effects of treatment or disease progression.

Neuropsychological tests can measure performance across different domains of cognition, including orientation and attention, language functions, visual motor constructional ability (praxis), memory, abstract and conceptional reasoning, and executive functions (formulating goals, planning, and executing plans). A person's pattern of performance across such tests can help in (a) identifying dementia among persons with high premorbid intellectual functioning, (b) discriminating patients with a dementing illness from those with focal cerebral disease, and (c) differentiating among certain causes of dementia.

Neuropsychological evaluation may be useful in certain circumstances: (a) when the mental status test is abnormal but the functional assessment is normal; (b) when a family member expresses concern or dementia is suspected and results of mental status tests are within the normal range and the patient has more than a high school education or an occupation that indicates high premorbid intelligence; and (c) when mental status test results indicate cognitive impairment and when any of the following circumstances apply to the patient:

- Low level of formal education.
- Evidence of long-term low intelligence (more than 10 years).
- Inadequate command of English for the test.
- Minority racial or ethnic background.
- Impairment in only one cognitive area on mental status tests.
- No evidence of cognitive impairment for more than 6 months.
- No evidence of functional impairments.

Neuropsychological evaluation must be interpreted within the context of other clinical information, such as informant-based history of cognitive decline; evidence of impairment in IADLs; educational background; assessment for depression; sensory impairment; and factors other than dementia that may account for impaired performance (see Confounding Factors).

Importance of Followup

Followup, with assessment of declining mental function, may be the most useful diagnostic procedure for differentiating Alzheimer's disease from normal aging. For this reason, repeat the mental status test over a period of 6 to 12 months and note change or stability of scores. (For the MMSE, a change of four points per year is expected in scores of persons with Alzheimer's disease.) In cases of referral, make sure test results and medical records follow the patient from the specialist back to the referring clinician.

When a diagnosis of dementia is made, the patient and family members have serious issues to consider. The progressive nature of cognitive impairment makes followup especially important for persons with Alzheimer's disease or a related disorder; however, followup cannot be ensured. For this reason, the visit during which the diagnosis is given is an appropriate time for the clinician to discuss relevant issues with the patient and family or close friends, for example:

- The patient's competence to drive and carry out other routine functions that raise issues of safety (e.g., cooking); manage finances; supervise or care for grandchildren.

- Financial, legal, and medical planning, including execution of a durable power of attorney for health care.

The list of resources provided can be helpful to families when they are ready to confront the many implications of a diagnosis of dementia.

Resources for Health Professionals, Patients, and Families

Federal Resources

Administration on Aging
330 Independence Avenue, SW
Washington, DC 20201
(202) 619-1006
Fax: (202) 619-7586
Internet: http://www.aoa.dhhs.gov

The Administration on Aging (AoA) coordinates delivery of services specified by the Older Americans Act. Services are coordinated and provided through 57 State agencies and 657 areas. The range of services provided by these Agencies on Aging (AAA) varies, but all include nutrition, access, in-home, and community services. Addresses and phone numbers of State and local AAAs are available from the national office. The Elder Care Locator (800-677-1166) provides a toll-free access number to locate State agency networks.

Alzheimer's Association
919 North Michigan Avenue
Suite 100
Chicago, IL 60611-1676
(312) 335-8700
800-272-3900 for information and local chapter referrals nationwide
(24-hour telephone line)
Internet: http://www.alz.org

The Alzheimer's Association is a national voluntary organization with 220 local chapters and more than 2,000 support groups. The Alzheimer's Association funds research, promotes public awareness, advocates legislation for patients and families, and provides support services, including support groups, adult day care programs, respite care programs, and telephone helplines through its national, chapter, and volunteer network.

Alzheimer's Disease Centers
(access through ADEAR; see next entry)

The National Institute on Aging, part of the National Institutes of Health, supports 28 Alzheimer's Disease Centers across the country. This program provides clinical services, conducts basic and clinical research, disseminates professional and public information, and sponsors educational activities. A growing number of satellite clinics associated with this program are helping to expand diagnostic and treatment services in rural and minority communities and collect research data from a more diverse population.

Alzheimer's Disease Education and Referral Center
P.O. Box 8250
Silver Spring, MD 20907-8250
800-438-4380
Fax: (301) 495-3334
Internet: adear@alzheimers.org

The Alzheimer's Disease Education and Referral (ADEAR) Center, a service of the National Institute on Aging, provides information and publications on Alzheimer's disease for health professionals, people with Alzheimer's disease and their families, and the public. The ADEAR Center serves as a national resource for information on diagnosis, treatment issues, patient care, caregiver needs, long-term care, education, research, and ongoing programs. In addition, the Center provides referrals to national and State resources.

The Corporation for National Service
Office of Public Liaison
1201 New York Avenue, NW
Washington, DC 20525
(202) 606-5000
Fax: (202) 565-2794

The Corporation for National and Community Service is a public corporation that administers Federal service programs, including AmeriCorps, the Foster Grandparent Program, and the Senior Companion Program (SCP), which provides supportive services to adults with physical, emotional, and health limitations. A major SCP emphasis is preventing or delaying institutionalization. Foster Grandparent volunteers work with children, including those with disabilities. AmeriCorps members address a range of local health issues.

Other Resources

American Association of Retired Persons (AARP)
Washington, DC
(202) 434-2277
800-424-3410

AARP Pharmacy Price Quote Center
800-456-2226 (open 24 hours a day)

American Bar Association Commission on Legal Problems of the Elderly
Washington, DC
(202) 662-8690

Children of Aging Parents
Levittown, PA
(215) 945-6900

Consortium to Establish a Registry for Alzheimer's Disease (CERAD)
Durham, NC
(919) 286-6406 or 6405

Insurance Consumer Helpline
Washington, DC
800-942-4242

Medicare Beneficiaries Defense Fund
New York, NY
(212) 869-3850
800-333-4114

Medicare Hotline
Baltimore, MD
800-638-6833

National Association for Continence
Spartanburg, SC
800-BLADDER
(800-252-3337)

National Citizen's Coalition for Nursing Home Reform
Washington, DC
(202) 332-2275

National Hospice Organization
Arlington, VA
(703) 243-5900
800-658-8898

National Parkinson's Foundation
East Coast: Miami, FL
800-327-4545
West Coast: Encino, CA
800-522-8855

National Stroke Association
Englewood, CO
(303) 771-1700
800-STROKES

Social Security Information
800-772-1213 (open 7 am-7 pm in all time zones)

U.S. Department of Veterans Affairs
Regional Office, Veterans Assistance
Washington, DC
(202) 418-4343
800-827-1000

Selected Bibliography

American Psychiatric Association. *Diagnostic and statistical manual of mental disorders. 4th ed. (DSM-IV)*. Washington (DC): American Psychiatric Association; 1994. 886 p.

Bleecker ML, Bolla-Wilson K, Kawas C, et al. Age-specific norms for the Mini-Mental State Exam. *Neurology* 1988;38: 1565-8.

Crum RM, Anthony JC, Bassett SS, et al. Population-based norms for the Mini-Mental State Examination by age and educational level. *JAMA* 1993;269:2386-91.

Folstein MF, Folstein SE, McHugh PR. "Mini-Mental State": a practical method for grading the cognitive state of patients for the clinician. *J Psychiatr Res* 1975; 12:189-98.

Katzman R, Brown T, Fuld P, et al. Validation of a short orientation-memory-concentration test of cognitive impairment. *Am J Psychiatry* 1983; 140:734-9.

Kokmen E, Naessens JM, and Offord KP. A short test of mental status: description and preliminary results. *Mayo Clin Proc* 1987:62;281-8.

Morrison RL, Katz IR. Drug-related cognitive impairment: current progress and recurrent problems. *Annu Rev Gerontol Geriatr* 1989;9:232-79.

Pfeffer RI, Kurosaki TT, Harrah C, et al. Measurement of functional activities in older adults in the community. *J Gerontol* 1982 37:323-9.

White H, Davis PB. Cognitive screening tests: an aid in the care of elderly outpatients. *J Gen Intern Med* 1990;5:438-45.

Assessing for Delirium

Albert MS, Levkoff SE, Reilly C, et al. The delirium symptoms interview: an interview for the detection of delirium symptoms in hospitalized patients. *J Geriatr Psychiatry Neurol* 1992;5:14-21.

Anthony JC, LeResche LA, Von Korff MR, et al. Screening for delirium on a general medical ward: the tachistoscope and a global accessibility rating. *Gen Hosp Psychiatry* 1985;7:36-42.

Gottlieb GL, Johnson J, Wanich C, et al. Delirium in the medically ill elderly: operationalizing the DSM-III criteria. *Int Psychogeriatr* 1991;3:181-96.

Inouye SK, van Dyck CH, Alessi CA, et al. Clarifying confusion: the Confusion Assessment Method—a new method for detection of delirium. *Ann Intern Med* 1990;113:941-8.

Inouye SK, Viscoli CM, Horwitz RI, et al. A predictive model for delirium in hospitalized elderly medical patients based on admission characteristics. *Ann Intern Med* 1993; 119:474-81.

Assessing for Depression

Brink TL, Yesavage JA, Lum 0, et al. Screening tests for geriatric depression. *Clin Gerontologist* 1982; 1:37-43.

National Institutes of Health. Consensus Development Panel on Depression in Late Life. Diagnosis and treatment of depression in late life. *JAMA* 1992;268:1018-24.

Radloff LS. The CES-D scale: a self-report depression scale for research in the general population. *Appl Psychol Measurement* 1977;1:385-401.

Rush JA, Golden WE, Hall GW, et al. *Depression in primary care: Volume 1.* Detection and diagnosis. *Clinical Practice Guideline No. 5.* AHCPR Publication No. 93-0550. Rockville, MD: Agency for Health Care Policy and Research, Public Health Service, U.S. Department of Health and Human Services. April 1993.

Yesavage JA. Geriatric depression scale. *Psychopharmacol Bull* 1988:24:709-11.

Further Evaluation

American Academy of Neurology. Practice parameters for diagnosis and evaluation of dementia (summary statement): report of the Quality Standards Subcommittee of the American Academy of Neurology. *Neurology* 1994;44:2203-6.

Clarfield AM. *Canadian consensus conference on the assessment of dementia,* 5-6 October 1989. Montreal, Quebec: *Canadian Consensus Conference on the Assessment of Dementia;* 1991.

McKhann G, Drachman D, Folstein M, et al. Clinical diagnosis of Alzheimer's disease: report of the NINCDS-ADRDA Work Group under the auspices of Department of Health and Human Services Task Force on Alzheimer's Disease. *Neurology* 1984;34:939-44.

National Institutes of Health. Differential diagnosis of dementing diseases. *Consensus Development Conference Statement* 1987 (July);6(11):1-9.

U.S. Department of Veterans Affairs. *Dementia: guidelines for diagnosis and treatment, 1989* (revised). VA Publication No. 1B 18-3. 107 p.

Part Two

Other Dementias and Related Disorders

Chapter 9

Multi-Infarct Dementia

Serious forgetfulness, mood swings, and other behavior changes are not a normal part of aging. Some of these changes are caused by problems that can be treated or corrected, like a poor diet or lack of sleep. Sometimes too many medicines cause these symptoms in older people. Feelings of loneliness, boredom, or depression also can cause a person to be forgetful. These problems are serious and should be treated. Often, though, they can be reversed.

Sometimes mental changes cannot be treated easily because they are caused by diseases that permanently damage brain cells. The term dementia is used to describe symptoms that are usually caused by changes in the normal activity of very sensitive brain cells. Dementia seriously interferes with a person's ability to carry out daily activities. Two common causes of dementia in older people are Alzheimer's disease and multi-infarct dementia.

Alzheimer's disease is the most common cause of dementia in older persons. Alzheimer's disease develops when nerve cells in the brain die. Symptoms begin slowly and become steadily worse. At this time, no one knows what causes the nerve cells to die, and there is no cure for the disease.

The second most common cause of dementia in older people is multi-infarct dementia. Multi-infarct dementia usually affects people between the ages of 60 and 75. Men are slightly more likely than women to have multi-infarct dementia. Multi-infarct dementia is

Alzheimer's Disease Education & Referral Center, National Institute on Aging, NIH Pub. No. 93-3433, January 1994.

105

caused by a series of strokes that damage or destroy brain tissue. A stroke occurs when blood cannot get to the brain. A blood clot or fatty deposits (called plaques) can block the vessels that supply blood to the brain, causing a stroke. A stroke also can happen when a blood vessel in the brain bursts. The main causes of strokes are untreated high blood pressure, high blood cholesterol, diabetes, and heart disease. Of these, the most important risk factor for multi-infarct dementia is high blood pressure. It is rare for a person without high blood pressure to develop multi-infarct dementia.

Symptoms

Symptoms that begin suddenly may be a sign of multi-infarct dementia. In addition to confusion and problems with recent memory, symptoms of multi-infarct dementia may include wandering or getting lost in familiar places; moving with rapid, shuffling steps; loss of bladder or bowel control (incontinence); emotional problems, such as laughing or crying inappropriately; difficulty following instructions; and problems handling money.

Multi-infarct dementia is often the result of a series of small strokes, called ministrokes or TIAs (transient ischemic attacks). The symptoms of a TIA often are very slight. They may include mild weakness in an arm or leg, slurred speech, and dizziness. The symptoms generally do not last for more than a few days. Several TIAs may occur before the person notices any symptoms of multi-infarct dementia. People with multi-infarct dementia may improve for short periods of time, then decline again upon having further strokes.

Diagnosis

People who show signs of dementia or who have a history of strokes should have a complete physical exam. The doctor will ask the patient and the family about the person's diet, medications, sleep patterns, personal habits, past strokes, and other medical problems. The doctor will ask about recent illnesses or stressful events like the death of someone close and problems at home or work that may account for the symptoms. To look for signs of stroke, the doctor will check for weakness or numbness in the arms or legs, difficulty with speech, or dizziness. To check for other health problems that could cause symptoms of dementia, the doctor may order office or laboratory tests. These tests may include a blood pressure reading, an electroencephalogram (EEG), a test of thyroid function, and blood tests.

106

The doctor also may ask for x-rays or special tests such as a computerized tomography (CT) scan or a magnetic resonance imaging (MRI) test. Both CT scans and MRI tests take pictures of sections of the brain. The pictures are then displayed on a computer screen to allow the doctor to see inside the brain. CT scans and MRI tests are painless and do not require surgery. Specialists called radiologists and neurologists interpret these tests. In addition, the doctor may send the patient to a psychologist or psychiatrist to test reasoning, learning ability, memory, and attention span.

Sometimes multi-infarct dementia is difficult to distinguish from Alzheimer's disease. It is possible for a person to have both multi-infarct dementia and Alzheimer's disease, making it hard for the doctor to diagnose either.

Treatment

While no treatment can reverse damage that has already been done, treatment to prevent additional strokes is very important. High blood pressure, the primary risk factor for multi-infarct dementia, can be treated successfully. Diabetes also is a treatable risk for stroke. To prevent additional strokes, doctors may prescribe medicines to control high blood pressure, high cholesterol, heart disease, and diabetes. They will counsel patients about good health habits such as exercising and avoiding smoking and drinking alcohol. The patient may require a special diet.

Doctors sometimes prescribe aspirin or other drugs to prevent clots from forming in the small blood vessels. Drugs also can be prescribed to relieve restlessness or depression or to help the patient sleep better. Sometimes doctors recommend a type of surgery known as carotid endarterectomy. This surgery is done to remove blockage in the carotid artery, the main blood vessel to the brain. Studies are under way to see how well this surgery works in treating patients with multi-infarct dementia. Some scientists also are studying drugs that increase the flow of blood to the brain.

Helping Someone with Multi-Infarct Dementia

Family members and friends can help someone with multi-infarct dementia cope with mental and physical problems. They can encourage patients to keep up their daily routines and regular social and physical activities. By talking with them about events and daily activities, family members can help patients use their mental abilities

107

as much as possible. Some families find it helpful to use reminders such as lists, alarm clocks, and calendars to help the patient remember important times and events.

A person with multi-infarct dementia should be under the regular care of a doctor. If the patient has health problems such as diabetes, other specialists may be consulted as well.

Help and advice for home caregivers are available from a variety of sources, including nurses, family doctors, social workers, and physical and occupational therapists. Home health care and respite or day care services in some neighborhoods can provide much-needed relief to caregivers. A State or local health department, a local hospital, or the patient's doctor may be able to provide a telephone number to call for such services.

Support groups offer emotional support for family members caring for a person with dementia. A State or local health department, government agency on aging, or local hospital can provide information about support groups in the community.

Additional Help

The organizations listed below offer more information about some of the topics mentioned in this chapter.

Additional copies of this text and single copies of the *Age Pages* "Stroke Prevention and Treatment," "Memory Loss and Confusion in Old Age: It's Not What You Think," and "Depression: A Serious But Treatable Illness" are available from:

Alzheimer's Disease Education and Referral (ADEAR) Center
P.O. Box 8250
Silver Spring, MD 20907-8250
800-438-4380

A free information packet about multi-infarct dementia and information about support groups for families are available from:

Alzheimer's Association
919 North Michigan Avenue
Suite 1000
Chicago, IL 60611
800-272-3900

Information about stroke and current research on stroke-related conditions is available from:

National Institute of Neurological Disorders and Stroke
Building 31, Room 8A06
9000 Rockville Pike
Bethesda, MD 20892
301-496-5751

Information about stroke and support for stroke survivors and their families is available from:

National Stroke Association
Suite 240
300 East Hampden Avenue
Englewood, CO 80110
303-762-9922

Information about preventing stroke, including information about risk factors such as high blood pressure, high cholesterol, heart disease, and smoking, is available from:

National Heart, Lung, and Blood Information Center
P.O. Box 30105
Bethesda, MD 20824-0105
301-951-3260

Information about controlling diabetes, an important risk factor for stroke, is available from:

National Diabetes Information Clearinghouse
Box NDIC
9000 Rockville Pike
Bethesda, MD 20892
301-468-2162

Information about services and resources in your area, such as adult day care programs, transportation, and meal services, is available from:

Eldercare Locator Service
Administration on Aging
800-677-1116

Chapter 10

Forms of Cerebral Atrophy

In the not too distant past Alzheimer's disease was considered sufficiently ubiquitous to permit its diagnosis in the elderly demented, once cerebrovascular disease, cerebral trauma, and alcohol abuse had been excluded. An attempt to use inclusion rather than exclusion criteria for "probable" or "possible" Alzheimer's disease is contained in the *Diagnostic Statistical Manual III*. The latter now serves as holy writ in the search for clinical confirmation of Alzheimer's disease to the neglect of forms of cerebral atrophy which may be clinically and pathologically distinct from Alzheimer's disease and yet meet its descriptive psychiatric diagnostic criteria.

The last few years have witnessed a directional change in the investigation of primary cerebral atrophy with qualitative neuropsychological analysis of clinical syndromes allied to more functional brain imaging techniques and histological verification. Some new and distinct cerebral disorders have emerged, which are much more common than previously supposed and those reviewed here comprise dementia frontal-lobe type (DFT), DFT and motor neuron disease (MND), lobar atrophy, and diffuse Lewy body disease.

Dementia of Frontal-Lobe Type (DFT)

Studies from Manchester, United Kingdom[1] and Lund, Sweden[2] have delineated the form of non-Alzheimer's disease dementia designated as dementia of frontal-lobe type (DFT). Two further studies from

Journal of Neurology, Neurosurgery, and Psychiatry 1990; 53:929-931; reprinted with permission.

these centers[3,4] have independently confirmed that DFT, as a form of cerebral atrophy distinct from Alzheimer's disease, is more common than previously supposed. This disorder occurs at an earlier age than Alzheimer's disease and approximately half the patients have a parent with dementia. No sexual preponderance is seen, as in Alzheimer's disease, and in the British series, the ratio of the incidence of DFT to Alzheimer's disease was estimated at 1:4.

Patients present with a striking change in personality and social conduct, followed by progressive impairment of speech, with preservation of visuo-spatial abilities until the end stages of the disease. Stereotyped behavior and hyper-oral tendencies are characteristic. Neurological signs are minimal and confined to the emergence of primitive reflexes. Formal neuropsychological testing confirms a "frontal lobe syndrome." The electroencephalogram is normal and regional cerebral blood flow is selectively reduced in the anterior cerebral hemispheres.[5]

Biopsy tissue examination excludes Alzheimer's disease, and necropsy[6] reveals striking atrophy of the frontal and temporal lobes with loss of large cortical neurons, cortical spongiform change and both cortical and sub-cortical astrocytic gliosis. Neurofibrillary tangles and senile plaques are absent; in only four out of 20 patients with the syndrome were balloon cells and neuronal inclusion bodies, compatible with Pick's disease, observed. The precise status of DFT in relationship to Pick's disease requires clarification, but it is a disorder distinct from Alzheimer's disease on clinical, neurophysiological, pathological and demographic grounds.

Dementia of Frontal-Lobe Type and Motor Neuron Disease

In general, patients with DFT survive for many years and some have survived for over fifteen years from onset. However, four patients have been described,[7] in whom a profound and rapidly progressive dementia occurred in association with clinical features of motor neuron disease. Mental changes occurred first and the pattern of dementia indicated impaired frontal lobe function, confirmed by reduced tracer uptake in the frontal lobes on single photon emission computerized tomography (SPECT). Later weakness, wasting and fasciculations of limb muscles emerged and progressive bulbar palsy led to death within two years of onset. Electrophysiological studies confirmed widespread muscular denervation compatible with motor neuron disease.

Pathological examination of the brains of three patients revealed fronto-temporal lobe atrophy, with loss of large pyramidal neurons, mild gliosis and spongiform change. Similar changes were found in the corpus striatum and thalamus and also there was significant cell loss and gliosis in the substantia nigra. Depletion of neurons in the hypoglossal nuclei and anterior horns of the spinal cord was not accompanied by significant changes in the cortico-bulbar and cortico-spinal tracts. The pathological findings mirror closely those of Japanese patients with dementia and motor neuron disease.[8]

Previous studies have failed to define the precise clinical characteristics of the associated dementia. However in this most recent study both the clinical picture and pathological findings resembled those of DFT and were distinct from those of Alzheimer's disease.

It is clear that the high familial incidence of DFT demands further cytogenetic studies to shed light on the associated motor neuron disease and other forms of primary degenerative dementia.

Lobar Atrophy

Awareness of DFT and other cerebral degenerations with non-Alzheimer's pathology such as the syndrome of slowly progressive aphasia,[9,10] ought to awaken investigators to the possibility of additional forms of focal atrophy. Slowly progressive aphasia first described by Wechsler[14] consists of speech reduction progressing to mutism in the relative absence of other neuropsychological deficits. Imaging studies indicated a selective disorder of the left dominant cerebral hemisphere, confirmed pathologically and demonstrated to be due to a loss of large cortical neurons with spongiform change and astrocytic gliosis asymmetrically involving the dominant hemisphere.

Case reports have proliferated.[12-16] However, descriptions of the language disorder vary and the extent to which other deficits emerge with disease progression appears not to be uniform. Although a minority of cases has come to necropsy,[17-20] debate regarding the etiological status of progressive aphasia remains unresolved: specifically whether the cases represent focal representations of Alzheimer's disease,[14,21] or Pick's disease,[17,18,20] or constitute a distinct disease entity.[9,19]

The relatively large number of cases of progressive aphasia in the literature, presumably reflects the vulnerability of language functions to cerebral disease and it is predicted that selective neuropsychological deficits will be associated with focal degenerations in the right cerebral hemisphere. Pathological evidence will be required to bring unity to increasing numbers of clinically based observations.

Benson *et al.*[22] have described the clinical syndrome of "posterior cortical atrophy" which is likely to represent lobar atrophy of the parieto-occipital cortex. Five patients presented with early and severe ataxia, agraphia, acalculia, anomia, visual agnosia and disorientation, disorders of ocular fixation and a transcortical sensory aphasia. Memory, insight, and personal conduct were strikingly preserved and the neurological examination was normal. Computerized tomography and magnetic resonance imaging revealed cerebral atrophy most marked in the posterior hemispheres. Pathological verification indicates non-Alzheimer's disease in some cases, and in others forms of Alzheimer's disease in which the pathological changes appear preferentially to affect the parietal occipital association cortex in the early stages of progression.

A case has been described of progressive apraxia in the absence of any other neuropsychological deficits[23] and atrophy localized to the superior parietal lobules has been demonstrated on SPECT. Progressive apraxia has also been described in association with apperceptive visual agnosia.[24] Unfortunately, pathological characterization was lacking from these case descriptions.

Lewy Body Disease

Japanese investigators described the syndrome of dementia and rigidity in which Lewy bodies occurred in mid-line nuclei with or without cortical neuro-fibrillary tangles and senile plaques.[25,26] Unfortunately, clinical psychological descriptions were meager. Interest in "Lewy body disease" was kindled by a description of patients initially thought to have Parkinson's disease because of akinesia and rigidity but who had striking and early fluctuating mental changes of a subacute confusional state with behavioral disorder and hallucinations. Necropsy revealed Lewy bodies not only in the substantia nigra but widespread throughout the cerebral cortex.[27]

The Nottingham group went on to demonstrate the superiority of anti-ubiquitin immunocytochemistry over conventional techniques in the detection of diffuse Lewy bodies.[28] Utilizing the technique, they described the clinical and pathological features of fifteen cases of diffuse Lewy body disease.[29,30] Fifteen brains with the pathological hallmarks of diffuse Lewy body disease had been collected in one center in one year. The patients had been longitudinally studied, neurologically and psychologically with sufficient cognitive measures to permit the rating of severity of dementia on a five point scale. Of equal incidence were patients who had presented with Parkinson's disease

114

and later developed dementia, and patients who had presented with dementia and who later developed Parkinson's disease. The form of Parkinson's disease was indistinguishable from idiopathic Parkinson's disease and the motor symptoms were responsive to levodopa. The dementia was "cortical" in type with amnesia, aphasia, visuo-spatial disorientation and apraxia running a fluctuating course and complicated by hallucinations, agitation and confusion.

Pathologically, Lewy bodies were identified profusely in the cerebral cortex and their numbers were highly correlated with the severity of dementia. There was neuronal loss in the substantia nigra with Lewy bodies in the surviving neurons, but there was no correlation with these sub-cortical changes and the severity of dementia. This was true for similar changes in the nucleus basalis. Of considerable interest was the presence of large numbers of cortical senile plaques, the density of which correlated with that of cortical Lewy bodies. Only a few brains were found to contain neurofibrillary tangles and their numbers did not correlate with those of senile plaques or the severity of dementia. Similar clinical pathological findings have been documented by Perry et al.[31] who have chosen the title "Senile Dementia of Lewy body type", to designate this group of patients, thought to rank second in frequency to Alzheimer's disease as the cause of primary cerebral atrophy in the elderly. Previously the patients had been clinically diagnosed as forms of vascular encephalopathy because of the fluctuating clinical course.

It is suggested that Parkinson's disease and diffuse Lewy body disease represent clinical syndromes determined by the distribution of Lewy bodies in the brain stem and cerebral cortex. Senile plaques must be seen as non-specific changes which do not necessarily denote the presence of Alzheimer's disease. This view is supported by the studies of Gibb et al.[32] where again the clinical syndrome of Parkinson's disease and "cortical dementia" was associated with a distribution of Lewy bodies in the brain stem and cerebral cortex and significant changes of Alzheimer's disease were absent.

Conclusion

It is evident from a survey of recent investigations into dementia that not all primary cerebral atrophy represents Alzheimer's disease and it is likely that fresh clinical pathological designations will proliferate. Such progress will be made by adopting neuropsychological analytical techniques which specify the qualitative nature of clinical syndromes rather than submerging differences under a weight of numbers generated by standard clinical psychological battery tests. The quantification and rating of the severity of dementia should follow the specification of the dementia syndrome. Distinct neurological syndromes can now be evaluated in life using functional imaging such as SPECT and PET which are capable of generating topographical cerebral correlates of behavior. The pathological evaluation of brains, using morphometric histological analyses and the new dynamic techniques is bound to be most informative when correlated with quantitative neuropsychological measures made during life.

Principally, conceptual progress is likely to be furthered by rejecting the notion that dementia represents a nonspecific breakdown in intellect and memory, rather than distinct neuropsychological syndromes characterizing particular cerebral disorders and their pathological and functional differentiation within the brain.

Notes

1. Neary D, Snowden JS, Bowen DM, *et al*. Neuro-psychological syndromes in presenile dementia due to cerebral atrophy. *J Neurol Neurosurg Psychiatry* 1986;49:163-74.

2. Gustafson L, Brun A, Frank Holmvist A, Risberg J. Regional cerebral blood flow in degenerative frontal lobe dementia of non-Alzheimer's type. *J Cereb Blood Flow Metab* 1985;S(suppl 1):141-2.

3. Gustafson L. Frontal lobe degeneration of non-Alzheimer type. II. Clinical picture and differential diagnosis. *Arch Gerontol Geriatr* 1987;6:209-23.

4. Neary D, Snowden JS, Northen B, *et al*. Dementia of frontal lobe type. *J Neurol Neurosurg Psychiatry* 1988;51:353-61.

5. Risberg J. Frontal lobe degeneration of non-Alzheimer type. III. Regional cerebral blood flow. *Arch Gerontol Geriatr* 1987;6:225-33.

6. Brun A. Frontal lobe degeneration of non-Alzheimer type. I. Neuropathology. *Arch Gerontol Geriatr* 1987;6:193-208.

7. Neary D, Snowden JS, Mann DMA, *et al*. Frontal lobe dementia and motor neuron disease. *J Neurol Neurosurg Psychiatry* 1990;53:23-32.

8. Morita K, Kaiya H, Ikeda T, Namba M. Presenile dementia combined with amyotrophy: a review of 34 Japanese cases. *Arch Gerontol Geriatr* 1987;6:263-77.

9. Mesulam MM. Slowly progressive aphasia without generalized dementia. *Ann Neurol* 1982;11:592-8.

10. Kirshner HS, Webb WG, Kelly MP, Wells CE. Language disturbance—an initial symptom of cortical degenerations and dementia. *Arch Neurol* 1984;41:491-6.

11. Wechsler AF. Presenile dementia presenting as aphasia. *J Neurol Neurosurg Psychiatry* 1977;40:303-5.

12. Heath PD, Kennedy P, Kapur N. Slowly progressive aphasia without generalized dementia. *Ann Neurol* 1983;13:687-8.

13. Chawluk JB, Mesulam MM, Hurtig H, *et al*. Slowly progressive aphasia without generalized dementia: studies with positron emission tomography. *Ann Neurol* 1986;19:68-74.

14. Poeck K, Luzzatti C. Slowly progressive aphasia in three patients. *Brain* 1988;111:151-68.

15. Goulding PJ, Northen B, Snowden JS, *et al*. Progressive aphasia with right sided extrapyramidal signs: another manifestation of localized cerebral atrophy. *J Neurol Neurosurg Psychiatry* 1989;52:128-30.

16. Snowden JS, Goulding PJ, Neary D. Semantic dementia: a form of circumscribed cerebral atrophy. *Behav Neurol* 1989;2:167-82.

17. Wechsler AF, Verity A, Rosenschein S, *et al*. Pick's disease. A clinical computed tomographic and histologic study with golgi impregnation observations. *Arch Neurol* 1982;39:287-90.

18. Holland AL, McBurney DH, Moossy J, Reinmuth OM. The dissolution of language in Pick's disease with neurofibrillary tangles: a case study. *Brain Lang* 1985;24:36-58.

19. Kirshner HS, Tanridag O, Thurman L, Whetsell WO. Progressive aphasia without dementia: two cases with focal spongiform degeneration. *Ann Neurol* 1987;22:527-32.

20. Graff-Radford NR, Damasio AR, Hyman BT, *et al*. Progressive aphasia in a patient with Pick's disease: a neuropsychological, radiologic and anatomic study. *Neurology* 1990;40:620-6.

21. Green J, Morris JC, Sandson J, *et al*. Progressive aphasia a precursor of global dementia? *Neurology* 1990;40:423-9.

22. Benson DF, Davis RJ, Snyder BD. Posterior cortical atrophy. *Arch Neurol* 1988;45:789-93.

23. Dick JPR, Snowden JS, Northen B. *et al*. Slowly progressive apraxia. *Behavioral Neurology* 1989;2:101-14.

24. De Renzi E. Slowly progressive visual agnosia or apraxia without dementia. *Cortex* 1986;22:171-80.

25. Kosaka K. Lewy bodies in cerebral cortex. Report of 3 cases. *Acta Neuropathol* 1978;42:127-34.

26. Kosaka K, Tsuchiya K, Yoshimura M. Lewy body disease with and without dementia: a clinicopathological study of 35 cases. *Clin Neuropathol* 1988;7:299-305.

27. Byrne EJ, Lowe J, Godwin-Austen RB. Dementia and Parkinson's disease associated with diffuse cortical Lewy bodies. *Lancet* 1987;i:501.

28. Lennox G, Lowe J, Morrell K, *et al*. Anti-ubiquitin immunocytochemistry is more sensitive than conventional techniques in the detection of diffuse Lewy body disease. *J Neurol Neurosurg Psychiatry* 1989;52:67-71.

29. Byrne EJ, Lennox G, Lowe J. *et al*. Diffuse Lewy body disease: clinical features in fifteen cases. *J Neurol Neurosurg Psychiatry* 1989;52:709-17.

30. Lennox G, Lowe J, Landon M, *et al*. Diffuse Lewy body disease: correlative neuropathology using anti-ubiquitin immunocytochemistry. *J Neurol Neurosurg Psychiatry* 1989;52:1236-47.

31. Perry RH, Irving D, Blessed G, *et al*. Clinically and neuropathologically distinct form of dementia in the elderly. *Lancet* 1989;i:166.

32. Gibb WRG, Luthert PJ, Janota I, *et al*. Cortical Lewy body dementia, clinical features and classification. *J Neurol Neurosurg Psychiatry* 1989;52:185-92.

—by D. Neary, Department of Neurology, Manchester Royal Infirmary, Manchester

Chapter 11

Huntington's Disease

This text was written by the National Institute of Neurological Disorders and Stroke (NINDS), the United States' leading supporter of research on disorders of the brain and nervous system, including Huntington's disease. NINDS, one of the U.S. Government's 17 National Institutes of Health in Bethesda, Maryland, is part of the Public Health Service within the U.S. Department of Health and Human Services.

Introduction

In 1872, the American physician George Huntington wrote about an illness that he called "an heirloom from generations away back in the dim past." He was not the first to describe the disorder, which has been traced back to the Middle Ages at least. One of its earliest names was chorea—which as in "choreography" is the Greek word for dance. The term chorea describes how people affected with the disorder writhe, twist, and turn in a constant, uncontrollable dance-like motion. Later, other descriptive names evolved. "Hereditary chorea" emphasizes how the disease is passed from parent to child. "Chronic progressive chorea" stresses how symptoms of the disease worsen over time. Today, physicians commonly use the simple term Huntington's disease (HD) to describe this highly complex disorder that causes untold suffering for thousands of families.

National Institute of Neurological Disorders and Stroke (NINDS), April 7, 1998.

In the United States alone, about 30,000 people have HD; estimates of its prevalence are about 1 in every 10,000 persons. At least 150,000 others have a 50 percent risk of developing the disease and thousands more of their relatives live with the possibility that they, too, might develop HD.

Until recently, scientists understood very little about HD and could only watch as the disease continued to pass from generation to generation. Families saw the disease destroy their loved ones' ability to feel, think, and move. In the last several years, scientists working with support from the National Institute of Neurological Disorders and Stroke (NINDS) have made a significant number of breakthroughs in the area of HD research. With these advances, our understanding of the disease continues to improve.

This chapter presents information about HD, and about current research progress, to health professionals, scientists, caregivers, and, most importantly, to those already too familiar with the disorder: the many families who are affected by HD.

What Causes Huntington's Disease?

HD results from genetically programmed degeneration of brain cells, called neurons, in certain areas of the brain. This degeneration causes uncontrolled movements, loss of intellectual faculties, and emotional disturbance. Specifically affected are cells of the basal ganglia, structures deep within the brain that have a number of important functions, including coordinating movement. Within the basal ganglia, HD especially targets neurons of the striatum, particularly those in the caudate nuclei and the pallidum. Also affected is the brain's outer surface, or cortex, which controls thought, perception, and memory.

How Is HD Inherited?

HD is found in every country of the world. It is a familial disease, passed from parent to child through a mutation or misspelling in the normal gene.

A single abnormal gene, the basic biological unit of heredity, produces HD. Genes are composed of deoxyribonucleic acid (DNA), a molecule shaped like a spiral ladder. Each rung of this ladder is composed of two paired chemicals called bases. There are four types of bases—adenine, thymine, cytosine, and guanine—each abbreviated by the first letter of its name: A, T, C, and G. Certain bases always "pair" together, and different combinations of base pairs join to form coded messages. A gene is a long string of this DNA that is composed of various combinations of A, T, C, and G. These unique combinations determine the gene's function, much like letters join together to form words. Each person has about 100,000 genes—three billion base pairs of DNA or bits of information repeated in the nuclei of human cells—which determine individual characteristics or traits.

Genes are arranged in precise locations along 23 rod-like pairs of chromosomes. One chromosome from each pair comes from an individual's mother, the other from the father. Each half of a chromosome pair is similar to the other, except for one pair, which determines the sex of the individual. This pair has two x chromosomes in females and one x and one y chromosome in males. The gene that produces HD lies on chromosome 4, one of the 22 non-sex-linked, or "autosomal," pairs of chromosomes, placing men and women at equal risk of acquiring the disease.

The impact of a gene depends partly on whether it is dominant or recessive. If a gene is dominant, then only one of the paired chromosomes is required to produce its called-for effect. If the gene is recessive, both parents must provide chromosomal copies for the trait to be present. HD is called an autosomal dominant disorder because only one copy of the defective gene, inherited from one parent, is necessary to produce the disease.

The genetic defect responsible for HD is a small sequence of DNA on chromosome 4 in which several base pairs are repeated many, many times. The normal gene has three DNA bases, composed of the sequence CAG. In people with HD, the sequence abnormally repeats itself dozens of times. Over time—and with each successive generation—the number of CAG repeats may expand further.

Each parent has two copies of every chromosome but gives only one copy to each child. Each child of an HD parent has a 50-50 chance of inheriting the HD gene. If a child does not inherit the HD gene, he or she will not develop the disease and cannot pass it to subsequent generations. A person who inherits the HD gene, and survives long enough, will sooner or later develop the disease. In some families, all the children may inherit the HD gene; in others, none do. Whether one child inherits the gene has no bearing on whether others will or will not share the same fate.

A small number of cases of HD are sporadic, that is, they occur even though there is no family history of the disorder. These cases are thought to be caused by a new genetic mutation—an alteration in the gene that occurs during sperm development and that brings the number of CAG repeats into the range that causes disease.

What Are the Major Effects of the Disease?

Early signs of the disease vary greatly from person to person. A common observation is that the earlier the symptoms appear, the faster the disease progresses.

Family members may first notice that the individual experiences mood swings or becomes uncharacteristically irritable, apathetic, passive, depressed, or angry. These symptoms may lessen as the disease progresses or, in some individuals, may continue and include hostile outbursts or deep bouts of depression.

HD may affect the individual's judgment, memory, and other cognitive functions. Early signs might include having trouble driving, learning new things, remembering a fact, answering a question, or making a decision. Some may even display changes in handwriting. As the disease progresses, concentration on intellectual tasks becomes increasingly difficult.

In some individuals, the disease may begin with uncontrolled movements in the fingers, feet, face, or trunk. These movements—which are signs of chorea—often intensify when the person is anxious. HD can also begin with mild clumsiness or problems with balance. Other persons develop choreic movements later on as the disease progresses. They may stumble or appear uncoordinated. Chorea often creates serious problems with walking, increasing the likelihood of falls.

The disease can progress to the point where speech is slurred and vital functions, such as swallowing, eating, speaking, and especially walking, continue to decline. Some individuals are unable to recognize others. Many, however, remain aware of their environment and are able to express emotions.

Some physicians have employed a recently developed Unified HD Rating Scale, or UHDRS, to assess the clinical features, stages, and course of HD. In general, the duration of the illness ranges from 10 to 30 years. The most common causes of death are infection (most often pneumonia), injuries related to a fall, or other complications.

At What Age Does HD Appear?

The rate of disease progression and the age of onset vary from person to person. Adult-onset or classic HD, with its disabling, uncontrolled movements, most often begins during middle age. There are, however, other variations of HD distinguished not just by age of onset but by a distinct array of symptoms. For example, some persons develop the disease as adults, but without chorea. They may appear rigid and move very little, or not at all, a condition called akinesia. These individuals are said to have akinetic-rigid HD or the Westphal variant of HD.

Some individuals develop symptoms of HD when they are very young—before age 20. The terms early-onset HD or juvenile HD are often used to describe HD that appears in a young person. A common sign of HD in a younger individual is a rapid decline in school performance. Symptoms can also include subtle changes in handwriting and slight problems with movement, such as slowness, rigidity, tremor, and rapid muscular twitching, called myoclonus. Several of these symptoms are similar to those seen in Parkinson's disease, and they differ from the chorea seen in individuals who develop the disease as adults. People with juvenile HD may also have seizures and mental disabilities. As mentioned previously, the earlier the onset of HD, the faster the disease seems to progress. The disease progresses most rapidly in individuals with juvenile or early-onset HD, and death often follows within 10 years.

It appears that individuals with juvenile HD have usually inherited the disease from their fathers. These individuals also tend to have the largest number of CAG repeats. Scientists believe that the reason for this may be found in the process of sperm production. Unlike eggs, sperm are produced in the millions. Because DNA is copied millions of times during this process, scientists theorize that there is an increased possibility for genetic mistakes to occur. To verify that there was a link between the number of CAG repeats in the HD gene and the age of onset of the disease, scientists studied a young boy who developed HD at the age of two, one of the youngest and most severe cases ever recorded. They found that he had the largest number of CAG repeats of anyone they had studied so far—nearly 100. The boy's case was central to the identification of the HD gene and at the same time helped confirm that juvenile patients with HD have the longest segments of CAG repeats, the only proven correlation between repeat length and age at onset.

A few individuals develop HD after age 55. Diagnosis in these persons can be very difficult. The symptoms of HD may be masked by other health problems, or the person may not display the severity of symptoms seen in individuals with an earlier onset of HD. These individuals may also show signs of depression rather than anger or irritability, or they may retain sharp control over their intellectual functions, such as memory, reasoning, and problem-solving.

There is also a related complex called senile chorea. Some elderly individuals display the symptoms of HD, especially choreic movements, but have a normal gene and lack a family history of the disorder. Some scientists believe that a different gene mutation may account for this small number of cases. Others, however, believe senile chorea is a late-onset form of HD.

How Is HD Diagnosed?

The great American folk singer and composer Woody Guthrie died on October 3, 1967, after suffering from HD for 13 years. He had been misdiagnosed, considered an alcoholic, and shuttled in and out of mental institutions and hospitals for years before being properly diagnosed. His case, sadly, is not extraordinary, although the diagnosis can be made easily by experienced neurologists.

The discovery of the HD gene in 1993 resulted in a direct genetic test to make or confirm a diagnosis of HD in an individual who is exhibiting HD-like symptoms. Using a blood sample, the genetic test analyzes DNA for the HD mutation by counting the number of repeats in the HD gene region. Individuals who do not have HD usually have 28 or fewer CAG repeats. Individuals with HD usually have 40 or more repeats. A small percentage of individuals, however, have a number of repeats that fall within a borderline region (see Table 11.1).

Table 11.1. Genetic Test for Huntington's Disease.

No. of CAG repeats	Outcome
≤ 28	Normal range; individual will not develop HD
29-34	Individual will not develop HD but the next generation is at risk
35-39	Some, but not all, individuals in this range will develop HD; next generation is also at risk
≥ 40	Individual will develop HD

The physician will interview the individual intensively to obtain the medical history and rule out other conditions. He or she will perform a neurological examination including tests of the person's hearing, eye movements, strength, sensation, reflexes, balance, movement, and mental status, and will probably order a number of laboratory tests as well. Together, these tests form the neurological examination. In addition, the physician will ask about recent intellectual or emotional problems, which may be indications of HD.

In addition to direct testing, another tool used by physicians to diagnose HD is to take the family history, sometimes called a pedigree or genealogy. It is extremely important for family members to be candid and truthful with a doctor who is taking a family history.

People with HD commonly have impairments in the way the eye follows or fixes on a moving target. Abnormalities of eye movements vary from person to person and differ depending on the stage and duration of the illness.

The physician may ask the individual to undergo a brain imaging test. The computed tomography (CT) scanner provides an excellent image of brain structures with little if any discomfort. Those with HD may show shrinkage of some parts of the brain—particularly two areas known as the caudate nuclei and putamen—and enlargement of cavities within the brain called ventricles. These changes do not definitely indicate HD however, because they can also occur in other disorders. In addition, a person can have early symptoms of HD and still have a normal CT scan. When used in conjunction with a family history and record of clinical symptoms, however, CT can be an important diagnostic tool.

Other technologies for brain visualization, such as magnetic resonance imaging (MRI) and positron emission tomography (PET), are an important part of HD research efforts, but their usefulness to physicians trying to diagnose HD has not yet been established.

What Is Presymptomatic Testing?

Presymptomatic testing is a method for identifying persons carrying the HD gene before symptoms appear. In the past, no laboratory test could positively identify people carrying the HD gene—or those fated to develop HD—before the onset of symptoms. That situation changed in 1983, when a team of scientists supported by the NINDS located the first genetic marker for HD—the initial step in developing a laboratory test for the disease.

A marker is a piece of DNA that lies near a gene and is usually inherited with it. Discovery of the first HD marker allowed scientists to locate the HD gene on chromosome 4. The marker discovery quickly led to the development of a presymptomatic test for some individuals, but this test required blood or tissue samples from both affected and unaffected family members in order to identify markers unique to that particular family. For this reason, adopted individuals, orphans, and people who had few living family members were unable to use the test.

Discovery of the HD gene has led to a less expensive, scientifically simpler, and far more accurate presymptomatic test that is applicable to the majority of at-risk people. The new test uses CAG repeat length to detect the presence of the HD mutation in blood. This is discussed further in the next section.

In a small number of individuals with HD—1 to 3 percent—no family history of HD can be found. Some individuals may not be aware of their genetic legacy, or a family member may conceal a genetic disorder from fear of social stigma. A parent may not want to worry children, scare them, or deter them from marrying. In other cases, a family member may die of another cause before he or she begins to show signs of HD. Sometimes, the cause of death for a relative may not be known, or the family is not aware of a relative's death. Adopted children may not know their genetic heritage, or early symptoms in an individual may be too slight to attract attention. These are among the many complicating factors that reflect the complexity of diagnosing HD.

How Is the Presymptomatic Test Conducted?

An individual who wishes to be tested should contact the nearest testing center. (A list of such centers can be obtained from the Huntington Disease Society of America at 1-800-345-HDSA.) The testing process should include several components. Most testing programs include a neurological examination, pretest counseling, and followup. The purpose of the neurological examination is to determine whether or not the person requesting testing is showing any clinical symptoms of HD. It is important to remember that if an individual is showing even slight symptoms of HD, he or she risks being diagnosed with the disease during the neurological examination, even before the genetic test. During pretest counseling, the individual will learn about HD, about his or her own level of risk, and about the testing procedure. The person will be told about the test's limitations, the accuracy of the test, and possible outcomes. He or she can then weigh the risks and benefits of testing and may even decide at that time against pursuing further testing.

If a person decides to be tested, a team of highly trained specialists will be involved, which may include neurologists, genetic counselors, social workers, psychiatrists, and psychologists. This team of professionals helps the at-risk person decide if testing is the right thing to do and carefully prepares the person for a negative, positive, or inconclusive test result.

Individuals who decide to continue the testing process should be accompanied to counseling sessions by a spouse, a friend, or a relative who is not at risk. Other interested family members may participate in the counseling sessions if the individual being tested so desires.

The genetic testing itself involves donating a small sample of blood that is screened in the laboratory for the presence or absence of the HD mutation. Testing may require a sample of DNA from a closely related affected relative, preferably a parent, for the purpose of confirming the diagnosis of HD in the family. This is especially important if the family history for HD is unclear or unusual in some way.

Results of the test should be given only in person and only to the individual being tested. Test results are confidential. Regardless of test results, followup is recommended.

In order to protect the interests of minors, including confidentiality, testing is not recommended for those under the age of 18 unless there is a compelling medical reason (for example, the child is exhibiting symptoms).

Testing of a fetus (prenatal testing) presents special challenges and risks; in fact some centers do not perform genetic testing on fetuses. Because a positive test result using direct genetic testing means the at-risk parent is also a gene carrier, at-risk individuals who are considering a pregnancy are advised to seek genetic counseling prior to conception.

Some at-risk parents may wish to know the risk to their fetus but not their own. In this situation, parents may opt for prenatal testing using linked DNA markers rather than direct gene testing. In this case, testing does not look for the HD gene itself but instead indicates whether or not the fetus has inherited a chromosome 4 from the affected grandparent or from the unaffected grandparent on the side of the family with HD. If the test shows that the fetus has inherited a chromosome 4 from the affected grandparent, the parents then learn that the fetus's risk is the same as the parent (50-50), but they learn nothing new about the parent's risk. If the test shows that the fetus has inherited a chromosome 4 from the unaffected grandparent, the risk to the fetus is very low (less than 1%) in most cases.

Another option open to parents is *in vitro* fertilization with pre-implantation screening. In this procedure, embryos are screened to determine which ones carry the HD mutation. Embryos determined not to have the HD gene mutation are then implanted in the woman's uterus.

In terms of emotional and practical consequences, not only for the individual taking the test but for his or her entire family, testing is enormously complex and has been surrounded by considerable controversy. For example, people with a positive test result may risk losing health and life insurance, suffer loss of employment, and other liabilities. People undergoing testing may wish to cover the cost themselves, since coverage by an insurer may lead to loss of health insurance in the event of a positive result, although this may change in the future.

With the participation of health professionals and people from families with HD, scientists have developed testing guidelines. All individuals seeking a genetic test should obtain a copy of these guidelines, either from their testing center or from the organizations listed in the back of this chapter. These organizations have information on sites that perform testing using the established procedures and they strongly recommend that individuals avoid testing that does not adhere to these guidelines.

How Does a Person Decide Whether to be Tested?

The anxiety that comes from living with a 50 percent risk for HD can be overwhelming. How does a young person make important choices about long-term education, marriage, and children? How do older parents of adult children cope with their fears about children and grandchildren? How do people come to terms with the ambiguity and uncertainty of living at risk?

Some individuals choose to undergo the test out of a desire for greater certainty about their genetic status. They believe the test will enable them to make more informed decisions about the future. Others choose not to take the test. They are at peace with being at risk and with all that that may entail. There is no right or wrong decision, as each choice is highly individual. The guidelines for genetic testing for HD, discussed in the previous section, were developed to help people with this life-changing choice.

Whatever the results of genetic testing, the at-risk individual and family members can expect powerful and complex emotional responses. The health and happiness of spouses, brothers and sisters, children, parents, and grandparents are affected by a positive test result, as are an individual's friends, work associates, neighbors, and others. Because receiving test results may prove to be devastating, testing guidelines call for continued counseling even after the test is complete and the results are known.

Is There a Treatment for HD?

Physicians may prescribe a number of medications to help control emotional and movement problems associated with HD. It is important to remember however, that while medicines may help keep these clinical symptoms under control, there is no treatment to stop or re verse the course of the disease.

Antipsychotic drugs, such as haloperidol, or other drugs, such as clonazepam, may help to alleviate choreic movements and may also be used to help control hallucinations, delusions, and violent outbursts. Antipsychotic drugs, however, are not prescribed for another form of muscle contraction associated with HD, called dystonia, and may in fact worsen the condition, causing stiffness and rigidity. These medications may also have severe side effects, including sedation, and for that reason should be used in the lowest possible doses.

For depression, physicians may prescribe fluoxetine, sertraline hydrochloride, nortriptyline, or other compounds. Tranquilizers can help control anxiety and lithium may be prescribed to combat pathological excitement and severe mood swings. Medications may also be needed to treat the severe obsessive-compulsive rituals of some individuals with HD.

Most drugs used to treat the symptoms of HD have side effects such as fatigue, restlessness, or hyperexcitability. Sometimes it may be difficult to tell if a particular symptom, such as apathy or incontinence, is a sign of the disease or a reaction to medication.

What Kind of Care Does the Individual with HD Need?

Although a psychologist or psychiatrist, a genetic counselor, and other specialists may be needed at different stages of the illness, usually the first step in diagnosis and in finding treatment is to see a neurologist. While the family doctor may be able to diagnose HD, and may continue to monitor the individual's status, it is better to consult with a neurologist about management of the varied symptoms.

Problems may arise when individuals try to express complex thoughts in words they can no longer pronounce intelligibly. It can be helpful to repeat words back to the person with HD so that he or she knows that some thoughts are understood. Sometimes people mistakenly assume that if individuals do not talk, they also do not understand. Never isolate individuals by not talking, and try to keep their environment as normal as possible. Speech therapy may improve the individual's ability to communicate.

It is extremely important for the person with HD to maintain physical fitness as much as his or her condition and the course of the disease allows. Individuals who exercise and keep active tend to do better than those who do not. A daily regimen of exercise can help the person feel better physically and mentally. Although their coordination may be poor, individuals should continue walking, with assistance if necessary. Those who want to walk independently should be allowed to do so as long as possible, and careful attention should be given to keeping their environment free of hard, sharp objects. This will help ensure maximal independence while minimizing the risk of injury from a fall. Individuals can also wear special padding during walks to help protect against injury from falls. Some people have found that small weights around the ankles can help stability. Wearing sturdy shoes that fit well can help too, especially shoes without laces that can be slipped on or off easily.

Impaired coordination may make it difficult for people with HD to feed themselves and to swallow. As the disease progresses, persons with HD may even choke. In helping individuals to eat, caregivers should allow plenty of time for meals. Food can be cut into small pieces, softened, or pureed to ease swallowing and prevent choking. While some foods may require the addition of thickeners, other foods may need to be thinned. Dairy products, in particular, tend to increase the secretion of mucus, which in turn increases the risk of choking. Some individuals may benefit from swallowing therapy, which is especially helpful if started before serious problems arise. Suction cups for plates, special tableware designed for people with disabilities, and plastic cups with tops can help prevent spilling. The individual's physician can offer additional advice about diet and about how to handle swallowing difficulties or gastrointestinal problems that might arise, such as incontinence or constipation.

Caregivers should pay attention to proper nutrition so that the individual with HD takes in enough calories to maintain his or her body weight. Sometimes people with HD, who may burn as many as 5,000 calories a day without gaining weight, require five meals a day to take in the necessary number of calories. Physicians may recommend vitamins or other nutritional supplements. In a long-term care institution, staff will need to assist with meals in order to ensure that the individual's special caloric and nutritional requirements are met. Some individuals and their families choose to use a feeding tube; others choose not to.

Individuals with HD are at special risk for dehydration and therefore require large quantities of fluids, especially during hot weather. Bendable straws can make drinking easier for the person. In some cases, water may have to be thickened with commercial additives to give it the consistency of syrup or honey.

What Community Resources Are Available?

Individuals and families affected by HD can take steps to ensure that they receive the best advice and care possible. Physicians and state and local health service agencies can provide information on community resources and family support groups that may exist. Possible types of help include:

Legal and social aid. HD affects a person's capacity to reason, make judgments, and handle responsibilities. Individuals may need help with legal affairs. Wills and other important documents should be drawn up early to avoid legal problems when the person with HD may no longer be able to represent his or her own interests. Family members should also seek out assistance if they face discrimination regarding insurance, employment, or other matters.

Home care services. Caring for a person with HD at home can be exhausting, but part-time assistance with household chores or physical care of the individual can ease this burden. Domestic help, meal programs, nursing assistance, occupational therapy, or other home services may be available from federal, state, or local health service agencies.

Recreation and work centers. Many people with HD are eager and able to participate in activities outside the home. Therapeutic work and recreation centers give individuals an opportunity to pursue hobbies and interests and to meet new people. Participation in these programs, including occupational, music, and recreational therapy, can reduce the person's dependence on family members and provides home caregivers with a temporary, much needed break.

131

Group housing. A few communities have group housing facilities that are supervised by a resident attendant and that provide meals, housekeeping services, social activities, and local transportation services for residents. These living arrangements are particularly suited to the needs of individuals who are alone and who, although still independent and capable, risk injury when they undertake routine chores like cooking and cleaning.

Institutional care. The individual's physical and emotional demands on the family may eventually become overwhelming. While many families may prefer to keep relatives with HD at home whenever possible, a long-term care facility may prove to be best. To hospitalize or place a family member in a care facility is a difficult decision; professional counseling can help families with this.

Finding the proper facility can itself prove difficult. Organizations such as the Huntington's Disease Society of America (see Information Resources below) may be able to refer the family to facilities that have met standards set for the care of individuals with HD. Very few of these exist however, and even fewer have experience with individuals with juvenile or early-onset HD who require special care because of their age and symptoms.

What Research Is Being Done?

Although HD attracted considerable attention from scientists in the early 20th century, there was little sustained research on the disease until the late 1960s when the Committee to Combat Huntington's Disease and the Huntington's Chorea Foundation, later called the Hereditary Disease Foundation, first began to fund research and to campaign for federal funding. In 1977, Congress established the Commission for the Control of Huntington's Disease and Its Consequences, which made a series of important recommendations. Since then, Congress has provided consistent support for federal research, primarily through the National Institute of Neurological Disorders and Stroke, the government's lead agency for biomedical research on disorders of the brain and nervous system. The effort to combat HD proceeds along the following lines of inquiry, each providing important information about the disease:

Basic neurobiology. Now that the HD gene has been located, investigators in the field of neurobiology—which encompasses the anatomy, physiology, and biochemistry of the nervous system—are continuing to study the HD gene with an eye toward understanding how it causes disease in the human body.

Clinical research. Neurologists, psychologists, psychiatrists, and other investigators are improving our understanding of the symptoms and progression of the disease in patients while attempting to develop new therapeutics.

Imaging. Scientific investigations using PET and other technologies are enabling scientists to see what the defective gene does to various structures in the brain and how it affects the body's chemistry and metabolism.

Animal models. Laboratory animals, such as mice, are being bred in the hope of duplicating the clinical features of HD and can soon be expected to help scientists learn more about the symptoms and progression of the disease.

Fetal tissue research. Investigators are implanting fetal tissue in rodents and nonhuman primates with the hope that success in this area will lead to understanding, restoring, or replacing functions typically lost by neuronal degeneration in individuals with HD.

These areas of research are slowly converging and, in the process, are yielding important clues about the gene's relentless destruction of mind and body. The NINDS supports much of this exciting work.

Molecular Genetics

For 10 years, scientists focused on a segment of chromosome 4 and, in 1993, finally isolated the HD gene. The process of isolating the responsible gene—motivated by the desire to find a cure—was more difficult than anticipated. Scientists now believe that identifying the location of the HD gene is the first step on the road to a cure.

Finding the HD gene involved an intense molecular genetics research effort with cooperating investigators from around the globe. In early 1993, the collaborating scientists announced they had isolated the unstable triplet repeat DNA sequence that has the HD gene. Investigators relied on the NINDS-supported Research Roster for Huntington's Disease, based at Indiana University in Indianapolis, to accomplish this work. First started in 1979, the roster contains data on many American families with HD, provides statistical and demographic data to scientists, and serves as a liaison between investigators and specific families. It provided the DNA from many families affected by HD to investigators involved in the search for the gene and was an important component in the identification of HD markers.

For several years, NINDS-supported investigators involved in the search for the HD gene made yearly visits to the largest known kindred with HD—14,000 individuals—who live on Lake Maracaibo in Venezuela. The continuing trips enable scientists to study inheritance patterns of several interrelated families.

The HD Gene and Its Product

Although scientists know that certain brain cells die in HD, the cause of their death is still unknown. Recessive diseases are usually thought to result from a gene that fails to produce adequate amounts of a substance essential to normal function. This is known as a loss-of-function gene. Some dominantly inherited disorders, such as HD, are thought to involve a gene that actively interferes with the normal function of the cell. This is known as a gain-of-function gene.

How does the defective HD gene cause harm? The HD gene encodes a protein—which has been named huntingtin—the function of which is as yet unknown. The repeated CAG sequence in the gene causes an abnormal form of huntingtin to be made, in which the amino acid glutamine is repeated. It is the presence of this abnormal form, and not the absence of the normal form, that causes harm in HD. This explains why the disease is dominant and why two copies of the defective gene—one from both the mother and the father—do not cause a more serious case than inheritance from only one parent. With the HD gene isolated, NINDS-supported investigators are now turning their attention toward discovering the normal function of huntingtin and how the altered form causes harm. Scientists hope to reproduce, study, and correct these changes in animal models of the disease.

Huntingtin is found everywhere in the body but only outside the cell's nucleus. Mice bred in the laboratory to produce no huntingtin fail to develop past a very early embryo stage and quickly die. Huntingtin, scientists now know, is necessary for life. Investigators hope to learn why the abnormal version of the protein damages only certain parts of the brain. One theory is that cells in these parts of the brain may be supersensitive to this abnormal protein.

Cell Death in HD

Although the precise cause of cell death in HD is not yet known, scientists are paying close attention to the process of genetically programmed cell death that occurs deep within the brains of individuals with HD. This process involves a complex series of interlinked events leading to cellular suicide. Related areas of investigation include:

- Excitotoxicity. Overstimulation of cells by natural chemicals found in the brain.

- Defective energy metabolism. A defect in the power plant of the cell, called mitochondria, where energy is produced.

- Oxidative stress. Normal metabolic activity in the brain that produces toxic compounds called free radicals.

- Trophic factors. Natural chemical substances found in the human body that may protect against cell death.

Several HD studies are aimed at understanding losses of nerve cells and receptors in HD. Neurons in the striatum are classified both by their size (large, medium, or small) and appearance (spiny or aspiny). Each type of neuron contains combinations of neurotransmitters. Scientists know that the destructive process of HD affects different subsets of neurons to varying degrees. The hallmark of HD, they are learning, is selective degeneration of medium-sized spiny neurons in the striatum. NINDS-supported studies also suggest that losses of certain types of neurons and receptors are responsible for different symptoms and stages of HD.

What do these changes look like? In spiny neurons, investigators have observed two types of changes, each affecting the nerve cells' dendrites. Dendrites, found on every nerve cell, extend out from the cell body and are responsible for receiving messages from other nerve cells. In the intermediate stages of HD, dendrites grow out of control. New, incomplete branches form and other branches become contorted. In advanced, severe stages of HD, degenerative changes cause sections of dendrites to swell, break off, or disappear altogether. Investigators believe that these alterations may be an attempt by the cell to rebuild nerve cell contacts lost early in the disease. As the new dendrites establish connections, however, they may in fact contribute to nerve cell death. Such studies give compelling, visible evidence of the progressive nature of HD and suggest that new experimental therapies must consider the state of cellular degeneration. Scientists do not yet know exactly how these changes affect subsets of nerve cells outside the striatum.

Animal Models for HD

As more is learned about cellular degeneration in HD, investigators hope to reproduce these changes in animal models and to find a way to correct or halt the process of nerve cell death. Such models serve the scientific community in general by providing a means to test the safety of new classes of drugs in nonhuman primates. NINDS-supported scientists are currently working to develop both nonhuman primate and mouse models to investigate nerve degeneration in HD and to study the effects of excitotoxicity on nerve cells in the brain.

Investigators are working to build genetic models of HD using transgenic mice. To do this, scientists transfer the altered human HD gene into mouse embryos so that the animals will develop the anatomical and biological characteristics of HD. This genetic model of mouse HD will enable in-depth study of the disease and testing of new therapeutic compounds.

Another idea is to insert into mice a section of DNA containing CAG repeats in the abnormal, disease gene range. This mouse equivalent of HD could allow scientists to explore the basis of CAG instability and its role in the disease process.

Fetal Tissue Research

A relatively new field in biomedical research involves the use of brain tissue grafts to study, and potentially treat, neurodegenerative disorders. In this technique, tissue that has degenerated is replaced with implants of fresh, fetal tissue, taken at the very early stages of development. Investigators are interested in applying brain tissue implants to HD research. Extensive animal studies will be required to learn if this technique could be of value in individuals with HD.

Clinical Studies

Scientists are pursuing clinical studies that may one day lead to the development of new drugs or other treatments to halt the disease's progression. Examples of NINDS-supported investigations, using both asymptomatic and symptomatic individuals, include:

- *Genetic studies on age of onset, inheritance patterns, and markers found within families.* These studies may shed additional light on how HD is passed from generation to generation.

- *Studies of cognition, intelligence, and movement.* Studies of abnormal eye movements, both horizontal and vertical, and tests of patients' skills in a number of learning, memory, neuropsychological, and motor tasks may serve to identify when the various symptoms of HD appear and to characterize their range and severity.

- *Clinical trials of drugs.* Testing of various drugs may lead to new treatments and at the same time improve our understanding of the disease process in HD. Classes of drugs being tested include those that control symptoms, slow the rate of progression of HD, and block effects of excitotoxins, and those that might correct or replace other metabolic defects contributing to the development and progression of HD.

Imaging

NINDS-supported scientists are using positron emission tomography (PET) to learn how the gene affects the chemical systems of the body. PET visualizes metabolic or chemical abnormalities in the body, and investigators hope to ascertain if PET scans can reveal any abnormalities that signal HD. Investigators conducting HD research are also using PET to characterize neurons that have died and chemicals that are depleted in parts of the brain affected by HD.

Like PET, a form of magnetic resonance imaging (MRI) called functional MRI can measure increases or decreases in certain brain chemicals thought to play a key role in HD. Functional MRI studies are also helping investigators understand how HD kills neurons in different regions of the brain.

Imaging technologies allow investigators to view changes in the volume and structures of the brain and to pinpoint when these changes occur in HD. Scientists know that in brains affected by HD, the basal ganglia, cortex, and ventricles all show atrophy or other alterations.

How Can I Help?

In order to conduct HD research, investigators require samples of tissue or blood from families with HD. Access to individuals with HD and their families may be difficult however, because families with HD are often scattered across the country or around the world. A research project may need individuals of a particular age or gender or from a certain geographic area. Some scientists need only statistical data while others may require a sample of blood, urine, or skin from family members. All of these factors complicate the task of finding volunteers. The following NINDS-supported efforts bring together families with HD, voluntary health agencies, and scientists in an effort to advance science and speed a cure.

Research Roster and DNA Bank

The NINDS-sponsored HD Research Roster at the Indiana University Medical Center in Indianapolis, which was discussed earlier, makes research possible by matching scientists with patient and family volunteers. The first DNA bank was established through the roster. Although the gene has already been located, DNA from individuals who have HD is still of great interest to investigators. Of continuing interest are twins, unaffected individuals who have affected offspring, and individuals with two defective HD genes, one from each parent — a very rare occurrence. Participation in the roster and in specific research projects is voluntary and confidential. For more information about the roster and DNA bank, contact:

Indiana University Medical Center
Department of Medical and Molecular Genetics
Medical Research and Library Building
975 W. Walnut Street
Indianapolis, IN 46202-5251
(317) 274-5744 (call collect)

Brain Tissue Donations

Brain tissue is also critical to the HD research effort, and many individuals are willing to donate their brains and other organs to research after they die. The NINDS supports two national human brain specimen banks, one at the Wadsworth Veterans Administration Medical Center in Los Angeles, and the other at McLean Hospital near Boston. These banks supply investigators around the world with tissue not only from individuals with HD but also from those with other neurological or psychiatric diseases. Both banks need brain tissue to enable scientists to study these disorders more intensely. Prospective donors should contact:

Wallace W. Tourtellotte, M.D., Ph.D.
Director, National Neurological Research Specimen Bank
VA Wadsworth Medical Center Neurology Research
Wilshire & Sawtelle Boulevards
Los Angeles, CA 90073
(310) 268-3536 (call collect)

Francine M. Benes, M.D., Ph.D.
Director, Harvard Brain Tissue Resource Center
Mailman Research Center, McLean Hospital
115 Mill Street
Belmont, MA 02178
(617) 855-2400 (call collect)
(800) 272-4622

What Is the Role of Voluntary Organizations?

Private organizations have been a mainstay of support and guidance for at-risk individuals, people with HD, and their families. These organizations vary in size and emphasis, but all are concerned with helping individuals and their families, educating lay and professional audiences about HD, and promoting medical research on the disorder. Some voluntary health agencies support scientific workshops and research and some have newsletters and local chapters throughout the country. These agencies enable families, health professionals, and investigators to exchange information, learn of available services and benefits, and work toward common goals. The organizations listed in the Information Resources section (below) welcome inquiries from the public.

Information Resources

National Institutes of Health

NIH Neurological Institute
P.O. Box 5801
Bethesda, MD 20824
(301) 496-5751; (800) 352-9424

The National Institute of Neurological Disorders and Stroke, a component of the National Institutes of Health, is the leading Federal supporter of research on disorders of the brain and nervous system. The Institute also sponsors an active public information program with staff who can answer questions about diagnosis and research related to Huntington's disease.

Private Organizations

Private voluntary organizations that provide the public with information on treatment, diagnosis, and services include the following:

Huntington's Disease Society of America (HDSA)
140 West 22nd Street, 6th Floor
New York, NY 10011-2420
(212) 242-1968
(800) 345-HDSA (345-4372)

The HDSA supports research, assists and educates families, trains professionals about Huntington's disease, and monitors testing guidelines. The Society publishes brochures, pamphlets, a newsletter, reprints, and listings of testing centers. It also sponsors conferences, training programs, and nationwide chapters and support groups.

Hereditary Disease Foundation
1427 Seventh Street, Suite 2
Santa Monica, CA 90401
(310) 458-4183

This foundation promotes research on genetic disorders and sponsors workshops and fellowship programs. The group provides additional support to the two brain banks noted above.

Chapter 12

AIDS-Related Dementia

Description

Acquired immune deficiency syndrome (AIDS) is the result of an infection with the human immunodeficiency virus (HIV). This virus attacks selected cells of the immune, nervous, and other systems impairing their proper function. HIV infection may cause damage to the brain and spinal cord, causing encephalitis (inflammation of the brain), meningitis (inflammation of the membranes surrounding the brain), nerve damage, difficulties in thinking (i.e., AIDS dementia complex), behavioral changes, poor circulation, headache, and stroke. AIDS-related cancers such as lymphoma and opportunistic infections (OI) may also affect the nervous system. Neurological symptoms may be mild in the early stages of AIDS, but may become severe in the final stages. Complications vary widely from one patient to another. Cerebral toxoplasmosis, a common OI in AIDS patients, causes such symptoms as headache, confusion, lethargy, and low-grade fever.

This chapter contains excerpts from "Neurological Manifestations of AIDS," National Institute of Neurological Disorders and Stroke, January 1997; "Dementia, Depression, and Quality of Life," by J. Hampton Atkinson, Lisa Capaldini, Jerome F. Levine, and Richard W. Price, *Patient Care*, May 15, 1996 v30 n9 p131(9), © 1996 Medical Economics Publishing, reprinted with permission; and "New Clues to Cause of Dementia in AIDS Patients," *AIDS Weekly Plus*, March 3, 1997 p7(2), © 1997 Charles Henderson, Publisher of *AIDS Weekly Plus* and *Alzheimer's Disease Weekly*, (800) 633-4931, (205) 995-1588 fax; reprinted with permission.

Other symptoms may include weakness, speech disturbance, ataxia, apraxia, seizures, and sensory loss. Progressive multifocal leukoencephalopathy (PML), a disorder that can also occur in AIDS patients, causes weakness, hemiparesis or facial weakness, dysphasia, vision loss, and ataxia. Some patients with PML may also develop compromised memory and cognition.

AIDS Dementia Complex (ADC)

It became apparent early in the AIDS epidemic that immune system compromise often was accompanied by cognitive and motor changes ranging from mild impairment to dementia approaching the severity of Alzheimer's disease. As researchers have sought to categorize various aspects of AIDS during the past 15 years, they have also worked to clarify the nature and impact of the so-called AIDS dementia complex (ADC). A staging scheme has been developed. [For a description of the stages, which range from Stage 0—Normal to Stage 4—End-Stage, see: Sidtis JJ, Price RW: Early HIV-1 infection and the AIDS dementia complex, *Neurology* 1990;40:323-326.]. Full-fledged dementia generally is associated only with advanced AIDS and severe immunosuppression and is a poor prognostic sign. The overall prevalence of dementia in people with frank AIDS is estimated at 5-15%.

ADC is in part a diagnosis of exclusion. Ruling out other causes of neuropsychological disturbance such as central nervous system (CNS) infection or lymphoma is, of course, important. The workup includes a good history and physical and careful neurologic examination; when indicated by the clinical findings and circumstances, laboratory tests such as serum VDRL and cryptococcal antigen assays also should be ordered. A lumbar puncture and MRI of the brain are sometimes indicated. Older patients appear to be more at risk for neurologic changes because of the aging brain's increasing vulnerability to injury. Children are also at particular risk—the developing brain is susceptible to vital damage that leads to encephalopathy.

Mild Impairment

Although frank dementia is not common, as many as one half of all symptomatic AIDS patients exhibit a mild degree of neurocognitive impairment known as minor cognitivemotor disorder. A typical observation is that patients have difficulty concentrating or completing tasks that had been routine. This may manifest as forgetfulness, feeling "spaced out," or having difficulty functioning efficiently at work.

Seropositive but asymptomatic patients may also experience minor cognitive-motor changes, but this is rare. This milder form of impairment may present a particular challenge to the primary care physician: When are the changes important? Do they suggest a need for more aggressive antiretroviral treatment? How often do they relate to depression rather than early ADC?

Evidence suggests that zidovudine (AZT) can be beneficial in reversing or slowing the progress of clinically overt dementia. Although there have been no controlled trials evaluating the clinical effects of other antiretroviral drugs on neurologic function, HIV infects the CNS. It is therefore reasonable to assume that lessening the systemic and CNS viral load would help preserve CNS functioning. The potential role of the new protease inhibitors also needs to be evaluated in HIV patients.

Optimal antiretroviral treatment is desirable because maintaining immune function can help improve cognitive and motor function. This can enhance emotional health and quality of life, which may, in turn, improve immune system function. Mortality also may be affected, with even milder impairment possibly being associated with shortened survival time.

It's important to keep in mind that mild or early cognitive impairment can be one of the most distressing aspects of HIV disease for patients and families. Patients may be acutely aware of what is happening to them—and what may lie ahead. In no facet of AIDS care is empathy more important, and your role is crucial. Let the patient know that you will continue to be available for support and help, regardless of what comes. Reassure the patient and family that mild cognitive or motor difficulties do not necessarily progress to full-blown dementia. Issues of dignity and autonomy may be very much on the patient's mind, and your influence can be great.

When Symptoms Worsen

The diagnosis of dementia as set out in the *Diagnostic and Statistical Manual of Mental Disorders, Fourth Edition (DSM-IV)* requires that the patient exhibit difficulties with memory and one other area of mental functioning, such as aphasia, apraxia, or a decrease in the executive functions of judgement, synthesis, and action. Diagnostic criteria for ADC also have been specified, and since 1986 dementia has been considered an AIDS-defining condition. The condition must have a significant impact on the patient's life, usually involving the inability to work and care for oneself adequately.

Various tests are used to evaluate dementia, but these are often time-consuming, requiring 2-6 hours of formal testing. To facilitate the diagnosis of HIV-related dementia, a group of investigators recently designed a quick bedside test, the Mental Alternation Test. The patient is asked to count to 20, recite the alphabet, and then alternate between the two: 1-A, 2-B, 3-C, etc. The investigators reported that the test was perhaps more sensitive than the Mini-Mental State Exam. Its specificity is lower than standard tests, but the investigators note that false positive results will be screened out by more extensive testing. They concluded that the Mental Alternation Test could be useful in primary care in determining the need for neurologic referral.

The patient's demeanor and behavior also may suggest worsening dementia, such as when a formerly reliable patient suddenly begins missing office appointments. The patient may seem unable to connect with you or the surroundings, and motor control and balance may be noticeably impaired. Symptoms of dementia tend to fluctuate, so keep in mind that the person who appears completely lucid may not always be so. Conversely, even the most demented-appearing person may have periods of lucidity. Any discussions therefore should be conducted with the assumption that the patient is aware of what is being said.

What Can Be Done

Along with optimal antiretroviral treatment, environmental and behavioral strategies can help the patient with mild to moderate cognitive impairment to maximize function. Simplifying routines and avoiding time pressures can help alleviate the frustration of cognitive impairment. Many people find that making lists helps keep them focused. The environment should be kept uncluttered and as familiar as possible. Numerous community resources such as social service agencies and AIDS programs are available for patients and caregivers.

With disease progression and worsening dementia, however, come more severe difficulties. The patient with end-stage AIDS and severe dementia may be too much for the family to cope with—or there may be no family support to enlist. Nursing homes often are unwilling to take these patients. They may linger in the acute care setting to little benefit and at great cost. Hospice involvement becomes all-important.

There is reason for optimism, however. Researchers are now looking at possible pharmacologic options for improving cognitive functioning in AIDS patients, and phase II studies are under way. The calcium channel blocker memantine HCI, for example, is being tested. This agent is not active against the virus itself, but *in vitro* it reverses HIV-induced disruptions in calcium metabolism and impedes cytokine activity that may destabilize neuronal function. Its clinical usefulness awaits farther study.

New Clues to Cause of Dementia in AIDS Patients.

Scientists investigating the cause of dementia in AIDS patients said they may have discovered how the virus gets into the brain. Dana Gabuzda, Dana-Farber Cancer Institute, Boston, Massachusetts, said the findings could have significant implications for the development of drugs to prevent or treat AIDS dementia.

More than 3.1 million people contracted AIDS in 1996, bringing the world total to around 30 million. Between 20 and 30 percent of patients develop some sort of brain disease after advanced AIDS sets in, suffering symptoms like memory loss and loss of bodily function, Gabuzda said.

Dementia is a relatively poorly understood aspect of the disease, though, she said, because research tends to focus on the immune system. Results from the five member Dana-Farber team, published in *Nature*, showed that both CCR3 and CCR5 receptors present in the brain could promote infection of the central nervous system by some strains of HIV. The scientists found that individuals with defective CCR5 exhibited resistance to HIV-1, suggesting that CCR5 plays an important role as a co-receptor in allowing the virus entry. This finding marked the first proof that CCR3 plays a role in HIV infection and is likely to pave the way for further study, Gabuzda said. Studies would now look at the possibility that CCR3 could be acting as a receptor elsewhere in the body, for example in the lungs or lymph nodes.

"The identification of CCR3 as a co-receptor contributing to efficient HIV-1 infection of microglia (the main target cells in the brain) may suggest new therapeutic strategies to inhibit HIV-1 replication in the central nervous system," the authors reported in *Nature*.

A recent study of 2,600 AIDS patients published in the *British Medical Journal* showed median survival after diagnosis to be 20 months. While a cure for AIDS remains a distant prospect, scientists say new drugs are delaying the development of advanced AIDS in HIV infected patients.

For Further Information

These articles, available from a medical library, are sources of in-depth information on the neurological manifestations of AIDS:

McArthur, J. "Neurologic Manifestations of Human Immunodeficiency Virus Infection." In *Diseases of the Nervous System: Clinical Neurobiology*, W.B. Saunders Co., Philadelphia, pp. 1312-1330 (1992).

Mintz, M, and Epstein, L. "Neurologic Manifestations of Pediatric Acquired Immunodeficiency Syndrome: Clinical Features and Therapeutic Approaches." *Seminars in Neurology*, 12:1; 51-56 (March 1992).

Newton, H. "Common Neurologic Complications of HIV-1 Infection and AIDS." *American Family Physician*, 51:2; 387-398 (February 1, 1995).

Pajeau, A, and Roman, G. "HIV Encephalopathy and Dementia." *Psychiatric Clinics of North America*, 15:2; 455-466 (June 1992).

Simpson, D, and Tagliati, M. "Neurologic Manifestations of HIV Infection." *Annals of Internal Medicine*, 121:10; 769-785 (November 1994).

Organizations

Additional information or services are available from the following organizations:

American Foundation for AIDS Research
733 Third Ave., 12th Flr.
New York, NY 10017
(212) 682-7440

Pediatric AIDS Foundation
1311 Colorado Avenue
Santa Monica, CA 90404
(310) 395-9051

CDC National AIDS Clearinghouse
P.O. Box 6003
Rockville, MD 20849-6003
(800) 458-5231

National Institute of Allergy & Infectious Diseases
Building 31, Room 7A50
Bethesda, MD 20892-2520
(301) 496-5717

National Association of People with AIDS
1413 K Street, NW
Washington, DC 20005
(202) 898-0414

AIDS Clinical Trials Information Service
P.O. Box 6421
Rockville, MD 20849-6421
(800) TRIALS-A

Chapter 13

Alcoholic Dementia and Wernicke-Korsakoff Syndrome

What Drinking Does to the Brain

Slurred speech. Moodiness. A lurching walk. These well-known signs of drunkenness may warn of an ongoing problem with alcoholism, if they occur frequently enough. Just as ominous, however, is when sober alcoholics have trouble thinking and remembering. Problems with higher mental functions, or cognition, can occur with excessive, long-term drinking. Finding out why these problems appear and what to do about them is a key goal for clinical researchers—a goal that is well worth the effort, according to Dr. Enoch Gordis, Dana Alliance member and Director of the National Institute on Alcohol Abuse and Alcoholism.

Two extreme results of long-term alcoholism are Wernicke-Korsakoff syndrome (WKS), a severe difficulty in remembering recent events, and a condition known as "alcoholic dementia," a precipitous decline of general intellectual abilities. Evidence shows that, for several million alcoholics who have not reached these extremes, the progression of mental deterioration can be halted. Research also offers hope that the effects of alcoholism on the brain can be at least partially reversed. Below, Dr. Gordis discusses some of the most promising findings.

"All addictive substances threaten the well-being of body and mind. Although alcohol abuse is widespread and the results can be devastating, many mysteries greet the scientists who investigate the ways that alcohol exerts its effects. The more we understand about how it leads to damage, the more successful courses of treatment we can find.

"WKS is a comparatively well understood cause of severe cognitive impairment in alcoholics. The condition first appears, usually in the emergency room, as confusion, irregular eye movement and unsteady gait (Wernicke syndrome). It often evolves into an inability to form memories based on new information (Korsakoff syndrome). For example, fifteen minutes after the start of a conversation, a Korsakoff patient may forget everything that has been said.

"Most scientists believe the cause to be a deficiency in vitamin B1 (thiamine). In developed countries, almost all WKS patients are chronic alcoholics. Thiamine deficiency can result from poor diet (common in alcoholics), alcohol's interference with the body's absorption of thiamine, and possibly a genetic susceptibility.

"WKS shows the importance of knowing the mechanism that leads to cognitive problems in alcoholics. If Wernicke syndrome is recognized as such, thiamine supplements, given in the emergency room and subsequently, can improve the symptoms. Thiamine also reduces the risk of developing the severe memory deficits associated with Korsakoff syndrome. In patients who already show these memory deficits, symptoms can improve with abstinence and with the medications clonidine and fluvoxamine.

"New research is providing a better understanding of WKS. One imaging study examined alcoholics with Korsakoff syndrome who had abstained from alcohol for up to two years. In these patients, in some brain areas associated with memory, use of glucose decreased in a way that correlates with the pattern of memory deficits characteristic of Korsakoff syndrome.

"Another study found an unusual brain wave in abstaining alcoholics with Korsakoff syndrome. Called the O-wave, it denotes a fundamental problem in the brain's ability to detect novel stimuli. According to Dr. Michael Eckardt, senior science adviser at NIAAA, continuing research on basic malfunctions, like inability to pay attention, could explain problems with higher thought processes, like memory.

"Dr. Marlene Oscar-Berman, professor of psychiatry and neurology at the Boston University School of Medicine, notes that WKS, a relatively rare disorder, is more a tantalizing model than an explanation for all of the cognitive impairments observed in alcoholics. Scientists are exploring other means by which the specific effects of alcohol can be targeted and, ideally, reversed.

"Evidence is mounting that some alcoholics without alcoholic dementia or Korsakoff syndrome have a distinct set of mental impairments. These include difficulty in learning new information, adapting to changing sets of rules, and thinking abstractly (e.g., determining the rules or principles behind new information and situations). In terms of breaking away from alcohol addiction, these impairments may hinder accepting the existence of the drinking problem, realizing that life must now be lived differently, and avoiding people or situations that may trigger the urge for a drink. An alcoholic's inability to change living and drinking patterns is often interpreted as denial or weakness. But it may result in part from subtle, yet specific, damage to the brain.

"These mental impairments show considerable improvement beginning two to three weeks after the last drink, particularly in those under 40. One approach to boost this recovery—particularly those mental skills crucial to staying sober—is known as 'cognitive rehabilitation therapy.' It may be that when patients who have stopped drinking practice repetitive mental tasks that reinforce new ways of thinking, they can recover their mental skills even faster.

"Recovery of these mental abilities parallels changes observed in recent brain-imaging studies. Some alcoholics have a shrinkage in the cortex (the outer, layered part of the brain, which plays a vital role in higher mental functioning). In several studies, patients received MRI scans on entering treatment and again up to one year later. Strikingly, after even three weeks' abstinence from alcohol, the cortex began to expand again; after six to 12 months of abstinence, it appeared almost normal.

"The reason for this recovery is not known, but it may be that the brain cells are simply rehydrating themselves, like sponges. In any event, alcohol-induced structural changes and cognitive impairments can often be reversed by abstaining from drinking.

"The first and most important treatment is to stop drinking alcohol. Alcoholics with Korsakoff syndrome, alcohol dementia, or other alcohol-related cognitive problems will grow steadily worse if the patient continues to drink. Quitting drinking can halt alcohol's terrible effects, as long as another damaging process is not going on at the same time. In addition, research into alcohol and the brain is raising hopes that the mind damaged by alcohol can be reclaimed."

Chapter 14

Other Less Common Dementias

Binswanger's Disease

Description

Binswanger's disease is an extremely rare form of dementia characterized by cerebrovascular lesions in the deep white-matter of the brain, loss of memory and cognition, and mood changes. Patients usually show signs of abnormal blood pressure, stroke, blood abnormalities, disease of the large blood vessels in the neck, and disease of the heart valves. Other prominent features of the disease include urinary incontinence, difficulty walking, parkinsonian-like tremors, and depression. These symptoms, which tend to begin after the age of 60, are not always present in all patients and may sometimes appear only as a passing phase. Seizures may also be present.

Treatment

There is no specific course of treatment for Binswanger's disease. Treatment is symptomatic, often involving the use of medications to control high blood pressure, depression, heart arrhythmias and low blood pressure.

National Institute of Neurological Disorders and Stroke (NINDS), "Binswanger's Disease," April 1998; "Metachromatic Leukodystrophy," October 1997; "Pick's disease," July 1997; and "Corticobasal Degeneration," October 1997.

Prognosis

Binswanger's disease is a slowly progressive condition for which there is no cure. The disorder is often marked by strokes and partial recovery. Patients with this disorder usually die within 5 years after its onset.

Research

The NINDS conducts and supports a wide range of research on dementing disorders, including dementias of old age such as Binswanger's disease. The goals of this research are to improve the diagnosis of dementias and to find ways to treat and prevent them. The National Institute on Aging and the National Institute of Mental Health also support research related to the dementias.

These articles, available from a medical library, may provide more in-depth information on Binswanger's disease:

Babikian, V, and Ropper, A. "Binswanger's disease: A review." *Stroke*, 18:1; 2-12 (January-February 1987).

Roman, G. "Senile dementia of the Binswanger type." *Journal of the American Medical Association*, 258:13; 1782-1788 (October 1987).

Metachromatic Leukodystrophy

Description

Metachromatic leukodystrophy (MLD) is a genetic disorder caused by a deficiency of the enzyme ***arylsulfatase A***. It is one of a group of genetic disorders called the ***leukodystrophies*** that affect growth of the myelin sheath, the fatty covering—which acts as an insulator—on nerve fibers in the brain. There are three forms of MLD: late infantile, juvenile, and adult. In the ***late infantile*** form, which is the most common, onset of symptoms begins between ages 6 months and 2 years. The infant is usually normal at birth, but eventually loses previously gained abilities. Symptoms include hypotonia (low muscle tone), speech abnormalities, loss of mental abilities, blindness, rigidity (uncontrolled muscle tightness), convulsions, impaired swallowing, paralysis, and dementia. Symptoms of the ***juvenile*** form begin between ages 4 and 14, and include impaired school performance, mental deterioration, ataxia, seizures, and dementia. In the ***adult*** form, symptoms, which begin after age 16, may include impaired concentration, depression, psychiatric disturbances, ataxia, tremor, and dementia. Seizures may occur in the adult form, but are less common than in the other forms. In all three forms mental deterioration is usually the first sign.

Treatment

There is no cure for MLD. Bone marrow transplantation may delay progression of the disease in some cases. Other treatment is symptomatic and supportive.

Prognosis

The prognosis for MLD is poor. Death generally occurs within 6 to 14 years after onset of symptoms. In the infantile form death may occur between 3 and 6 years after onset.

Research

The NINDS supports research on genetic disorders including leukodystrophies such as MLD. The goals of this research are to increase scientific understanding of these disorders, and to find ways to prevent, treat, and cure them.

These articles, available from a medical library, are sources of in-depth information on MLD:

Baumann, N, et al. "Adult Forms of Metachromatic Leukodystrophy: Clinical and Biochemical Approach." *Developmental Neuroscience*, 13; 211-215 (1991).

Bradley, W, et al. (eds). *Neurology in Clinical Practice: The Neurological Disorders*, vol. II, 2nd edition, Butterworth-Heinemann, Boston, pp. 1555-1556, 1910 (1996).

Krivitt, W, et al. "Treatment of Late Infantile Metachromatic Leukodystrophy by Bone Marrow Transplantation." *The New England Journal of Medicine*, 322:1; 28-32 (January 4, 1990).

Menkes, J. "The Leukodystrophies." *The New England Journal of Medicine*, 322:1; 54-55 (January 4, 1990).

Rowland, L (ed). *Merritt's Textbook of Neurology*, 9th edition, Williams & Wilkins, Baltimore, pp. 558-560 (1995).

Wenger, D. "Research Update on Lysosomal Disorders with Special Emphasis on Metachromatic Leukodystrophy and Krabbe Disease." *APMIS*, Suppl 40:101; 81-87 (1993).

Wyngaarden, J, et al. (eds). *Cecil Textbook of Medicine*, 19th edition, W.B. Saunders Co., Philadelphia, pp. 2200-2201 (1992).

Pick's Disease

Description

Pick's disease is a form of dementia characterized by a slowly progressive deterioration of social skills and changes in personality leading to impairment of intellect, memory, and language. Although the disease varies greatly in the way it affects individuals, there is a common core of symptoms among patients which may be present at different stages of the disease. These symptoms include loss of memory, lack of spontaneity, difficulty in thinking or concentrating, and disturbances of speech. Other symptoms include gradual emotional dullness, loss of moral judgment, and progressive dementia. Although the disease usually affects individuals between the ages of 40 and 60, the age of onset may range from 20 to 80. The cause of the disease is unknown.

Treatment

There is no cure or specific treatment for Pick's disease. Its progression cannot be slowed. However, some of the symptoms of the disease may be treated effectively.

Prognosis

The course of Pick's disease is an inevitable progressive deterioration. The length of progression varies, ranging from less than 2 years in some to more than 10 years in others. Death is usually caused by infection.

Research

The NINDS conducts and supports research to learn more about the cause, prevention, and treatment of dementing disorders such as Pick's disease. NINDS investigators are currently conducting a pathogenetic study of Pick's disease patients. The study includes cerebral imaging with positron emission tomography, and experimental therapeutic interventions. The National Institute on Aging also conducts research relevant to Pick's disease.

These articles, available from a medical library, may provide more in-depth information on Pick's disease:

Farrer, L, Abraham, C, Volicer, L, Foley, E, Kowall, N, McKee, A, and Wells, J. "Allele epsilon 4 of apolipoprotein E shows a dose effect on age at onset of Pick disease." *Experimental Neurology*, 136:2; 162-170 (December 1995).

Feany, M, Mattiace, L, and Dickson, D. "Neuropathologic overlap of progressive supranuclear palsy, Pick's disease, and corticobasal degeneration." *Journal of Neuropathology and Experimental Neurology*, 55:1; 53-67 (January 1996).

Hof, P, Bouras, C, Perl, D, and Morrison, J. "Quantitative analysis of Pick's disease cases: cortical distribution of Pick bodies and coexistence with Alzheimer's disease." *Acta Neuropathology*, 87:2; 115-124 (1994).

Terry, RD, Katzman, R, and Bick, KL. (eds). *Alzheimer's Disease.* Raven Press, New York (1994).

Corticobasal Degeneration

Description

Corticobasal degeneration is a progressive neurological disorder characterized by nerve cell loss and atrophy (shrinkage) of multiple areas of the brain including the **cerebral cortex** and the **basal ganglia**. Corticobasal degeneration progresses gradually. Initial symptoms, which typically begin at or around age 60, may first appear on one side of the body (unilateral), but eventually affect both sides as the disease progresses. Symptoms include signs of parkinsonism such as poor coordination, akinesia (an absence of movements), rigidity (a resistance to imposed movement), and disequilibrium (impaired balance); and limb dystonia (abnormal muscle postures). Other symptoms such as cognitive and visual-spatial impairments, apraxia (loss of the ability to make familiar, purposeful movements), hesitant and halting speech, myoclonus, and dysphagia (difficulty swallowing) may also occur. The patient is unable to walk. Symptoms vary among patients.

Treatment

There is no treatment available to slow the course of corticobasal degeneration, and the symptoms of the disease are generally resistant to therapy. Antiparkinsonian drugs do not produce any significant or sustained improvement. Clonazepam may help the myoclonus. Occupational, physical, and speech therapy may help in managing disability.

Prognosis

The course of corticobasal degeneration is one of inexorable progression until death, usually 6 to 8 years after diagnosis. Death is generally caused by pneumonia or other complications of severe debility such as sepsis or pulmonary embolism.

Research

The NINDS supports and conducts research studies on degenerative disorders such as corticobasal degeneration. The goals of these studies are to increase scientific understanding of these disorders and to find ways to prevent, treat, and cure them.

These articles, available from a medical library, are sources of in-depth information on corticobasal degeneration:

Bradley, W, et al. (eds). *Neurology in Clinical Practice: Principles of Diagnosis and Management*, vol. II, Butterworth-Heinemann, Boston, p. 1596 (1991).

Fahn, S. "Parkinson's Disease and Other Basal Ganglion Disorders." In *Diseases of the Nervous System: Clinical Neurobiology*, W.B. Saunders Co., Philadelphia, pp. 1144-1158 (1992).

Joynt, R (ed). *Clinical Neurology*, vol. 3, J.B. Lippincott Co., Philadelphia, p. 84 (1992).

Riley, D, and Lang, A. "Cortical-Basal Ganglionic Degeneration." In *Current Neurology*, vol. 12, Mosby-Year Book Inc., pp. 155-171 (1992).

Rinne, J, et al. "Corticobasal Degeneration: A Clinical Study of 36 Cases." *Brain*, 117 (Pt. 5); 1183-1196 (October 1994).

Other Resources

Further information on dementing disorders may be obtained from the organizations listed in *Part V: Additional Help and Information*.

Chapter 15

Delirium in the Elderly Patient

Diagnosing Delirium

Delirium is characterized by disorganized thinking and difficulty in focusing attention. This confusion occurs suddenly, with widely fluctuating symptoms. General medical conditions, substance intoxication, and substance withdrawal are common causal factors.

The frequent misdiagnosis of delirium, often as depression or dementia, and subsequent failure to recognize the etiology of delirium result in high morbidity and mortality. A high index of suspicion and early diagnosis are important to avert the complications associated with delirium.

Epidemiology and Risk Factors

Delirium occurs in approximately 10 percent of all hospitalized patients.[2] Elderly patients are especially susceptible to this disorder, with delirium rates ranging from 22 to 38 percent in hospitalized elderly patients.[3-9] Delirium rates increase significantly as the number of underlying risk factors increases.[3-6,8,10-13]

Any condition that compromises brain function can cause delirium. Anticholinergic medications, which block cholinergic transmitters in the brain, are thought to be the primary drug-related causes of delirium.[14,15]

"Delirium in the Elderly Patient," by Michael H. Bross and Nancy O. Tatum, *American Family Physician*, November 1, 1994 v50 n6 p1325(8) © 1994 American Academy of Family Physicians; reprinted with permission.

Fourteen of the 25 drugs most commonly prescribed for the elderly, including furosemide (Lasix), digoxin (Lanoxin), theophylline, and nifedipine (Adalat, Procardia), have detectable anticholinergic effects.[15] Alcohol withdrawal or sedative-hypnotic drug withdrawal may underlie delirium.

Infections, especially pyelonephritis and pneumonia, commonly cause delirium in the elderly, even in the absence of sepsis.[4,6] Fluid and electrolyte disturbances and major organ system failure often induce delirium.[3,6] Surgery or trauma can induce delirium as a result of hypovolemia, pain, analgesia, and anesthesia. For example, a 61 percent incidence of delirium has been reported among elderly patients undergoing surgery for hip fracture.[11] Hospitalization itself is stressful and can contribute to the development of delirium. When several potential etiologies coexist, the delirium rate is very high.

Clinical Presentation

Three clinical presentations of delirium have been described: hyperactive, hypoactive, and mixed.[16] Hyperactive patients show increased psychomotor activity, such as rapid speech, irritability, and restlessness. Hypoactive patients present with lethargy, slowed speech, decreased alertness, and apathy. Patients with hypoactive delirium are not disruptive to others and are often overlooked or misdiagnosed as being depressed. Patients with mixed delirium shift between hyperactive and hypoactive states.

A recent study of delirium subtypes found that 52 percent were mixed, 19 percent were hypoactive, 15 percent were hyperactive and 14 percent were neither (patients classified as "neither" did not demonstrate a cluster of hyperactive or hypoactive symptoms).[9] The patient in the following illustrative case exhibited a combination of hypoactive and hyperactive symptoms of delirium.

Illustrative Case

A 65-year-old woman was admitted to a hospital because of pneumonia. This was her third admission for pneumonia in the past year; she had a long history of chronic obstructive pulmonary disease. On admission, she was moderately short of breath; she was drowsy but cooperative when aroused.

During the second night in the hospital, she suddenly panicked. She pointed at the curtain and shouted that someone was coming in the window. She later mistook an aide for her husband, who had died

160

more than 30 years before. When her son tried to comfort her, she did not recognize him. After consultation, sedating medications were begun. The patient's condition worsened, with persistent daytime somnolence and nighttime agitation.

Her primary care physician began to suspect delirium. Aggressive pulmonary treatments, low-flow oxygen, and discontinuance of the sedating medications corrected her hypoxemia. As her medical condition stabilized, the delirium cleared completely.

Diagnostic Evaluation

History

The history is extremely helpful in establishing a diagnosis of delirium and finding the cause. The clinician should question family members and nursing staff regarding the patient's baseline level of function and any recent mental changes. When did the confusion begin? Does the condition change over a 24-hour period? Is there a change in the patient's sleep pattern? What specific thought problems have been noticed? Is there a history of mental illness or similar thought disturbance?

Since delirium has an organic etiology, the current history is also essential for identifying acute organic illness. New-onset urinary incontinence often occurs with delirium.[3,11] Knowing the patient's past medical history, medications and social habits, and reviewing systems helps the physician identify possible causes of delirium.

Physical Examination

The hallmark of delirium is the abnormal mental status examination. Physicians correctly diagnose delirium in fewer than 20 percent of cases.[3,17] Mental status screening tests are helpful in identifying cognitive defects and should be performed routinely in elderly patients.[4,6,14,18,19]

The Mini-Mental State examination[20] is most favored as a helpful screening test.[14,17,21,22] A score of 23 or less indicates cognitive disturbance.[23] Consideration should be given to advanced age and low education level in some patients with a low score.[24] If drawing is difficult for an elderly patient, the Short Portable Mental Status Questionnaire is appropriate.[18]

Further investigation of mental status helps to confirm suspected delirium. The letter recognition test may highlight attention problems:

161

after instructing the patient to raise his or her hand only when the letter "a" is heard, the examiner then begins saying letters from the alphabet randomly. Delirious patients have inconsistent responses.

Delirious speech is often rambling, with poorly connected thoughts, and may reveal misperceptions (i.e., distortions, illusions, and hallucinations). Speech and overall activity level may either be accelerated or slowed.

A comprehensive physical examination will usually identify the likely causes of delirium. Signs of infection include hypothermia and hyperthermia. Careful examination of the chest and abdomen may uncover infectious etiologies. Tachycardia may be a sign of infection, alcohol withdrawal, or congestive heart failure. Other signs of congestive heart failure include a third heart sound, basilar rales, and dependent edema. Suprapubic and rectal examination may reveal urinary retention and fecal impaction.

A neurologic examination might uncover the focal deficits of a cerebrovascular injury. Signs of meningitis, subarachnoid hemorrhage, subdural hemorrhage, and normal-pressure hydrocephalus may also be found. Tremor and restlessness suggest alcohol withdrawal. Asterixis and myoclonus are suggestive of a metabolic encephalopathy, such as that associated with liver failure.

Diagnostic Tests

The choice of diagnostic tests is based on the history and physical findings.[22,25] Baseline laboratory studies include a complete blood count, urinalysis, and determination of electrolyte, calcium, blood urea nitrogen, creatinine, glucose, albumin, and liver enzyme levels. Electrocardiography and chest radiographs are also indicated.

Thyroid function tests, determination of vitamin B$_{12}$ and folic acid levels, and screening for syphilis are warranted in patients with chronic mental status changes. To detect toxic ingestions, it is helpful to obtain drug and heavy-metal screens and determine drug levels. When central nervous system trauma or vascular injury is suspected, computed tomographic scanning or magnetic resonance imaging is beneficial. Signs of infection call for appropriate culture, and lumbar puncture is indicated if meningitis is a diagnostic consideration. If cardiac or pulmonary disease is a possibility, determination of cardiac isoenzymes and arterial blood gases should be performed.

When it is difficult to differentiate delirium from an acute psychotic state, electroencephalography is helpful. The electroencephalogram reveals diffuse slowing in most cases of delirium, fast activity in cases of delirium related to drug withdrawal and normal patterns in patients with acute functional psychosis.[14]

Differential Diagnosis

The clinical history, physical examination and laboratory studies usually differentiate delirium from other causes of confusion.[16] The chronic confusion of dementia occurs gradually, persists for greater than one month and is usually irreversible. Although both patients with dementia and those with delirium have cognitive impairment, most demented patients are alert and able to maintain attention. Sudden deterioration of a patient with dementia suggests that delirium has become superimposed.

Depression with apathy, slowed speech and mood disturbance may mimic hypoactive delirium. Acute functional psychosis can also resemble delirium. Functional psychosis usually has its onset before age 40, and most elderly patients with functional psychosis have a history of psychiatric illness. In patients with functional psychosis, hallucinations tend to be auditory and delusions are more elaborate than those associated with delirium. Consultation with a psychiatrist or a neurologist may be necessary in difficult cases.

Management

Effective management of delirium requires prompt treatment of the underlying conditions and creation of a maximally supportive environment. In some cases, control of agitation is necessary. Attention should be paid to prevention of the complications of associated immobility.

Immediate medical treatment is imperative because further deterioration may occur rapidly. Medications should be reduced to the minimum. Adequate nutrition and hydration are essential, since many delirious patients present in a malnourished state, with a low serum albumin level.[12] When oral feeding is not tolerated, enteral tube feeding or parenteral hyperalimentation may be necessary. Treatment of the underlying pathology typically results in rapid improvement of the delirium.[6]

The importance of a supportive environment cannot be overemphasized in the care of the delirious patient. The presence of family members or friends provides needed reassurance, relieves anxiety, and helps prevent disorientation. Familiar items from home, such as clothing, photographs, and a favorite pillow, are comforting. Sensory losses that contribute to misperceptions can be minimized by having the patient use eye-glasses and hearing aids. A night light and minimal noise can provide a soothing environment for sleep. Sleep should not be interrupted for checking of vital signs or medication administration unless absolutely necessary.

Placing a delirious patient near the nursing station makes it easier to monitor frequently for changes in the patient's behavior. Specific nursing interventions, such as techniques to reinforce the patient's orientation and increase continuity of care, have been shown to decrease the incidence of delirium after hip fracture.[13] Having someone stay with the patient allows constant supervision to prevent injury and provides respite for family members.

Significant agitation may occur in spite of supportive efforts. Controlling the agitated patient may require medical and physical restraints in some cases. However, restraints must not be used as a substitute for prompt medical evaluation and treatment of the underlying condition, where applicable. Inappropriate use of restraints may delay diagnosis, or increase morbidity and mortality.

For medical restraint, most clinicians favor a high-potency neuroleptic agent such as haloperidol (Haldol).[14,16,22] Haloperidol, with its low anticholinergic and hypotensive effects, is well tolerated by critically ill elderly patients.[26] An appropriate starting dose is 0.5 to 2 mg, given intramuscularly or intravenously for rapid onset of action. The dose may be doubled every 30 minutes to control severe agitation.[26] Extrapyramidal side effects (such as dystonic reactions, akathisia, and tardive dyskinesia) and neuroleptic malignant syndrome are associated with the use of neuroleptics.

If haloperidol is not effective, a short-acting benzodiazepine, such as lorazepam (Ativan), is indicated. Lorazepam can be given intramuscularly or intravenously, starting with a dose of 0.5 to 1 mg. For delirious patients suffering from alcohol or sedative withdrawal, benzodiazepines are the agents of choice. Benzodiazepines and neuroleptic agents both have the potential to cause or worsen delirium and must be used with caution.

Physical restraints are rarely indicated and can cause harm.[27] If restraints are absolutely necessary, care should be taken to restrain as few limbs as possible. Reassessment should be frequent until restraints are removed. Constant observation may be a more appropriate control measure and obviates the need for restraints.

Care must be taken to avoid the complications of immobility. Skin breakdown can be minimized by frequently turning the patient, providing appropriate bedding ,and keeping the patient's skin dry. Bowel and bladder problems, especially constipation, diarrhea, and urinary incontinence, warrant prompt attention. Pulmonary care is often necessary to avoid atelectasis and pneumonia. If the patient is able to cooperate, strengthening exercises and early ambulation help preserve function.

Prognosis

The prognosis of elderly hospitalized patients with delirium is worse than the prognosis of those without delirium.[3-8,11,12,28] Delirious patients are sicker[3,4,6,28] and have longer periods of hospitalization.[3,5,8,11,12] Hospital mortality rates are high, ranging from 6 to 35 percent.[3,4,6,7,9,12,21] After hospitalization, delirious patients show more cognitive impairment[5,7,28] and have greater rates of institutionalization.[3-5,11,28] Mortality rates after hospitalization are also high: 14 to 26 percent at six months,[3,5,9] 39 percent at two years,[28] and 66 percent at four years.[21]

Prevention

Preventing delirium in elderly patients requires addressing all the components of sound geriatric care. Community support systems, such as home health care and geriatric day care, can assist family and friends in the care of frail elderly patients. Immunizations for influenza and pneumococcal pneumonia may prevent a serious illness leading to delirium in these patients. Frequent evaluations for early treatment of medical illness can also prevent hospitalizations that contribute to delirium. If hospitalization is required, efforts can be made to ensure rapid diagnosis and treatment of medical illness. Medications known to precipitate or worsen delirium, especially anticholinergics, sedative-hypnotics, and narcotics, should be used sparingly. Stressful situations should be addressed, such as the control of pain and avoidance of unnecessary intensive care settings. Family and community support must be enlisted to help detect delirium in the early stages and quickly reorient patients. Prevention of delirium rests on the recognition of risk factors and the rapid treatment of the underlying organic causes.

References

1. American Psychiatric Association. *Diagnostic and statistical manual of mental disorders*. 4th ed. Washington, D.C.: American Psychiatric Association, 1994:129-33.

2. Brown MM, Hachinski VC. Acute confusional states and delirium. In: Wilson JD, Braunwald E, Isselbacher KJ, Petersdorf RG, Martin JB, Fauci AS, et al, eds. *Harrison's Principles of internal medicine*. 12th ed. New York: McGraw-Hill, 1991:186-8.

3. Francis J, Martin D, Kapoor WN. A prospective study of delirium in hospitalized elderly. *JAMA* 1990;263:1097-101.

4. Jitapunkul S, Pillay I, Ebrahim S. Delirium in newly admitted elderly patients: a prospective study. *Q J Med* 1992;83:307-14.

5. Levkoff SE, Evans DA, Liptzin B, Cleary PD, Lipsitz LA, Wetle TT, et al. Delirium. The occurrence and persistence of symptoms among elderly hospitalized patients. *Arch Intern Med* 1992;152:334-40.

6. Rockwood K. Acute confusion in elderly medical patients. *J Am Geriatr Soc* 1989;37:150-4.

7. Rockwood K. The occurrence and duration of symptoms in elderly patients with delirium. *J Gerontol* 1993;48:M162-6.

8. Schor JD, Levkoff SE, Lipsitz LA, Reilly CH, Cleary PD, Rowe JW, et al. Risk factors for delirium in hospitalized elderly. *JAMA* 1992;267:827-31.

9. Liptzin B, Levkoff SE. An empirical study of delirium subtypes. *Br J Psychiatry* 1992;161:843-5.

10. Williams-Russo P, Urquhart BL, Sharrock NE, Charlson ME. Post-operative delirium: predictors and prognosis in elderly orthopedic patients. *J Am Geriatr Soc* 1992;40:759-67.

11. Gustafson Y, Berggren D, Brannstrom B, Bucht G, Norberg A, Hansson LI, et al. Acute confusional states in elderly patients treated for femoral neck fracture. *J Am Geriatr Soc* 1988;36:525-30.

12. Levkoff SE, Safran C, Cleary PD, Gallop J, Phillips RS. Identification of factors associated with the diagnosis of delirium in elderly hospitalized patients. *J Am Geriatr Soc* 1988;36:1099-104.

13. Williams MA, Campbell EB, Raynor WJ, Mlynarczyk SM, Ward SE. Reducing acute confusional states in elderly patients with hip fractures. *Res Nurs Health* 1985;8:329-37.

14. Francis J. Delirium in older patients. *J Am Geriatr Soc* 1992;40:829-38.

15. Tune L, Carr S, Hoag E, Cooper T. Anticholinergic effects of drugs commonly prescribed for the elderly: potential means for assessing risk of delirium. *Am J Psychiatry* 1992;149:1393-4.

16. Lipowski ZJ. Delirium in the elderly patient. *N Engl J Med* 1989;320:578-82.

17. Johnson JC, Kerse NM, Gottlieb G, Wanich C, Sullivan E, Chen K. Prospective versus retrospective methods of identifying patients with delirium. *J Am Geriatr Soc* 1992;40:316-9.

18. Kallman H, May HJ. Mental status assessment in the elderly. *Prim Care* 1989;16:329-47.

19. Jarvik LF, Lavretsky EP, Neshkes RE. Dementia and delirium in old age. In: Brocklehurst JC, Tallis RC, Fillit HM, eds. *Textbook of geriatric medicine and gerontology*. 4th ed. New York: Churchill Livingstone, 1992:326-48.

20. Folstein MF, Folstein SE, McHugh PR. "Minimental state." A practical method for grading the cognitive state of patients for the clinician. *J Psychiatr Res* 1975;12:189-98.

21. Koponen HJ, Riekkinen PJ. A prospective study of delirium in elderly patients admitted to a psychiatric hospital. *Psychol Med* 1993;23:103-9.

22. O'Brien JG. Evaluation of acute confusion (delirium). *Prim Care* 1989;16:349-60.

23. Tombaugh TN, McIntyre NJ. The mini-mental state examination: a comprehensive review. *J Am Geriatr Soc* 1992;40:922-35.

24. Crum RM, Anthony JC, Bassett SS, Folstein MF. Population-based norms for the Mini-Mental State Examination by age and educational level. *JAMA* 1993;269:2386-91.

25. Johnson JC. Delirium in the elderly. *Emerg Med Clin North Am* 1990;8:255-65.

26. Fish DN. Treatment of delirium in the critically ill patient. *Clin Pharm* 1991;10:456-66.

27. Evans LK, Strumpf NE. Tying down the elderly. A review of the literature on physical restraint. *J Am Geriatr Soc* 1989;37:65-74.

28. Francis J, Kapoor WN. Prognosis after hospital discharge of older medical patients with delirium. *J Am Geriatr Soc* 1992;40:601-6.

— by Michael H. Bross, M.D. and Nancy O. Tatum, M.D.

Michael H. Bross, M.D. is associate professor and director of community and rural medicine, Department of Family Medicine, at the University of Mississippi Medical Center, Jackson. He graduated from the University of Oklahoma Health Sciences Center, Oklahoma City, and completed a residency in family medicine at the University of Arkansas Area Health Education Center, Pine Bluff.

Nancy O. Tatum, M.D. is assistant professor and codirector of clinical ethics, Department of Family Medicine, at the University of Mississippi Medical Center. She graduated from and completed a family medicine residency at the University of Mississippi Medical Center.

Chapter 16

Confusional States

Confusion

Confusion is prevalent in the aging population and yet it is frequently misdiagnosed and thus mismanaged. Because confusion is socially disabling and makes unusually high demands on medical, nursing, and social resources, it is important for health care providers to understand the condition. However, confusion is rarely discussed by itself; rather, it is often viewed only as a symptom of another problem, such as dementia. As Nagley and Dever (1989) point out, "While there may be a shared understanding of confusion among practitioners, a clear and concise definition of confusion for scientific study is lacking" (p. 80). Anything that interrupts or violates the homodynamic equilibrium between man, body, self, and the environment can precipitate confusion. Aged persons are particularly vulnerable to disequilibrium due to losses associated with the aging process and various sociocultural factors that enhance the perception of stress (Hall, 1986).

Wolanin and Phillips (1981) delineated five sources of confusion: 1) compromised brain support; 2) sensoriperceptual problems; 3) disruption in pattern and meaning; 4) alterations in normal physiologic states; and 5) the true dementias. These sources provided the conceptual framework for a study of the knowledge and opinions of nursing home personnel regarding reversible and irreversible types of

Excerpted from *Long-Term Care for Older Adults*, National Institute of Nursing Research (NINR), 1994.

confusion (Lincoln, 1984). Findings suggested that nursing staff were not very knowledgeable about the irreversible dementias although a positive correlation was noted between amount of formal education of the staff and knowledge of the sources of confusion. As suggested by Wolanin and Phillips (1981), a distinction should be made between confusional states with reversible and irreversible etiologies; with reversible etiologies medical and nursing interventions can often restore normal function. Although conceptually fuzzy, confusional states with reversible etiologies will here be referred to as acute confusional states, or delirium, and those with irreversible etiologies will be referred to as chronic confusional states, or dementias.

The total number of indexed publications related to confusional states in older adults grew from 87 in 1976 to over 600 less than a decade later. However, nurses have begun to study acute and chronic confusional states only recently. Although nursing studies in this area are increasing rapidly, the number of nurse-initiated research projects is still small in comparison to biomedical research efforts that focus on the causes and cures for confusion. Until recently, nursing research questions related to confusion have received significantly less attention and funding than biomedical research efforts, in spite of the tremendous need to develop knowledge about care for the millions of Americans who suffer from acute and chronic confusional disorders (Cross & Gurland, 1986), and the need to delineate effective strategies to promote quality of life for both victims and their families (Buckwalter, Abraham, & Neundorfer, 1988).

Nursing studies related to acute and chronic confusional states cover a wide range of topics with only a few reports addressing the same or similar clinical issues (Maas & Buckwalter, 1991). The high number of isolated studies prohibits an integrated review of nursing research on confusion. The notable exception is studies of caregiver stress/burden among families when persons with chronic confusional states such as Dementia of the Alzheimer's type (DAT) are cared for in the home. The interaction of cognitive function and environmental characteristics appears to be a central concept in the theoretical orientations that guide research on care of confused patients (Maas & Buckwalter, 1991). The nurse's role in management of confusional states has evolved to the point where nursing now assumes major responsibility for the assessment, diagnosis, and management of nursing problems along the continuum of care from diagnosis to death (Maas & Buckwalter, 1991). Nursing research in these areas must keep pace with the increased clinical responsibilities.

State of the Science

Acute Confusional States (Delirium)

Acute confusional states are characterized by global impairment, and most often caused by pathophysiological changes of organic etiology that can be treated and reversed. They most commonly present as a transient delirium of rapid onset. According to the *Diagnostic and Statistical Manual of Mental Disorders, Third Edition, Revised (DSMIII-R)* (American Psychiatric Association, 1987), the symptoms of delirium may fluctuate, but commonly include clouding of consciousness, disorientation, memory impairment, and at least two of the following: perceptual disturbance, incoherent speech, disrupted sleep-wakefulness cycle, or psychomotor alterations.

In older persons, delirium or acute confusional syndromes may coexist with or lead to chronic confusional states making diagnosis complex and treatment more difficult. For example, Mullally, Ronthal, Huff, and Geschwind (1989) reported case studies of acute confusional states after infarction of the right middle cerebral artery. They noted that although patient recovery was usually excellent, some patients did not improve, resulting in chronic confusional states. Koponen, Hurri, Stenback, and Riekkinen (1987) discuss the marked predisposing role of structural brain diseases (e.g., primary degenerative and multi-infarct dementias, Parkinsonism) in the development of acute confusional states in older persons. Infections, medication interactions, toxic-metabolic conditions, intracranial lesions, trauma, hypoxia or hypoglycemia secondary to metabolic, cardiovascular or endocrine disorders such as Chronic Obstructive Pulmonary Disease (COPD) or diabetes, social isolation, sensory deprivation, and stress are common causes of confusion (Zisook, 1988). Behaviors often associated with reversible confusional states include: disorientation, inattentiveness, withdrawal, belligerence, impaired communication, and wandering (Hall, 1991; Wolanin & Phillips, 1981; Zarit, 1980). Fawdry and Berry (1989) suggest that agitated and unsafe behaviors represent an attempt by the confused elderly person to maintain self-image and physical and psychological integrity.

Much of the nursing literature in this area is devoted to the management of delirium (Batt, 1989; Hahn, 1981; Weymouth, 1968), the differentiation of delirium from dementia (Gomez & Gomez, 1989), or the prediction and prevention of delirium in the hospitalized elderly (Williams, Campbell, Raynor, Musholt, Mlynarczyk, & Crane, 1985). In general, nursing interventions are designed to reestablish

171

normal physiological status, or assist elderly persons to accurately understand and interpret their environment. For example, Williams, Campbell, Raynor, Mlynarczyk, and Ward (1985) found that the most effective interventions in reducing acute confusional states in elderly patients with hip fractures included those that provided orientation and clarification, corrected sensory deficits, and increased continuity of care. Almost all nursing research related to acute confusional states has focused on patients in acute care, rather than long-term care settings (Adams & Hanson, 1978; Chisolm & Deniston, 1982; Foreman, 1986, 1989; Nagley, 1986; Neelon & Champagne, 1986; Roslaniec & Fitzpatrick, 1979; Williams et al., 1985a, Williams, et al., 1985a, b). These studies and several recent medical investigations suggest the incidence of confusion among the hospitalized elderly is quite high and of great concern in that it compromises recovery and increases morbidity and mortality (Fields, MacKenzie, Charlson, & Sax, 1986; Rockwood, 1989). For example, Foreman (1989) found that 38 percent of 71 non-surgical elderly patients experienced confusion during their hospitalization. Confused patients were hypernatremic, hypokalemic, hyperglycemic, hypotensive, had elevated blood levels of creatinine and urea nitrogen, received more medications, and had fewer interactions with significant others than non-confused subjects. Other studies suggest that the incidence of acute confusional states in elderly persons undergoing surgery is even higher, ranging from 42 percent to 61 percent (Brannstrom, Gustafson, Norberg, & Winblad, 1989; Gustafson, Berggren, Brannstrom, Bucht, Norberg, Hansson, & Winblad, 1988).

Adequate treatment of delirium presupposes that its underlying causes have been identified. It is essential that clinicians establish whether older persons patient has delirium, dementia, or both, through review of history, clinical features, and a mental-status examination (Lipowski, 1989). Because the management of associated behaviors for acute and chronic confusional states can be very different, there is a real need to conduct nursing research on the phenomenon of delirium in long-term care settings, and to investigate assessment and management strategies when the two conditions coexist in the long-term care resident.

Sundown Syndrome

Sundown syndrome is confusion that occurs or increases in the late afternoon and early evening hours (Evans, 1987). This phenomenon is similar to delirium in its symptoms of confusion, agitation, restlessness, and wandering, although delirium is typically of a short duration. Few nurse researchers have investigated sundown syndrome. Evans (1987) studied 59 demented and 30 nondemented institutionalized elderly in an effort to describe this syndrome, determine its prevalence among nursing home residents, and define related psychosocial, physiologic, and environmental factors; she developed a Confusion Inventory for this research. Results showed increased restlessness and verbal behavior around sunset was associated with greater cognitive impairment, dehydration, nighttime awakenings for care, recent admission to the facility, and residing in their present room for less than 1 month. Interestingly, 85 percent of the demented subjects showed no symptoms related to sundowning, and there was no statistically significant relationship with morale, medications, demographic variables, use of restraints, or medical disorders. There is a need for further research in this area using round-the-clock observations of sleep/wake cycles and exacting indicators of psychological, physical, and biorhythm variables. At present, it is unclear whether "sundowning" in persons with irreversible dementias is a specific type of delirium with a unique etiology. More research is needed to determine if sundown syndrome is distinguishable from other types of confusion. In addition, the effects of nursing interventions on sundown syndrome deserve attention.

Chronic Confusional States (The Irreversible Dementias)

Although there are 70 different conditions that can cause dementia in the middle and later years (Blass, 1982, Katzman, 1986), DAT is the most common, representing 60 percent of older persons who are irreversibly demented. Most nursing research devoted to chronic confusional states focuses on DAT. This progressive disorder is characterized by losses of memory, intellectual and language ability, and general competency over a period averaging 6-15 years and ending in death. Although the most commonly cited figure is that 4 percent to 7 percent of persons ages 65-75 suffer from some form of dementia (Cross & Gurland, 1986), recent epidemiological evidence from the East Boston studies of Evans and colleagues (1989) suggests that the percentage may be almost twice that high. The percentage increases dramatically to 25 percent for those over age 85. A study of older community residents of a five-county region in North Carolina has suggested that the prevalence of dementia among blacks may be distinctly greater than among whites and that black women are particularly affected. Clearly, more research on the epidemiology and impact of this disorder in ethnic populations is needed (National Institute on Aging, 1990).

The costs associated with caring for persons with chronic confusion, both monetary and human, are enormous. Estimates average $48 billion annually, and are projected to grow as the percentage of older Americans rises to 21.6 percent by the year 2040, increasing the number of cases of DAT fivefold! These sociodemographic trends alone suggest that DAT (sometimes referred to as the "disease of the century") and other chronic, irreversible dementias are important areas for nursing research (Maas & Buckwalter, 1991).

Alzheimer's Disease and Related Dementias

As noted earlier, DAT, a progressive degenerative disorder of unknown etiology, is the most common of the chronic, irreversible confusional states. The diagnosis of DAT is made by exclusion of other possible causes of dementia (McKhann, Drachman, Folstein, Katzman, Price, & Stadlan, 1984). Several other degenerative brain diseases present with behaviors similar to those found in DAT, although their etiologies are quite different. Multi-infarct dementia (MID) accounts for about 10 percent of all dementing illnesses. When infarcts occur, cognitive and functional abilities diminish in abrupt, step-like fashion. MID and DAT coexist in another 17 percent of the cases of irreversible dementia (Heston & White, 1983). Other rare conditions account for 13 percent of the dementias, including Pick's disease, Creutzfeldt-Jakob disease, Parkinson's disease, Huntington's disease, normal pressure hydrocephalus, and Acquired Immune Deficiency Syndrome (AIDS).

The onset of DAT is usually slow and gradual. A number of other cognitive, psychiatric, and physical conditions can mimic DAT. Thus, observed changes in client status must be carefully evaluated so as to avoid inappropriate diagnosis. Hall (1991) has described three types of behavior that may be present throughout the course of the disease: 1) baseline or normative behavior where the client is still cognitively and socially accessible; 2) anxious behavior, which is a response to stress; and 3) dysfunctional behavior, when excess stress is not reduced and the DAT victim cannot process the amount, complexity, or intensity of stimuli. More research is needed to validate these behaviors and to test Hall's Progressively Lowered Stress Threshold Model (Hall & Buckwalter, 1987).

Assessment Measures Used by Nurses In Research on Confusion

Relatively few systematic studies have described the signs and symptoms of acute and chronic confusional states, or distinguished among the several types of dementias and other changes that accompany the aging process (Maas & Buckwalter, 1991). Some notable exceptions include the recent work of Neelon, Champagne and colleagues at the University of North Carolina. They developed the NEECHAM Confusion Scale (Champagne, Neelon, McConnell, & Funk, 1987) to permit rapid bedside documentation of normal information processing, early subtle cues of acute confusion behavior, and acute confusion. The tool has been tested in comparison to clinical indicators of acute confusion in nursing home residents and with 158 hospitalized elderly. A NEECHAM score of 24 or below predicted confusion with a sensitivity of 0.95 and a specificity of 0.78. Thus, the NEECHAM scale promises to be a useful instrument in the prediction and monitoring of confused older persons. Booth and Whall (1987) conducted a three-phase study designed to: 1) use case histories to describe the onset and progression of DAT; 2) develop a health history profile (called the Life Factor Profile) to discriminate between DAT and other disorders; and 3) test the discriminate validity of the case history instrument. Psychiatric symptoms, especially depression, are often associated with dementing illness. Because standardized instruments designed specifically to measure depressive symptoms in the demented population are lacking, Kumar, Peterson, Kumar, and Fulk (1989) conducted a comparative study of 38 community dwelling dementia patients to assess: 1) the usefulness of existing instruments to discern psychiatric illness that could be treated; 2) the ability of the relationship between various measures of cognitive function and behavioral changes to predict the course of the psychiatric illnesses; and 3) the ability of various measures to predict institutionalization. Results indicated a high level of depression that increased over time, and contradicted the belief that depression is more common in mildly demented persons than in severely demented persons. Similar research, evaluating common psychiatric and cognitive tools, should be conducted on confused patients residing in long-term care settings.

Although assessment tools are reported in the literature that profess to assist the nurse in accurately describing the behavioral manifestations of confusion and distinguishing specific etiologies, few nursing assessment tools have been rigorously evaluated in terms of their psychometric properties and clinical usefulness. For example,

Nagley (1986) found that the Short Portable Mental Status Questionnaire, used in many studies of confusion, did not adequately capture the phenomenon of confusion. She recommended that nurses use a combination of cognitive and behavioral responses in their assessment, and that confusion is best studied through daily or continuous observation and testing of mental status. McCartney and Palmateer (1985a; 1985b) compared assessment techniques of physicians and nurses using the Cognitive Capacity Screening Examination (CCSE) in a sample of hospitalized medical-surgical patients. They found that assessments did not routinely include either formal cognitive testing or enough precise behavioral descriptions and that both physicians and nurses failed to identify a significant number of cognitively impaired elderly. Studies of this nature should be replicated with long-term care populations.

The development and testing of comprehensive functional assessment instruments that incorporate perceptual, cognitive, and environmental components have received little attention in the nursing research literature. Noting that instruments to measure activities of daily living (ADL) were developed to assess physical function and were not designed to assess cognitive dysfunctions that influence self-care abilities, Beck (1988) designed and tested a Dressing Performance Scale for use with persons with dementia. Following a task analysis of dressing behavior based on multiple observations of demented persons and caregivers, a hierarchy of types of caregiver assistance required was defined. These types of assistance include: 1) no assistance; 2) stimulus control; 3) initial verbal prompt; 4) gestures or modeling; 5) occasional physical guidance; 6) complete physical guidance; and 7) complete assistance. Beck is currently using the Dressing Performance Scale in a study funded by the Alzheimer's Disease and Related Disorders Association to teach caregivers to use behavioral strategies as interventions for the demented to carry out ADL's.

Sandman, Norberg, Adolfsson, Axelsson, and Hedly, (1986) studied five hospitalized patients in different stages of DAT to describe the behaviors of patients and nurses during morning care. All of the DAT patients were severely demented and required some assistance with morning care, defined as a procedure involving a series of actions that are combined into meaningful wholes, for example, washing, showering, combing, tooth-brushing, shaving, and dressing in a special environment. A 12-step classification was developed as a guide to understand and determine abilities essential for performance of morning care for demented patients. The study found that missing abilities could be determined, that highest level of performance varied from day to day, and that the nurse could compensate for the DAT patient's fragmented behavior. Apraxia was identified as the critical factor in morning care. Paratonia (increasing muscle tone during passive movements of different strength) was observed frequently and could be falsely interpreted as conscious resistance or refusal to participate, indicating the need for nurses to continuously assess the DAT patient's abilities and the assistance required throughout morning care.

In an experimental study to evaluate the effects of a Special Alzheimer's Care Unit (SCU) on DAT patients' functional status, Maas and Buckwalter (1986) developed and tested a Functional Abilities Checklist (FAC). The instrument was developed because existing measures did not address all of the behaviors characteristic of demented patients that influence their abilities to function in their environment. The areas of functional abilities included in the scale are: self-care abilities (7 items); inappropriate behaviors (4 items); cognitive status (6 items); mobility status (6 items); communication behaviors (3 items); and emotional status (7 items). This instrument is undergoing psychometric evaluation. Interrater reliability yielded a Pearson r = 0.92 for the total scale among registered nurse raters. Internal consistency reliability coefficients (Cronbach's Alpha) by subscale have ranged from 0.63 to 0.86. Data for the instrument have been correlated with data collected using the Geriatric Rating Scale (GRS) (Plutchik & Conte, 1972) as estimates of concurrent and construct validity. Pearson correlations were determined among the subscales of both instruments yielding statistically significant coefficients of 0.52 or greater for self-care and mobility dimensions and small or inverse correlations for inappropriate behavior, cognitive status, communication, and emotional status.

Institutional Settings

Special Alzheimer's Care Units

Although the use of specially designed environments has been recognized as a needed intervention for persons with chronic confusional states such as DAT, research to evaluate the effects on patients, families, staff caregivers, and cost has only been reported within the past 5 years. Among the proposed environmental interventions, Special Alzheimer's Care Units (SCU) have been the most popular. Nursing homes have tended to believe that SCU's are effective in the care of chronically confused patients, although most information that exists regarding cost effectiveness is anecdotal (Maas & Buckwalter, 1986).

There are only a few reports of nursing studies to evaluate the effects of SCU's and most designs have not used enough controls to rule out alternative explanations of the findings (Benson, Cameron, Humbach, Servino, & Gambert, 1987; Cleary, Clamon, Price, & Shullaw, 1988; Greene, Asp, & Crane, 1985; Hall, Kirshchling, & Todd, 1986; Matthew, Sloan, Kilby, & Flood, 1988). Also, the studies reported have examined the effects of single SCU's. Because individual SCU's vary widely in philosophy, design, staffing, admission criteria, and treatment modalities used, results from these studies are difficult to compare or integrate. Only the Maas and Buckwalter (1986) study used random assignment of DAT patients to experimental (SCU) and control (traditional nursing units) environments and pretest and posttest repeated measures to assess the effects of the SCU strategy. Matthew et al. (1988) studied 13 dementia patients in one SCU and 34 patients in two comparison settings, that is, other wards in the nursing home with the SCU and another nursing home. Data were collected from observations, existing clinical records, and clinical examinations. More SCU than comparison patients were private pay, had a specific diagnosis of DAT, had fewer additional medical diagnoses, had less frequent use of physical restraints, and had families with high satisfaction with care. There was a trend toward more SCU patients being Caucasian, receiving more psychotropic medications, having more documented injuries and falls, and developing fewer decubiti. No differences were found in cognitive or functional status between the demented SCU patients and the comparison patients. Greene et al. (1985) reported behavioral characteristics of six DAT patients before and after care on a SCU in a 180-bed nursing home. An average of 43 percent negative behaviors (e.g., hostile, agitated, incontinent, combative) were reported while the patients were living on traditional units, compared to three percent with negative behaviors while living on the SCU.

Reduced Stimulation Units

Cleary et al. (1988) reported an evaluation of the effects of a Reduced Stimulation Unit (RSU) on patients, staff, and family members in a nonprofit life-care center. A pretest-posttest design with multiple measures was used, with pretest measures obtained in the three months prior to the opening of the unit and posttest measures obtained in the three months following the opening of the unit. All patients transferred to the RSU had been cared for previously on the same traditional nursing care unit. Patients showed a statistically significant improvement in performance of ADL's, but no significant improvement in emotional and mental characteristics. There was a statistically significant increase in patients' average weight, a significant reduction in use of physical restraints, no significant change in sleep patterns, and no differences in the levels of tranquilizing medications. There was significant improvement in family member satisfaction with care, although family satisfaction was already quite high prior to opening of the RSU. Neither staff knowledge nor satisfaction changed significantly.

Low Stimulus Units

Hall et al. (1986) studied 12 DAT patients after they were moved to a Low Stimulus Unit (LSU) in an 89-bed nursing home. The DAT patients were followed for three months post transfer to the LSU and the following changes were observed: 1) interaction and social support increased among the DAT patients; 2) socialization at mealtime increased; 3) either weight increased or weight loss decreased for all but one patient; 4) prescription of tranquilizers decreased; 5) all patients slept at night without sedation; 6) PRN sedation decreased; and 7) agitation, combative behavior, and wandering episodes decreased.

References

Adams, M., & Hanson, R. (1978). The confused patient: Psychological responses in critical care units. *American Journal of Nursing*, 9, 1504-1520.

American Psychiatric Association: *Diagnostic and Statistical Manual of Mental Disorders-Revised (1987)*. Washington, D.C., pp.100-103.

Batt, L.J. (1989). Managing delirium. *Journal of Psychosocial Nursing*, 27(5), 22-25.

Beck, C. (1988). Measurement of dressing performance in persons with dementia. *The American Journal of Alzheimer's Care and Related Disorders & Research*, May/June, 21-25.

Benson, D.M., Cameron, E., Humbach, E., Servino, L., & Gambert, S. (1987). Establishment and impact of a dementia unit within the nursing home. *Journal of the American Geriatrics Society*, 35, 319-323.

Blass, J.P. (1982). Dementia. *Medical Clinics of North America*, 66, 1143-1160.

Booth, D., & Whall, A. (1987). Understanding progressive dementia: Making a case for the case study. In H.J. Altman (Ed.) *Alzheimer's Disease: Problems, Prospects and Perspectives* (pp. 209-212). (Proceedings of the National Conference on Alzheimer's Disease and Dementia, April 1986), New York: Plenum Press.

Brannstrom, B., Gustafson, Y., Norberg, A., & Winblad, B. (1989). Problems of basic nursing care in acutely confused and non-confused hip fracture patients. *Scandinavian Journal of Caring Sciences*, 3(1), 27-34.

Buckwalter, K.C. (1989). Applied services research: Clinical issues and directions. E. Light and B. Lebowitz (Eds.). *Alzheimer's disease treatment and family stress: Directions for research*, (pp. 434-458). Washington, D.C: U.S. Department of Health and Human Services.

Champagne, M.T., Neelon, V.J., McConnell, E., & Funk, S.G. (1987). The NEECHAM Confusional Scale: Assessing acute confusion in the hospitalized and nursing home elderly. *The Gerontologist*, 27, 4A (Abstract).

Chisholm, S., & Deniston, O. (1982). Prevalence of confusion in elderly hospitalized patients. *Journal of Gerontological Nursing*, 8, 87-96.

Cleary, T.A., Clamon, C., Price, M., & Shullaw, G. (1988). A reduced stimulus unit: effects on patients with Alzheimer's disease and related disorders. *The Gerontologist*, 28(4), 511-514.

Cross, P.S., & Gurland, B.J. (1986). *The epidemiology of dementing disorders*. Contract report prepared for the Office of Technology Assessment, U.S. Congress.

Evans, D.A., Funkenstein, H.H., Albert, M.S., Scherr, P.A., Cook, N.R., Chown, M.J., Hebert, L.E., Hennekens, C.H., & Taylor, J.O. (1989). Prevalence of Alzheimer's disease in a community population of older persons. *Journal of the American Medical Association*, 262(18), 2551-2557.

Fawdry, K., & Berry, M.L. (1989). Fear of senility: the nurse's role in managing reversible confusion. *Journal of Gerontological Nursing*, 15(4), 17-21.

Fields, S.D., MacKenzie, C. R., Charlson, M.E., & Sax, F. L. (1986). Cognitive impairment: Can it predict the course of hospitalized patients? *Journal of the American Geriatrics Society*, 34, 579-585.

Foreman, M. (1986). Acute confusional states in the hospitalized elderly: A research dilemma. *Nursing Research*, 35(1), 34-37.

Foreman, M.D. (1989). Confusion in the hospitalized elderly: Incidence, onset, and associated factors. *Research in Nursing and Health*, 12, 21-29.

Gomez, G., & Gomez, E. (1989). Dementia? Or Delirium? *Geriatric Nursing*, 10(3), 141-142.

Greene, J., Asp, J., & Crane, N. (1985). Specialized management of a Alzheimer's patient: does it make a difference? A preliminary progress report. *Journal of the Tennessee Medical Association*, 78(9), 58-63.

Gustafson, Y., Berggren, D., Brannstrom, B., Bucht, G., Norberg, A., Hansson, L, & Winblad, B. (1988). Acute confusional states in elderly patients treated for femoral neck fractures. *Journal of the American Geriatrics Society*, 36(6), 525-30.

Hahn, K. (1981). Using 24 hour reality orientation. *Journal of Gerontological Nursing*, 6(3), 130-135.

Hall, G.R., Kirschling, M., & Todd, S. (1986). Sheltered freedom: The creation of an Alzheimer's unit in an intermediate care facility. *Geriatric Nursing*, 7, 132-136.

Hall, G., & Buckwalter, K. (1987). Progressively lowered stress threshold: a conceptual model for care of adults with Alzheimer's Disease. *Archives of Psychiatric Nursing*, 1(6), 309-406.

Hall, G. (1991). Altered thought processes: Dementia. In M. Maas, K. Buckwalter, & M. Hardy (Eds). *Nursing diagnoses and interventions for the elderly*, (pp. 322-347). Menlo Park, CA: Addison Wesley.

Heston, L., & White, J. (1983). *Dementia: A practical guide to Alzheimer's disease and related illnesses*. New York: Freeman & Co.

Katzman, R. (1986). Alzheimer's Disease. *New England Journal of Medicine*, 314, 964-973.

Koponen, H., Hurri, L. Stenback, U., & Riekkinen, P.J. (1987). Acute confusional states in older persons: A radiologic evaluation. *Acta Psychiatrica Scandinavica*, 76(6), 726-731.

Kumar, V., Peterson, K., Kumar, N., & Fulk, L. (1989). Measuring cognitive and behavior changes in community dwelling Alzheimer's disease patients. *The American Journal of Alzheimer's Care and Related Disorders & Research*, Jan/Feb., 13-18.

Lincoln, R. (1984). What do nurses know about confusion in the aged? *Journal of Gerontological Nursing*, 10(8), 26-29.

Lipowski, Z.J. (1989) Delirium in older persons patient. *The New England Journal of Medicine*, 320(9), 578-582.

Maas, M., & Buckwalter, K.C. (1986). Evaluation of a special Alzheimer's unit. Unpublished manuscript, University of Iowa, Iowa City, IA.

Maas, M., & Buckwalter, K.C. (1991). Alzheimer's Disease. In J.J. Fitzpatrick, R.L. Taunton & A.K. Jacox, (Eds.). *Annual Review of Nursing Research*, (pp. 19-55). New York: Springer Publishing Co.

Matthew, L., Sloan, P., Kilby, M., & Flood, R. (1988). What's different about a special care unit for dementia patients: a comparative study and research. *The American Journal of Alzheimer's Care and Related Disorders*, March/April, 16-23.

McCartney, J.R., & Palmateer, L.M. (1985a). Do nurses know when patients have cognitive deficits? *Journal of Gerontological Nursing*, 11(2), 6-16.

McCartney, J.R., & Palmateer, L.M. (1985b). Assessment of cognitive deficit in geriatric patients. *Journal of the American Geriatric Society*, 33(7), 467-471.

McKhann, G., Drachman, D., Folstein, M., Katzman, R., Price, D., & Stadlan, E. (1984). Clinical diagnosis of Alzheimer's disease: Report of the NINCDS-ADRDA Work Group under the auspices of Department of Health and Human Services Task Force on Alzheimer's Disease. *Neurology*, 34, 939-944.

Mullally, W.J., Ronthal, M. Huff, K., & Geschwind, N. (1989). Chronic confusional state. *New Jersey Medicine*, 86(7), 541-544.

Nagley, S.J. (1986). Predicting and preventing confusion in your patients. *Journal of Gerontological Nursing*, 12(3), 27-31.

Nagley, S.J., & Dever, A. (1989). What we know about treating confusion. *Journal of Applied Nursing Research*, 1(2), 80-83.

Neelon, V.J., & Champagne, M.T. (1986). Acute confusion in hospitalized elderly: Patterns and early diagnosis. *Journal of Gerontological Nursing*, 8, 396-401.

National Institute of Aging (1990). *Progress Report on Alzheimer's Disease*. Washington, DC: U.S. Department of Health and Human Services.

Plutchik, R., & Conte, H. (1972). Change in social and physical functioning of geriatric patients over a one year period. *The Gerontologist*, 12(2), 181-184.

Roslaniec, A., & Fitzpatrick, J.J. (1979). Changes in mental status in older adults with four days hospitalization. *Research in Nursing and Health*, 2, 117-189.

Sandman, P.O., Norberg, A., Adolfsson, R., Axelsson, K., & Hedly, V. (1986). Morning care of patients with Alzheimer-type dementia: A theoretical model based on direct observations. *Journal of Advanced Nursing*, 11, 369-378.

Weymouth, L.T. (1968). Nursing care of the so-called confused patient. *Nursing Clinics of North America*, 3, 709-715.

Williams, M., Campbell, E., Raynor, W., Musholt, M., Mlynarczyk, S., & Crane, R. (1985). Predictors of acute confusional states in hospitalized elderly patients. *Research in Nursing and Health*, 8, 31-40.

Williams, M., Campbell, E. Raynor, W., Mlynarczyk, S., & Ward, S.E. (1985). Reducing acute confusional states in elderly patients with hip fractures. *Research in Nursing and Health*, 8, 329-337.

Wolanin, M., & Phillips, L. (1981). *Confusion: Prevention and care*. St. Louis: CV Mosby Co.

Zarit, S. (1980). *Aging and Mental Disorders: Psychological Approaches to Assessment and Treatment*. New York: The Free Press.

Zisook, S. (1988) Delirium. *Psychiatric Medicine*, 6,(4), 8-22.

Part Three

Prevention and Treatment Research

Chapter 17

Alzheimer's Disease: The Search for Causes

The brain has hundreds of billions of neurons, any one of which can have thousands, even hundreds of thousands, of connections with other neurons. Within and among their extensive branches travel dozens of chemical messengers—neurotransmitters, hormones, growth factors, and more—linking each neuron with others in a vast communications network.

Somewhere in this complex signaling system lies the cause of Alzheimer's disease. In the past two decades, neuroscientists have combed through it in search of defects that might explain what goes wrong in this disease. One of their earliest findings came from studies of neurotransmitters, the chemicals that relay messages between neurons.

Neurotransmitters

Neurotransmitters reside in tiny sacs at the ends of axons, the long tube-like extensions of neurons. Released when electrical impulses pass along the axon, the chemicals cross a minute space called the synapse and bind to a molecule (a receptor) sitting in the membrane of the next neuron. The neurotransmitters then either break down or pass back into the first neuron, while other substances inside the second neuron take up and relay the message.

In the mid 1970's, scientists discovered that levels of a neurotransmitter called acetylcholine fell sharply in people with Alzheimer's

Excerpted from "*Alzheimer's Disease: Unraveling the Mystery*," National Institute an Aging, NIH Pub. No. 96-3782, October 1996.

187

disease. The discovery was intriguing for several reasons. Acetylcholine is a critical neurotransmitter in the process of forming memories. Moreover, it is the neurotransmitter used commonly by neurons in the hippocampus and cerebral cortex—regions devastated by Alzheimer's disease.

Since that early discovery, which was one of the first to link Alzheimer's disease with biochemical changes in the brain, acetylcholine has been the focus of hundreds of studies. Scientists have found that its levels fall somewhat in normal aging but drop by about 90 percent in people with Alzheimer's disease. They have turned up evidence linking this decline to memory impairment. And they have looked for ways to boost its levels as a possible treatment for Alzheimer's disease.

Other neurotransmitters have also been implicated in Alzheimer's disease. For example, serotonin, somatostatin, and noradrenaline levels are lower than normal in some Alzheimer's patients, and deficits in these substances may contribute to sensory disturbances, aggressive behavior, and neuron death. Most neurotransmitter research, however, continues to focus on acetylcholine because of its steep decline in Alzheimer's disease and its close ties to memory formation and reasoning.

On the Other Side of the Synapse

Once the message carried by a neurotransmitter has crossed the synapse it passes into another territory, where neuroscientists are beginning to find more clues to Alzheimer's disease. The gateways to this new territory are the receptors, coil-shaped proteins embedded in neuron membranes. They interest Alzheimer's researchers for two reasons.

First, these molecules have chemical bonds with molecules of fat, called phospholipids, that lie next to them in the membrane. Several studies have detected phospholipid abnormalities in neurons affected by Alzheimer's disease. These abnormalities might change the behavior of neighboring receptors and garble the message as it passes from neuron to neuron.

Second, researchers have uncovered several types of receptors for acetylcholine and are now exploring their different effects on message transmission. It may be that the shapes and actions of the receptors themselves, independent of their neighboring phospholipids, play a role in Alzheimer's.

188

But the receiver is just the starting point of the cell's communications system. When a neurotransmitter binds to a receptor, it triggers a cascade of biochemical interactions that relay the message to the neuron's nucleus, where it activates certain genes, or to the end of the axon, where it passes to other cells.

This messaging system involves a number of proteins, and abnormalities in these proteins or dysfunction at the relay points could block or garble the message. So could other events and processes in the cell, such as problems with the system that turns food into energy (metabolism) or the mechanisms that keep calcium levels in balance.

Drug therapies aimed at these various postsynaptic events are now being explored, although most are still in the very earliest phases of testing. Two of them, vitamin E and deprenyl, are currently in clinical trials (studies of people).

The Proteins

Beta Amyloid

When Alois Alzheimer observed the plaques now known as a hallmark of this disease, he could say little about them. No one knows still what role they play in the disease process, but scientists have learned that plaques are composed of a protein fragment called beta amyloid mixed with other proteins. Beta amyloid is a string of 40 or so amino acids snipped from a larger protein called amyloid precursor protein or APP.

Scientists also know something about how beta amyloid is formed. Its parent protein, APP, protrudes through the neuron membrane, part inside and part outside the cell. There only for a moment, it is continually replaced by new APP molecules manufactured in the cell. While it is embedded in the membrane, enzymes called proteases snip or cleave it in two, creating the beta amyloid fragment.

What happens to the beta amyloid segment once it separates from APP is less clear. A number of studies have centered on how beta amyloid is processed, searching for abnormalities that could explain what goes wrong. Others are seeking clues in the environment surrounding the protein.

For instance, certain other substances in the neighborhood of beta amyloid protein may normally bind to it and thus keep it in solution. But in Alzheimer's disease, according to one theory, something causes the beta amyloid to drop out of solution and form the insoluble plaques.

Other areas of research center on how beta amyloid affects neurons—if at all. In one laboratory study, hippocampal neurons died when beta amyloid was added to the cell culture, suggesting that the protein is toxic to neurons. Another recent study suggests that beta amyloid breaks into fragments, releasing free radicals that attack neurons.

The precise mechanism by which beta amyloid might cause neuron death is still a mystery, but one recent finding suggests that beta amyloid forms tiny channels in neuron membranes. These channels may allow uncontrolled amounts of calcium into the neuron, an event that can be lethal in any cell.

Other recent studies suggest that beta amyloid disrupts potassium channels, which could also affect calcium levels. Still another study links beta amyloid to reduced choline concentrations in neurons; since neurons need choline to synthesize acetylcholine, this finding suggests a link between beta amyloid and the death of cholinergic neurons.

Tau

Another set of clues centers on a protein called tau, the major component of neurofibrillary tangles.

Neurofibrillary tangles resisted analysis until the late 1980's, when researchers discovered they were associated with neurons' internal structures, called microtubules. In healthy neurons, microtubules are formed like train rails, long parallel tracks with crosspieces, that carry nutrients from the body of the cells down to the ends of axons. In cells affected by Alzheimer's, this structure has collapsed. Tau normally forms the crosspieces between microtubules, but in Alzheimer's it twists into paired helical filaments, like two threads wound around each other. These are the basic constituents of neurofibrillary tangles.

Having identified beta amyloid and tau, researchers would now like to find out what they do in the brain and in Alzheimer's disease. Some ideas about their functions may come from studies of certain genes.

The Genes

Located along the DNA in the nucleus of each cell, genes direct the manufacture of every enzyme, hormone, growth factor, and other protein in the body. Genes are made up of four chemicals, or bases, arranged in various patterns. Each gene has a different sequence of bases, and each one directs the manufacture of a different protein.

Even slight alterations in the DNA code of a gene can produce a faulty protein. And a faulty protein can lead to cell malfunction and eventually disease.

Genetic research has turned up evidence of a link between Alzheimer's disease and genes on three chromosomes—14, 19, and 21. The apoE4 gene on chromosome 19 has been linked to late-onset Alzheimer's disease, which is the most common form of the disease.

ApoE4 and Alzheimer's Disease

The apoE4 gene came to light through long, patient detective work topped off by the serendipity that sometimes occurs in science. Alzheimer's researchers knew there were families in which many members developed the disease late in life. And therefore they knew there had to be a gene that the affected family members had in common. Searching for this gene, they combed through the DNA from these families and by 1992 had narrowed the search down to a region on chromosome 19.

In the same laboratory, another group of researchers were looking for proteins that bind to beta amyloid. They were disappointed at first. One version of a protein called apolipoproteinE (apoE) did bind quickly and tightly to beta amyloid, but apolipoproteinE was well known as a carrier of cholesterol in blood. No one suspected that it could have anything to do with Alzheimer's disease.

But by coincidence, or so it seemed, the gene apoE, which produces the protein, was also on chromosome 19. Moreover, it was on the same region of chromosome 19 as the Alzheimer's gene for which they had been searching.

The two groups of scientists decided to see if the apoE gene and the still missing Alzheimer's gene could be one and the same, and what they found made headlines: The apoE gene was identical to the gene they had been seeking. ApoE, it turned out, is much more common among Alzheimer's patients than among the general population.

More precisely, one version of apoE is more common among Alzheimer's patients. Like some other genes, the one that produces apoE comes in several forms or alleles. The apoE gene has three different forms—apoE2, apoE3, and apoE4. ApoE3 is the most common in the general population. But apoE4 occurs in approximately 40 percent of all late-onset Alzheimer's patients. Moreover, it is not limited to people whose families have a history of Alzheimer's. Patients with no known family history of the disease, cases of so-called sporadic Alzheimer's disease, are also more likely to have an apoE4 gene.

Since that finding, dozens of studies around the world have confirmed that the apoE4 allele increases the risk of developing Alzheimer's disease. People who inherit two apoE4 genes (one from the mother and one from the father) are at least eight times more likely to develop Alzheimer's disease than those who have two of the more common E3 version. The least common allele, E2, seems to lower the risk even more. People with one E2 and one E3 gene have only one-fourth the risk of developing Alzheimer's as people with two E3 genes.

What does the apoE4 gene do? On one level, all genes function by transcribing their codes into proteins, so when we ask what a gene does, we are really asking what its protein product does. Many laboratories are now exploring what the apoE4 product does, and they have several clues.

Some of these clues point to beta amyloid. While the apoE4 protein binds rapidly and tightly to beta amyloid, the apoE3 protein does not. Normally beta amyloid is soluble, but when the apoE4 protein latches on to it, the amyloid becomes insoluble. This may mean that it is more likely to be deposited in plaques. Studies of brain tissue suggest that apoE4 increases deposits of beta amyloid and that it directly regulates the APP protein from which beta amyloid is formed.

Other clues, however, point to tau as the pivotal protein. As the crosspiece in the microtubule, tau's function seems to be to stabilize the microtubule structure. One hypothesis suggests that the apoE4 protein allows this structure to come undone in some way, leading to the neurofibrillary tangles.

While still controversial and far from proven, the hypotheses surrounding apoE4 are driving new research. One next step is to see how tau and beta amyloid react with apolipoprotein in its several forms in living cells. Other experiments will attempt to determine the actions and role of the protein. Once these are clear, it should be easier to see how they might be affected by drugs. For instance, if apoE2 does turn out to be beneficial, then substances that mimic its effects might be designed to help prevent or slow the progress of Alzheimer's disease.

The theories surrounding apoE4 are not confined to the proteins. One finding that intrigues neuroscientists is that Alzheimer's patients with the apoE4 gene have neurons with shorter dendrites—the branchlike extensions that receive messages from other neurons. Researchers speculate that the dendrites have been pruned back by some unknown agent, limiting the neuron's ability to communicate with other neurons. Although this pruning can also occur in people without the apoE4 allele, it happens 20 or 30 years earlier in people with apoE4.

Will the genetic information available now ever be used in screening for Alzheimer's disease? Probably not. One of the puzzles surrounding apoE4 is why some people with the gene do not develop Alzheimer's disease and why, conversely, many people develop the disease even though they do not have the gene. ApoE4, in other words, is not a consistent marker for Alzheimer's.

This is one reason that few people advocate widespread screening for apoE4. Screening would miss a large percentage of those who will develop Alzheimer's and falsely identify others as future Alzheimer's patients. Some scientists suggest, however, that testing for the gene may someday help in the diagnosis of Alzheimer's.

Genes in Early-Onset Alzheimer's Disease

Two families in Belgium can count back six or seven generations in which some members developed Alzheimer's disease in their 30's and 40's. A Japanese family has 5 members who developed the disease in middle age; a Hispanic family has 12 members; a French-Canadian family, 23; a British family, 8. In families descended from Volga Germans—a group of German families that settled in the Volga River valley in Russia in the 1800s—dozens of descendants have developed Alzheimer's disease in middle age.

Alzheimer's strikes early and fairly often in these and other families around the world—often enough to be singled out as a separate form of the disease and given a label: early-onset familial Alzheimer's disease or FAD. Combing through the DNA of these early-onset families, researchers have found a mutation in one gene on chromosome 21 that is common to a few of the families. And they have linked a much larger proportion of early-onset families to a recently-identified gene on chromosome 14. The gene on chromosome 21 occurs less often in people with FAD than the chromosome 14 gene, which codes for a membrane protein whose function is not yet known.

The chromosome 21 gene carries the code for a mutated form of the amyloid precursor protein, APP, the parent protein for beta amyloid. The discovery of this gene supports the theory that beta amyloid plays a role in Alzheimer's disease, although the mutation occurs in only about 5 percent of early-onset families.

The chromosome 21 gene intrigues Alzheimer's researchers also because it is the gene involved in Down syndrome. People with Down syndrome have an extra version of chromosome 21 and, as they grow older, usually develop plaques and tangles like those found in Alzheimer's disease.

Few researchers think that the search for Alzheimer's genes is over. The Volga Germans, for one thing, have neither the chromosome 14 nor the chromosome 21 abnormality. Most investigators are convinced that there are several genes involved in Alzheimer's disease and, moreover, that other conditions must also be present for the disease to develop. One of these conditions may be a problem with the way in which neurons turn sugar, or glucose, into energy, a process known as glucose metabolism.

Metabolism

Every few months, Alzheimer's patients travel to the National Institutes of Health outside of Washington, D.C., and to other centers around the country to take part in research studies. One of the tests they take measures brain activity using special techniques, such as PET (short for positron emission tomography).

PET works on a simple principle. Brain activity, whether one is looking at a picture, working out a problem in calculus, or simply observing the surroundings, requires energy. Neurons produce energy through metabolism, a chain of biochemical reactions that uses large amounts of glucose and oxygen. PET can track the flow of glucose and oxygen molecules in the bloodstream to the parts of the brain producing energy, thus revealing which areas are active.

A patient having a PET scan rests on a long low platform as the scanner tracks the flow of glucose or oxygen. The data the scanner collects are fed into a computer program which translates it into multicolor images: red and orange for areas of high activity, yellow for medium, blue and black for little or none.

By deciphering these patterns, Alzheimer's researchers can chart the progress of the disease. Glucose metabolism declines dramatically as neurons degenerate and die. Scientists are also using PET to learn how changes in brain activity match up with changes in skills, such as the ability to do arithmetic or to remember names of objects.

No one knows whether the decline in glucose metabolism causes neurons to degenerate or whether neuron degeneration causes metabolism to decline. In the effort to find out, scientists have examined glucose molecules at every step of the way from bloodstream to neuron.

The route is complex. It begins as glucose-laden blood flows through the capillaries, the tiny blood vessels that carry the blood past neurons.

Specialized molecules capture glucose molecules from blood and shuttle them into the neurons.

These transporter molecules come in several forms. One recent study found that levels of two of them, GLUT1 and GLUT3, were low in the cerebral cortex of people with Alzheimer's disease. These reductions could be one reason glucose metabolism drops in Alzheimer's.

Another key element in this scenario could be the condition of the capillaries. The transport system could break down because of thickening of the capillary walls, deposits of minerals, cholesterol, and amyloid, or some injury to these microvessels.

Once inside the cell, glucose molecules are delivered to inner structures, called mitochondria, where they are turned into energy through metabolism. This process involves various enzymes and other proteins, as well as glucose and oxygen. An alteration in any of the ingredients could have a profound effect on the end result, so investigating these enzymes is another important area in Alzheimer's research. Studies have found, for instance, that the enzyme cytochrome oxidase, important in glucose metabolism, is produced at lower levels in cells affected by Alzheimer's. Since its decline matches the declines in glucose metabolism, it may play a role in the disease.

While the glitch in glucose metabolism has yet to be pinpointed, its results are known to be devastating. Neurons depend wholly on glucose for their sustenance and when glucose metabolism falters, they suffer in various ways. For example, they cannot manufacture as much acetylcholine as normal cells, which may be one reason this neurotransmitter declines in Alzheimer's.

In addition, neurons having a problem with metabolism react abnormally to another neurotransmitter, called glutamate. When these neurons are stimulated by glutamate—even normal amounts of glutamate—their regular mechanisms go awry and they are flooded by calcium, with deadly consequences.

The Calcium Hypothesis

Calcium is an important substance in certain cells of the body, the so-called excitable cells in muscles and the nervous system. Muscle cells need calcium to contract, neurons to transmit signals. Normally, the amount of calcium in a cell at any one time is carefully regulated; calcium channels allow in certain amounts of calcium at certain times, other proteins store the calcium within the cell or remove it.

Too much calcium can kill a cell, and some neuroscientists suspect that in the end, a rise in calcium levels may be precisely what is killing neurons in Alzheimer's disease. According to one hypothesis, an abnormally high concentration of calcium inside a neuron is the final step in cell death. Several different series or cascades of biochemical events could lead up to this last, fatal step.

What events might these be? One possibility is that an increase in calcium channels could allow an excess of calcium into the cell. Another possibility is that a defect develops in the structures that store calcium inside the cell or those that pump it out of the cell.

Still another hypothesis suggests that calcium levels rise because of an "energy crisis" in the neuron. In this scenario, chronically high levels of the neurotransmitter glutamate disrupt energy metabolism, leading to an influx of calcium. Glutamate is an excitatory neurotransmitter; it triggers action in a neuron, stimulating the flow of calcium into the cell. If it is produced in higher-than-normal levels, it can overexcite a neuron, driving in too much calcium. Moreover, glutamate can be dangerous to a neuron even at normal levels if glucose levels are low. Thus a problem with glucose metabolism could allow glutamate to overexcite the cell, allowing an influx of calcium.

Another hypothesis, involving the hormones called glucocorticoids, ties in with this theory. Glucocorticoids normally enhance the manufacture of glucose and reduce inflammation in the body. They came to the attention of Alzheimer's researchers when studies in older animals showed that long exposure to glucocorticoids contributed to neuron death and dysfunction in the hippocampus. Now several laboratories are exploring mechanisms by which glucocorticoids might lead to neuron death through their effect on glucose metabolism.

Environmental Suspects

No one doubts that genetic and other biological factors are important in Alzheimer's disease, but environmental factors could also contribute to its development. The most studied of these are aluminum, zinc, foodborne poisons, and viruses.

Aluminum

One of the most publicized and controversial hypotheses in this area concerns aluminum, which became a suspect in Alzheimer's disease when researchers found traces of this metal in the brains of Alzheimer's patients. Many studies since then have either not been able to confirm this finding or have had questionable results.

Aluminum does turn up in higher amounts than normal in some autopsy studies of Alzheimer's patients, but not in all. Further doubt about the importance of aluminum stems from the possibility that the aluminum found in some studies did not all come from the brain tissues being studied. Instead, some could have come from the special substances used in the laboratory to study brain tissue.

Aluminum is a common element in the Earth's crust and is found in small amounts in numerous household products and in many foods. As a result, there have been fears that aluminum in the diet or absorbed in other ways could be a factor in Alzheimer's. One study found that people who used antiperspirants and antacids containing aluminum had a higher risk of developing Alzheimer's. Others have also reported an association between aluminum exposure and Alzheimer's disease.

On the other hand, various studies have found that groups of people exposed to high levels of aluminum do not have an increased risk. Moreover, aluminum in cooking utensils does not get into food and the aluminum that does occur naturally in some foods, such as potatoes, is not absorbed well by the body. On the whole, scientists can say only that it is still uncertain whether exposure to aluminum plays a role in Alzheimer's disease.

Zinc

Zinc has been implicated in Alzheimer's disease in two ways. Some reports suggest that too little zinc is a problem, others that too much zinc is at fault. Too little zinc was suggested by autopsies that found low levels of zinc in the brains of Alzheimer's disease patients, especially in the hippocampus.

On the other hand, a recent study suggests that too much zinc might be the problem. In this laboratory experiment, zinc caused soluble beta amyloid from cerebrospinal fluid to form clumps similar to the plaques of Alzheimer's disease. Current experiments with zinc are pursuing this lead in laboratory tests that more closely mimic conditions in the brain.

Foodborne Poisons

Toxins in foods have come under suspicion in a few cases of dementia. Two amino acids found in seeds of certain legumes in Africa, India, and Guam may cause neurological damage. Both enhance the action of the neurotransmitter glutamate, also implicated in Alzheimer's disease.

In Canada, an outbreak of a neurological disorder similar to Alzheimer's occurred among people who had eaten mussels contaminated with demoic acid. This chemical, like the legume amino acids, is a glutamate stimulator. While these toxins may not be a common cause of dementia, they could eventually shed some light on the mechanisms that lead to neuron degeneration.

The Search for a Virus

In some neurological diseases a virus is the culprit, lurking in the body for decades before a combination of circumstances stirs it to action. So for years researchers have sought a virus or other infectious agent in Alzheimer's disease.

This line of research has yielded little in the way of hard evidence so far, although one study in the late 1980's did provide some data that have kept the possibility alive. A larger investigation is now under way.

A Disease with Many Causes?

The trails of clues that Alzheimer's leaves in its wake have so far not converged. When they do, some scientists think that this detective story will turn out to have a number of culprits. One theory suggests that several factors act in sequence or in combination to cause Alzheimer's disease, even though no single factor is sufficient by itself. To explain this idea, scientists use the metaphor of a light that requires several switches.

There might, for example, be just two switches, such as a gene mutation and another event to trigger the gene. Or there might be several. According to this idea, called the AND gate theory, these events do not have to occur at the same time, but their effects would have to linger and eventually coincide to bring about Alzheimer's disease.

Further Reading

Cotton P. Constellation of Risks and Processes Seen in Search for Alzheimer's Clues, *Journal of the American Medical Association* 271:89-91, 1994.

Pennis E. A Molecular Whodunit: New Twists in the Alzheimer's Mystery, *Science News* 145:8-11, 1993.

Neurotransmitters and Signaling

Davies P and Maloney AJ. Selective Loss of Central Cholinergic Neurons in Alzheimer's Disease, *Lancet* 2:1403, 1976.

Geula C and Mesulam M. Cholinergic Systems and Related Neuropathological Predilection Patterns in Alzheimer Disease. In Terry RD, Katzman R, and Bick KL eds. *Alzheimer Disease*, New York: Raven Press, 1994; pp 263-292.

Horsburgh K and Saitoh T. Altered Signal Transduction in Alzheimer Disease. In Terry RD, Katzman R, and Bick KL eds. *Alzheimer Disease*, New York: Raven Press, 1994; pp 387-404.

The Proteins

Kosik KS. Alzheimer's Disease: A Cell Biological Perspective, *Science* 256:780-783, 1992.

Lee VM, Balin BJ, Otvos L, and Trojanowski JQ. A68: A Major Subunit of Paired Helical Filaments and Derivatized Forms of Normal Tau, *Science* 251:675-678, 1991.

Cotman CW and Pike CJ. Beta-Amyloid and Its Contributions to Neurodegeneration in Alzheimer Disease. In Terry RD, Katzman R, and Bick KL eds. *Alzheimer Disease*, New York: Raven Press, 1994; pp 305-316.

Kosik K and Greenberg SM. Tau Protein and Alzheimer Disease. In Terry RD, Katzman R, and Bick KL eds. *Alzheimer Disease*, New York: Raven Press, 1994; pp 335-344.

The Genes

Hooper C. Research in Focus: Encircling a Mechanism in Alzheimer's Disease, *The Journal of NIH Research* 4:48-54, 1992.

St. George-Hyslop PH. The Molecular Genetics of Alzheimer Disease. In Terry RD, Katzman R, and Bick KL eds. *Alzheimer Disease*, New York: Raven Press, 1994; pp 345-352.

Metabolism

Beal MF. Energy, Oxidative Damage, and Alzheimer's Disease: Clues to the Underlying Puzzle, *Neurobiology of Aging* 15(Suppl. 2):S171-S174, 1994.

Rapoport SI and Grady CL. Parametric In Vivo Brain Imaging During Activation to Examine Pathological Mechanisms of Functional Failure in Alzheimer Disease, *International Journal of Neurosciences* 70:39-56, 1993.

Calcium

Landfield PW, Thibault O, Mazzanti ML, et al. Mechanisms of Neuronal Death in Brain Aging and Alzheimer's Disease: Role of Endocrine-Mediated Calcium Dyshomeostasis, *Journal of Neurobiology* 23:1247-1260, 1992.

Khachaturian ZS. The Role of Calcium Regulation in Brain Aging: Reexamination of a Hypothesis, *Aging* 1:17-34, 1989.

Khachaturian ZS. Calcium Hypothesis of Alzheimer's Disease and Brain Aging, *Annals of the New York Academy of Sciences* 7471-7481, 1994.

Environmental Suspects

Markesbery WR and Ehmann WD. Brain Trace Elements in Alzheimer Disease. In Terry RD, Katzman R, and Bick KL eds. *Alzheimer Disease*, New York: Raven Press, 1994; pp 353-368.

Gatz M, Lowe B, Berg S, et al. Dementia: Not Just a Search for the Gene, *The Gerontologist* 34:251-255, 1994.

Chapter 18

Alzheimer's Disease: Searching for Answers

Research Directions

Alzheimer's disease (AD) research is divided into three broad, overlapping areas: causes/risk factors, diagnosis, and treatment/caregiving. Research into the basic biology of the aging nervous system is critical to understanding what goes wrong in the brain of a person with AD. Understanding how nerve cells lose their ability to communicate with each other and the reasons why some nerve cells die is at the heart of scientific efforts to discover what causes AD.

Many researchers are working to slow AD's progression, delay its onset, or eventually, prevent it altogether. In looking for better ways to diagnose AD, investigators strive to identify diagnostic markers (indicators) of dementias, develop and improve ways to test patients, determine causes and assess risk factors, and improve case-finding and sampling methods for population studies. Scientists also seek better ways to treat AD, improve a patient's ability to function, and support caregivers of people with AD.

National Institute on Aging

The National Institute on Aging (NIA) is part of the Federal Government's National Institutes of Health (NIH). The NIA has primary responsibility for research aimed at finding ways to prevent,

Excerpted from *Progress Report on Alzheimer's Disease: 1997*, National Institute on Aging, NIH Pub. No. 97-4014, November 1997.

treat, and cure AD. One of NIA's main goals is to enhance the quality of life of older people by expanding knowledge about the aging brain and nervous system.

NIA's AD research has important implications for public policy. Changes in the way the brain works are associated with many age-related losses that lead to institutional care. Changes in the brain that significantly affect the senses, movement, and the ability to think influence the quality of life of older people. For people with AD, decline in these abilities limits independence, affects self-image, and influences the attitudes of others. Ultimately, these attitudes determine the nature and quality of health care services AD patients receive.

AD research can identify early treatments that may change the disease's course or reduce its severity. Although no cure exists yet for AD, there is reason to be optimistic. Many researchers are working hard to find what causes this devastating illness and how to treat it effectively.

This chapter highlights recent progress in AD research conducted or supported by the NIA and other components of the NIH, including the following:

- National Heart, Lung, and Blood Institute
- National Institute of Diabetes and Digestive and Kidney Diseases
- National Institute of Neurological Disorders and Stroke
- National Institute on Deafness and Other Communication Disorders
- National Institute of Mental Health
- National Human Genome Research Institute
- National Center for Research Resources
- National Institute of Nursing Research

Other smaller AD research projects not summarized in this report are supported by the National Cancer Institute, National Eye Institute, National Institute of Allergy and Infectious Diseases, National Institute of Arthritis and Musculoskeletal and Skin Diseases, National Institute of Child Health and Human Development, National Institute of Dental Research, National Institute of Environmental Health Sciences, and Fogarty International Center.

National Heart, Lung, and Blood Institute

How AD develops has attracted the attention of investigators from diverse disciplines funded by the National Heart, Lung, and Blood (NHLBI). When a protease(s) cuts APP apart, a peptide may form that is 1 of 2 lengths: a chain of 40 amino acids or 42 amino acids. Amino acids are organic compounds needed for forming proteins and pieces of proteins. The shorter beta-amyloid is very soluble and aggregates slowly. The longer beta-amyloid rapidly forms insoluble aggregates and appears to play a critical role in the initial buildup of plaque and in the onset of AD.

Proteases generally are controlled by their inhibitors. One NHLBI grantee at the Scripps Research Institute in La Jolla, California, has been studying APP processing by certain proteases in platelets (disk-shaped blood cells that play a role in blood clotting) and large bone marrow cells. Since inhibitors control the activity of proteases, NHLBI researchers are trying to identify inhibitors of APP processing associated with platelets and bone marrow. So far, they have found one inhibitor related to platelets and one related to bone marrow.

A disease of blood vessels in the brain, called cerebral amyloid angiopathy (CAA), is common in patients with AD. CAA appears to be associated with the buildup of beta-amyloid peptide within the network of blood vessels in the body. In hereditary cerebral hemorrhage with amyloidosis-Dutch type (HCHWA-D) (bleeding in the brain with amyloid buildup), the pathology tends to be more severe, and patients develop frequently recurring bleeding within the brain when they are about 50 years of age. Amyloidosis is a generic term for a group of diverse diseases, all of which involve amyloid buildup in various organs and tissues to a degree that normal body function is altered. People with HCHWA-D have a mutation in their APP gene that is at a different place from those causing AD. As a result, the beta-amyloid peptide produced in these patients has an amino acid substitution within it.

An NHLBI grantee at the State University of New York in Stony Brook reported this year that the longer, not the shorter, beta-amyloid peptide caused damaging responses (including cell decay) in laboratory cultures of muscle cells surrounding blood vessels in the human brain. Recent results show that the mutation in the shorter beta-amyloid peptide from HCHWA-D patients converts the normally harmless peptide to a highly destructive form. In fact, the shorter beta-amyloid peptide containing the mutation caused more damage to these muscle cells in laboratory cultures than the longer beta-amyloid peptide. These findings on the altered properties of the mutated peptide may help explain the severe damage found in blood vessels of the brain observed in this disorder.

National Institute of Diabetes and Digestive and Kidney Diseases

The National Institute of Diabetes and Digestive and Kidney Diseases (NIDDK) conducts and supports research on molecular and biochemical mechanisms of cell signaling, including the roles of neurotransmitters and ion channels; and mechanisms involved in abnormal metabolic processes.

This year, scientists at the NIDDK reported progress in understanding how beta-amyloid affects ion channels in cells. Investigators found that beta-amyloid, when added to artificial membranes, spontaneously formed pores (openings) or ion channels. To understand how these pores for amyloid are formed, researchers performed a molecular modeling study and developed three basic types of channel models. Two of these models showed how adding a certain substance to the channel pore complex can affect whether the channel reacts to atoms that have positive or negative charges. These models were then used to design experiments to test the binding of zinc, a metal ion that some scientists think may play a role in the formation of amyloid plaques in AD. Researchers found that addition of zinc to the pore complex had a strong effect on how the channel worked, essentially blocking pore activity.

To determine whether beta-amyloid could form ion channels in natural membranes, investigators studied the buildup of beta-amyloid molecules in a nerve cell line. Once again, they found that exposing the membrane to beta-amyloid caused pores to form, and that addition of zinc blocked channel activity. These results support the idea that amyloid damages nerve cells by forming these channels.

NIDDK-funded scientists also are interested in amyloidosis; the most common form of amyloidosis is AD. In this disease, the amyloid is a fragment of APP. Recent studies have shown that beta-amyloid exists as a soluble protein in many body fluids, linking AD more closely to other amyloidoses such as transthyretin (TTR) amyloidoses, where a fragment of the TTR protein forms the insoluble amyloid. These diseases, like AD, are late-onset diseases and affect a large number of families in the United States.

Collaborating NIDDK-supported researchers at the Richard L. Roudebush Veterans Administration Medical Center at Indiana University/Purdue University of Indianapolis and Texas A&M University in College Station are studying the structure of normal and abnormal TTR proteins to understand the factors needed for protein processing that leads to amyloid formation. The goal of this research is to identify methods of interfering with the formation of amyloid fibrils and, thereby, preventing this abnormal buildup of protein fragments.

In other studies, NIDDK-supported researchers at the University of California at San Francisco and the Joslin Diabetes Center in Boston, Massachusetts, which is affiliated with the Harvard Medical Center, are studying the role of islet amyloid polypeptide (IAPP) in non-insulin-dependent (type 2) diabetes, which also is an age-dependent disease. IAPP is the major component of amyloid deposits in islets (isolated clusters of cells or tissue) in the pancreas and is thought to play a role in the development of type 2 diabetes.

Information gained studying TTR and IAPP proteins will contribute to the overall understanding of the mechanisms underlying amyloid and associated protein buildup. Increased understanding can lead to the design of treatments to: reduce the effects of tissue damage, increase the rate of recovery from tissue damage, and ultimately, prevent disease.

National Institute of Neurological Disorders and Stroke

The National Institute of Neurological Disorders and Stroke (NINDS) supports a broad array of studies directed toward understanding how AD develops. In studying the cause(s) of AD, NINDS-funded researchers are looking at the organization of the memory system in the cerebral cortex of mammals, the structure and function of neurons in this system, the pathology of these neurons including plaques and tangles, and genetic factors. They also seek to develop and use animal models of the disorder.

The pace of discovery in AD research has been most impressive in genetic studies. Scientists supported by the NIA and the NINDS found two genes linked to FAD, presenilins 1 and 2.

The two genes produce similar proteins with unknown functions. In analyzing gene sequences, scientists recently have shown that proteins produced by these two genes have chemical structures that are similar to that of a protein involved in the signaling and development of cells in a species of worm. The powerful genetic techniques that can be applied in this species may help researchers understand the function of these proteins. Additional recent studies suggest that these proteins are made by neurons throughout the brain and that they play a role in the processing of other proteins such as APP.

Until recently, there has been no good animal model for AD. The discovery of three defective genes that underlie inherited forms of AD has presented the opportunity to develop transgenic animal models.

Newer imaging studies, particularly PET scans and magnetic resonance imaging (MRI), have made it possible for researchers to study the selective abnormalities in brain functioning in AD patients. These studies give scientists a research baseline for use in finding ways to develop diagnostic measures, define the metabolic defect involved, and evaluate the effects of treatments.

The NINDS Laboratory of Adaptive Systems is determining whether a laboratory test they have developed may be a useful diagnostic test for AD. This test is not available outside the laboratory or research setting. It is based on drug-induced light signals that are missing in single skin or smell-receptor cells of AD patients but not healthy controls. The same test also may be useful for cells obtained from a simple blood sample. Beta-amyloid was found to produce the defects in the cells of healthy people. A simple laboratory diagnosis for AD would eliminate the cost of lengthy exams and procedures (e.g., computerized tomography (CT) scans, metabolic tests, etc.) as well as guide family members and clinicians for future decisions concerning patient care. Further biochemical studies will explore the relationship of the observed changes to the cause(s) of AD.

NINDS's Experimental Therapeutics Branch has initiated a clinical trial of a new anti-dementia medication, CX 516 (Ampakine), for patients with mild to moderate dementia. Scientists are studying CX 516 for properties that improve thinking and memory.

The identification of more genes for FAD should foster a better understanding of how FAD and sporadic AD develop, much as recent findings in familial breast cancer are leading to a better understanding of all breast cancer.

National Institute on Deafness and Other Communication Disorders

Investigators funded by the National Institute on Deafness and Other Communication Disorders (NIDCD) at the University of Pennsylvania in Philadelphia studied the understanding of subject-predicate sentences independent of their truth value by asking a group of AD patients to judge the coherence of statements such as "The tulip is tall" or "The tulip is jealous." The results suggest that these AD patients were significantly more impaired than healthy volunteers in judging the coherence of these simple sentences. Moreover, AD patients in the study were more successful at judging the coherence of statements that contained attributes with a narrow scope of reference compared to attributes with a broad scope of reference. These findings suggest that AD patients have impaired semantic (related to the meaning of words or language) memory and have trouble processing the network of semantic relations underlying word meaning in semantic memory.

Superoxide dismutases are among a cell's major enzyme-related defenses against toxic reactive oxygen molecules and oxidative stress. Reactive oxygen molecules, which induce these enzymes to work, have been implicated in the nerve cell decline associated with AD. As some people with AD show early, severe deficits in their olfactory ability (related to the sense of smell), NIDCD-supported scientists at the University of Kentucky in Lexington studied the location and activity of two enzymes, manganese and copper-zinc superoxide dismutases, within certain nose cells. Participants were young, middle-aged, and older people without dementia, and people with AD. Tissues were obtained at autopsy from people ranging in age from 19 to 98 years old. These researchers studied how each enzyme reacted with cells from different regions of the nose.

Manganese and copper-zinc superoxide dismutases showed a lot more disease-fighting activity in people with AD than in older participants without dementia. This finding suggests that oxidative stress may be responsible, at least in part, for the smelling deficits in AD patients.

NIDCD-funded scientists at the University of Kentucky also are studying a calcium-binding protein, called S-35, in nose cells of people who ranged in age from 16 weeks of fetal development to 98 years of age, including some with AD. This protein binds calcium that is outside cells and helps prevent cell death related to cells having too much calcium. The disease-fighting activity of S-35 was observed in olfactory (smell) receptor neurons (ORNs) and olfactory nerve bundles that react with olfactory marker protein (OMP) and neuron-specific enolase (NSE), another enzyme. At all ages, the mean number of ORNs that reacted with OMP did not change significantly. However, the mean number of NSE-reactive and S-35-reactive ORNs declined markedly in postnatal infant, young, and old patients when compared with that of the fetuses. S-35-reactive ORNs decreased significantly in AD patients when compared with control patients. These results suggest that ORNs in humans express S-35, and that there is an age-related decrease in the expression of S-35. Furthermore, the marked decrease of S-35 expression in ORNs of AD patients suggests that cell excitability associated with calcium ions and the ability of cells to protect themselves from too many calcium ions decline in these patients.

National Institute of Mental Health

Research supported by the National Institute of Mental Health (NIMH) includes the etiology, pathogenesis, clinical course, and treatment of AD; the stresses caregivers face; and the services AD patients and their caregivers use.

The NIMH Alzheimer's Disease Genetics Initiative has established a national resource of clinical information and DNA samples from people with AD and their family members. The NIMH funds research at three universities (Harvard Medical School/Massachusetts General Hospital in Boston, the University of Alabama at Birmingham, and Johns Hopkins University) to collect data and conduct genetic analyses. As of February 1997, the data set included clinical/diagnostic data and DNA samples from 1,161 people in 362 family lineages, including 804 subjects with AD. This data set includes 441 affected sibling pairs, and is the largest for late-onset AD thus far collected. Six research groups currently are conducting genetic analyses of samples provided by the Initiative. Descriptive information for the sample (including tables that are updated daily), instructions for gaining access, and a copy of the Distribution Agreement that must be signed by investigators requesting access, are available on the Internet at http://www-srb.nimh.nih.gov/gi.html.

Analyses based on data collected through the NIMH Alzheimer Disease Genetics Initiative confirm the role of the apoE4 gene as a risk factor for AD. Among 679 people with AD in the sample, having 2 copies, but not 1 copy, of the apoE4 allele was associated with a lower age at onset. These results also show that apoE4 exerts its maximal effect on risk for AD in people in their sixties, although an effect also was observed at later ages. As with other studies of late-onset diseases, this finding suggests that genes other than the apoE4 gene also influence a person's risk for developing late-onset AD.

Researchers also are looking at whether AD patients with the E4 allele are more likely to have a faster rate of decline. NIMH-funded researchers at Stanford University have found apoE4 to be a poor predictor of decline in AD, consistent with other recent reports. However, the E4 allele was found to be related to several measures of behavioral disturbance.

NIA- and NIMH-supported researchers at the Albert Einstein College of Medicine in New York City have been conducting neurochemical analyses of AD to find biochemical events that occur very early in the development of the disease. By producing monoclonal antibodies that recognize protein abnormalities, these scientists can explore different neuronal sites for abnormal changes that occur with AD. Antibodies are substances that play a role in protecting the body from disease by binding to foreign proteins. They are used in research to identify the location and amount of AD-related proteins. In particular, the order of changes that take place in these proteins is crucial for detecting the very early stages of AD. For example, it appears that tau is altered in the AD brain before paired helical filaments and neurofibrillary tangles develop. If confirmed, early detection of altered tau could be used as a marker in drug trials aimed at stopping or preventing AD.

Through an NIMH Small Business Technology Transfer grant, researchers at Isolab, Inc., in Akron, Ohio, are developing a laboratory test based on cerebrospinal fluid (CSF) samples to determine the density of paired helical filaments of neurofibrillary tangles using antibody assays (tests). This diagnostic kit for monitoring CSF potentially will be developed to serve as one element of the physician's evaluation of dementia, and holds potential as a useful diagnostic tool.

Researchers at McLean Hospital in Belmont, Massachusetts, and the Massachusetts Institute of Technology's Clinical Research Center in Boston are examining the metabolic regulation of acetylcholine synthesis and function in the AD brain. Uptake of choline—a precursor of acetylcholine—into the brain declines with age and may be an important contributing factor in AD, where acetylcholine neurons are susceptible to loss. Oral administration of CDP-choline (cytidine diphosphocholine), a metabolic intermediate that completely dissociates to form choline and cytidine, increases brain levels of choline, phospholipids, and acetylcholine biosynthesis in rat brain. In humans, CDP-choline (citicholine) has been shown to improve memory functioning in older people with well-functioning memory, as well as improving verbal memory (delayed recall) in older people with inefficient memory processing. Future studies will investigate the potential role of CDP-choline treatment in delaying the onset of cognitive impairment.

Nerve cell decay that is related to aging may be caused or made worse by declines in circulating hormones such as estrogen, leading to the hypothesis that estrogen may have a protective effect in AD. NIA- and NIMH-funded researchers at Columbia University have been seeking to understand the molecular mechanisms through which hormones could affect brain function. They have shown that hormone receptors are heavily represented in some brain regions implicated in the pathology of AD, and that hormones act in combination with neurotrophic factors to promote cell survival.

Although memory problems and cognitive impairment often are considered the primary symptoms of AD, psychiatric symptoms such as delusions, mood lability, apathy, irritability, agitation, disinhibition, and aggression also are key symptoms of the disorder. These noncognitive symptoms are critical because they have been associated with more rapid disease course, caregiver distress, and earlier institutionalization. Patients with both AD and depression may have a more complicated course of AD and also may have other physical illnesses such as diabetes or heart disease.

NIMH-funded researchers at the University of California at Los Angeles have found structural and functional correlates of psychiatric symptoms in the brains of AD patients. At the University of Pittsburgh, studies of brains at autopsy have indicated that AD patients who had depression had reduced levels of a neurotransmitter, serotonin, in the hippocampus. In NIMH-funded research at Stanford University, community-residing AD patients with the apoE4 allele showed greater behavioral disturbances than non-carriers of the allele, even when the level of cognitive impairment was taken into account. Further studies are under way to determine the replicability of these initial findings, which suggest that genetic variations in apoE may have a broader significance for the clinical symptoms of AD than has previously been recognized. All these studies are important because both psychiatric symptoms of AD and coexisting psychiatric disorders currently are more treatable than the cognitive symptoms of the disease, and their treatment can enhance quality of life for both patients and family caregivers.

Neuroleptic medications (drugs that affect a person's thinking, behavior, and mood, which are designed to reduce agitation and confusion) remain a frequent treatment for AD patients who are agitated and/or exhibit psychotic symptoms of delusions and hallucinations. In addition to determining the efficacy of these medications, scientists are refining information about the risk of neuroleptic-induced tardive dyskinesia (TD)—a condition characterized by involuntary muscle rigidity and tremors. NIMH-supported researchers at the University of California at San Diego have studied older psychiatric patients, including AD patients, for their risk for TD. These scientists have found that cumulative exposure to neuroleptics, as well as advancing age, are among the greatest risk factors for TD. Older patients are six times more susceptible to developing TD compared to younger patients. Among middle-aged and older adults, cumulative exposure is the greatest risk for TD, regardless of dosage. These efforts have been refined to determine risk profiles for distinctive subtypes of TD (for example, facial rigidity versus body contortion and hand tremors).

Efforts to find alternatives to these neuroleptic medications for managing disruptive and psychotic behaviors in AD patients include pharmacologic studies. Researchers at the University of Pittsburgh are looking at the effects of two different neuroleptics—perphenazine and melperone—to see how neuroleptics lead to changes in dopaminergic functioning in AD patients. The effects and actions of these medications are examined through drug challenge paradigms, where differences due to age and disease state can be studied. In addition to learning how to avoid TD when treating psychotic and behavioral symptoms in AD, these efforts aimed at understanding the dopamine-related system also will help scientists develop new drugs to treat the broader symptoms of AD.

Over the past decade, a number of NIMH-supported researchers have documented the mental and physical health consequences of caregiving stress among family members with an AD patient. Family caregivers of loved ones with AD have been called the "second victims" due to their increased risk for depression, cardiovascular problems, and compromised immune (disease-fighting) function. Researchers at Ohio State University have found that stressed caregivers build up less antibodies in response to an influenza vaccination, indicating that they are at greater risk for influenza and its complications. Newer vaccine preparations now enable scientists to test whether repeated vaccinations may improve stressed caregivers' abilities to resist influenza. A second line of immune function studies by these researchers is examining how stress among caregivers affects cytokine production and wound healing. Cytokines are proteins that react with certain foreign substances to mediate activities between cells, such as fighting disease.

In an NIMH-supported long-term study at New York University, spousal caregivers of AD patients were randomly put in either a psychosocial intervention program designed to increase family involvement or a standard minimal support program (controls). The psychosocial intervention provided individual counseling and family counseling as well as participation in support groups. More than 40 percent of these caregivers had clinically significant levels of depressive symptoms at baseline. Over 12 months, those who took part in the intervention program remained stable, whereas control caregivers became more depressed. Caregiver gender and patients' severity of dementia did not significantly predict change in depression over time. On the other hand, the intervention program accounted for 23 percent of the explainable variance in caregivers' depression. These results suggest that while psychosocial programs may relieve some of the burdens of providing long-term care for chronically impaired AD patients, an effective intervention may need to use several strategies, be sustained over time, and involve families in the support process.

National Human Genome Research Institute

The National Human Genome Research Institute (NHGRI) (formerly the National Center for Human Genome Research) helps identify genes involved in human diseases and the function of these genes and their products. The Human Genome Project provides data, material resources, and technology that will improve the ability of scientists to conduct biological research rapidly, efficiently, and cost-effectively; and supports a vigorous research program on the ethical, legal, and social implications of human genome research.

In the laboratories of the Division of Intramural Research, using the tools produced by the Human Genome Project, scientists are developing and using the most advanced techniques to study the fundamental mechanisms of inherited and acquired genetic disorders.

The NHGRI supports researchers at Case Western Reserve University who are examining ethical and policy issues regarding current genetic susceptibility testing for late-onset AD, as well as the ethical aspects of ongoing genetic testing in families with early-onset AD.

A Community Advisory Board and National Study Group were established to:

- examine current testing developments in AD genetics, their applicability to people before symptoms arise, and clinical usefulness

- consider costs of testing, potential groups of participants for testing, and justice in access to testing

- address the potential effect of susceptibility testing on the private long-term care insurance industry

- develop ethics guidelines for apoE susceptibility testing and APP autosomal dominant mutation testing

- develop recommendations for the Alzheimer's Association in ensuring public understanding of test developments

In addition, a pilot questionnaire study of population attitudes toward apoE susceptibility testing, to be implemented in Chicago, Illinois, is included. This project proceeds in collaboration with the National Alzheimer's Association.

To date, a book, *The Moral Challenge of Alzheimer Disease*, was published by the Johns Hopkins University Press, in December 1995. A second book on the findings of the National Study Group on ethics, genetics, and AD is being developed. In addition, a consensus manuscript from the National Study Group has been published in the Journal of the American Medical Association (March 12, 1997).

National Center for Research Resources

National Center for Research Resources (NCRR)-funded investigators are conducting AD research in the following areas: the structures of tangles in AD and related dementias, use of MRI to study cerebral blood flow in AD, use of CT scans to predict the rate of cognitive decline in AD, the effect of estrogen during menopause on risk and age at onset of AD, the way hyperinsulinemia may improve memory in AD, the role of apoE in APP buildup, and amyloid-related brain disease in older monkeys.

The NCRR-supported resource center at the University of California at San Diego brought together neuroscientists from Japan and the Albert Einstein College of Medicine in an international collaborative effort to examine damaged regions of the hippocampus that are thought to play an important role in cognitive changes in AD and related disorders. Immunologically-based chemical and electron microscopic analyses of tissue from patients with primary degenerative dementias along with their age-matched controls were performed using a specially designed electron microscope to enable viewing of thick sections.

Some of the tissue from AD patients and patients with related disorders (such as Lewy body dementia and progressive supranuclear palsy), but not from age-matched controls, reacted positively to the antibodies used. These findings indicate that neurofibrillary changes in all three of these neurodegenerative disorders have similar internal support structures.

Investigators at the General Clinical Research Center (GCRC) at the New England Medical Center in Boston used a new imaging technique, called dynamic susceptibility contrast MRI, to discriminate older patients with AD. Older patients with AD had a much lower blood volume in some parts of their brains. These scientists concluded that this new MRI technique is a low-cost and safe method for evaluating AD.

Some brain structures, such as the hippocampus and the amygdala, are severely affected even early in the course of AD. CT scans have shown a relationship between enlargement of the suprasellar cistern (SSC), a fluid-filled area in the base of the brain, and decline in cognitive function in AD patients. Investigators at Johns Hopkins University used this technique to predict future rates of cognitive decline. Twenty patients with diagnoses of probable AD received initial CT scans and then returned every 6 months for evaluation of their cognitive function. The interval between the initial testing and the most recent evaluation ranged between 12 and 67 months (the mean was 40.5 months). The investigators found that the size of the SSC correlated with a decline in cognitive function as measured by several mental tests, indicating that CT measurement of the SSC can predict the rate of decline in cognitive function in AD patients.

Estrogen use by postmenopausal women has many health benefits, but its effects in women with AD are not clear. Researchers at the Columbia University GCRC explored whether the use of estrogen could lower the risk of AD in 1,124 older women.

Growing evidence suggests that disruption of glucose regulation accompanies AD and may contribute to the severe memory impairment associated with the disease. NIA- and NCRR-funded investigators at the Washington University GCRC in St. Louis, Missouri, studied the effects of insulin and glucose in 22 patients with AD and 13 healthy adults. They found that raising insulin levels in the blood stream improved memory in the AD patients even when glucose levels did not change. Higher levels of glucose in the blood stream also improved memory, but not to the same extent as the higher insulin levels. These scientists also report that patients with AD have abnormal levels of some hormones that regulate glucose, and suggest that neuroendocrine factors play an important role in the development of AD.

Researchers at the University of Alabama are using a laboratory cell culture system to study the effects of genetically-induced overexpression of apoE. The researchers have discovered that apoE overexpression in this cell system significantly inhibits the aggregation of a protein fragment of beta-amyloid, indicating that apoE may be involved in the regulation of amyloid buildup.

Brains from 81 rhesus monkeys were collected to study the incidence and cerebral regional distribution of beta-amyloid plaques and amyloid-related blood vessel disease in the brains of autopsied rhesus monkeys. Different age groups were collected from autopsy cases performed at the University of Wisconsin Regional Primate Research Center during the past 14 years. Beta-amyloid and APP in the plaques were detected by chemical staining.

No amyloid plaques were found in the brains of 16- to 19-year-old monkeys (8 cases). In aged groups, the average rates of the plaque or blood vessel lesions were 20.8 percent in the 20 to 25 year group (24 cases), 60.9 percent in the 26 to 31 year group (41 cases), and 100 percent in the 33 to 39 year group (8 cases). Among 38 cases showing amyloid plaque lesions, 10 were accompanied by amyloid-related damage in the cerebral and meningeal blood vessels. No neurofibrillary tangles were detected in these brain lesions. Twelve cases in the aged monkeys had an involvement of visceral amyloidosis in the liver, adrenal, or the islets in the pancreas; and 7 of 12 had cerebral amyloidosis. The amyloid in the visceral organs showed no cross reactivity with beta-amyloid and precursor proteins. It appears that there is no disease-based correlation between cerebral and visceral myloidosis. As in the aged human population, the aged monkey also spontaneously develops AD-type brain lesions.

National Institute of Nursing Research

The National Institute of Nursing Research (NINR) supports research on the biobehavioral aspects of AD and related dementias. The primary focus has been on dealing with behavioral, physical, and functional problems, such as wandering, agitation, and sleep disturbances.

NINR-supported researchers at the University of Iowa in Iowa City have developed a caregiver training protocol that focuses on the setting in which caring for people with AD occurs. The program is based on the need to deal with the caregiver's increasing inability to cope with both environmental and internal stressors because of the patient's progressive cerebral pathology and associated cognitive decline. The model, the Progressively Lowered Stress Threshold, seeks to reduce stress by changing environmental demands to promote adaptive behavior. The model can be used in a variety of settings, including the home, and can be taught to family caregivers.

The family caregiver training protocol consists of two 2-hour sessions and a 1-hour in-home followup session 1 week later. Preliminary data have shown increased socialization; stable weight or gain in weight; and a reduction of psychotropic or neuroleptic medications, sedatives, and tranquilizers among patients whose caregivers received training. In addition, agitation and wandering episodes were decreased.

Initial findings in another study at the University of Texas Health Sciences Center at San Antonio indicate an alternative approach for managing problem behaviors. The strategy was based on a cognitive functional age approach to dementia. It has been noted that patients seem to lose their cognitive and functional abilities in a reverse order to that followed during the acquisition of those abilities. Researchers designed the interventions using a Piagetian model for assessment of cognitive functioning in conjunction with existing staging and assessment models. Preliminary findings show a decrease in problem behaviors while reducing the number of psychotropic medications.

Outlook

Investigators do not know yet how the various factors that may play a role in AD interrelate. In the next year, researchers will continue to study known genes and other risk factors and look for other genes and risk factors that might be linked to AD. Epidemiology studies will compare and identify environmental and genetic risk factors in diverse populations. Scientists also will study other disorders, such as strokes, to see if they affect the development or symptoms of AD.

Identification of genes implicated in AD provides new opportunities for analysis of the initiating cellular events, how the protein products affect these events, as well as how the initiating events lead to the well-recognized pathology of AD.

For example, many questions exist about the relationships of presenilin mutations to the development and production of amyloid in AD. Current challenges include finding and understanding additional mutations; determining how presenilins 1 and 2 are produced and processed, how they interact with cellular systems, and whether they play a role in nerve cell death and the development of late-onset AD; learning the effect of different presenilin mutations on APP metabolism and other cellular events; and comparing how presenilin 1 and 2 levels in cells change over the lifespan of healthy people and those with AD.

Mutations in the APP gene were discovered prior to those in the presenilins, and the knowledge base on the regulation and function of this precursor of beta-amyloid is correspondingly greater. Now, important steps for AD researchers will be to search for more receptors affected by beta-amyloid; understand the pathways involved in and look for substances that fight oxidative stress and beta-amyloid

216

production; and determine the relationship between amyloid deposits and the other neuropathologies of AD. Much work also is being done to discover why cells stop functioning properly and die in AD.

Ongoing research to produce transgenic animal models (e.g., for the various genetic forms of FAD) will aid researchers' understanding of the molecular mechanisms involved in AD development and help them identify treatments to retard disease progression. For example, comparing behavioral and anatomical approaches, researchers will be able to determine if the appearance of the plaques in transgenic mice carrying human APP mutations comes before or after the learning and memory problems. Scientists also are trying to develop ways to stop plaque formation and determine whether plaque formation is linked causally to cognitive changes.

So far, older transgenic mice with defects in the presenilin genes have not developed plaques or memory impairment. The challenge is to breed mice that develop AD-like symptoms so that investigators can study the mechanisms underlying their development. Plausible theories and evidence link both the presenilins and apoE to ways the body handles APP. Whether this is solely linked to beta-amyloid deposition or is, as well, related to the biological activity of APP is being investigated. What researchers are able to learn from the mouse model may help bring all of these findings together to form a coherent explanation of what causes AD, both in FAD and in late-onset AD.

In the clinic, scientists working to improve the diagnosis of AD seek to: validate and refine current recommended procedures; establish if differences in disease patterns in AD reflect genetic- and gender-based factors; determine how age affects the clinical and pathological criteria; find tests to determine which people with mild cognitive impairment will progress to clinical AD; develop biochemical and molecular methods for quickly diagnosing AD and compare the results to data obtained from currently recommended methods; standardize diagnostic methods and agents used at autopsy; develop and standardize quantitative methods; and determine the nature and significance of white matter pathological changes in AD.

ADCS investigations of estrogen, anti-inflammatory agents, and AIT-082 are examples of many efforts to test promising new treatments for AD. Preliminary data suggest that AIT-082 stimulates the production of neurotrophins, natural proteins that protect nerve cells from damage and enhance the regrowth of damaged nerve tissue. AIT-082 also stimulates cognitive function and memory in aged animals. As with other promising agents, the effectiveness of AIT-082 will only become known after lengthy and costly clinical trials.

One future direction for ADCS scientists is to test the effectiveness of vitamin E in people with mild cognitive impairment to determine whether this vitamin can reduce the number of people who would otherwise progress to more advanced stages of AD. This will be the first study to identify people at risk and bring them into a clinical trial. Eventually, the goal is to identify people at risk before they develop any signs of the disease and treat them with a drug (or a combination of drugs) that will slow or halt development of clinical AD.

Studies also continue to aid people who currently have AD and their caregivers. The ADCS plans additional studies of drugs used to treat the behavioral symptoms of AD. Members of the consortium currently are analyzing data from a clinical trial of the effectiveness of trazodone, haldol, and behavioral management in preventing or reducing agitation.

In addition to further studies of SCUs in nursing homes and special care in other residential settings, researchers seek to develop a framework for evaluating non-institutional care. Two recently funded NIA studies are using measures similar to those developed in the original SCU Initiative to examine the outcomes of residential care for people with dementia.

Research also will continue into caring for special populations to understand factors that influence minority and ethnic families, rural caregivers, employed caregivers, and male caregivers. In addition, scientists will study changing care structures; the interplay among older people, their families, and care settings; and the effects of these factors on an older person's ability to stay mentally and physically healthy.

Major recent advances in our understanding of AD hold promise for an accelerated pace of discovery into the causes and processes of this tragic disease. Recent findings also increase our ability to delay the progression of symptoms and bring us closer to being able to prevent and perhaps cure AD.

For a free printed copy of this report or further information about Alzheimer's disease, please contact:

Alzheimer's Disease Education and Referral (ADEAR) Center
PO Box 8250
Silver Spring, Maryland 20907-8250
800-438-4380
301-495-3334 (fax)
http://www.alzheimers.org/adear

Chapter 19

Changes in the Brain in Alzheimer's Disease

Structure and Function of the Brain

The brain does many things to ensure our survival. It integrates, regulates, initiates, and controls functions in the whole body, with the help of motor and sensory nerves outside of the brain and spinal cord. The brain governs thinking, personality, mood, and the senses. We can speak, move, and remember because of complex chemical processes that take place in our brains. The brain also regulates body functions that happen without our knowledge or direction, such as digestion of food.

The human brain is made up of billions of nerve cells, called neurons, that share information with one another through a large array of biological and chemical signals. Even more numerous (between 10 and 50 times the number of neurons) are glial cells, which surround, support, and nourish neurons. Each neuron has a cell body, an axon, and many dendrites. The nucleus, which contains deoxyribonucleic acid (DNA), controls the cell's activities. The axon, which extends from the cell body, sends messages from axons of other nerve cells or from specialized sense organs. Axons and dendrites collectively are called neurites.

Neurons communicate with each other and with sense organs by producing and releasing chemicals. An electrical charge (nerve impulse) builds up within the sending neuron as it receives messages

Excerpted from *Progress Report on Alzheimer's Disease, 1997*, National Institute on Aging, NIH Pub. No. 97-4014, November 1997.

219

from surrounding cells. The charge travels down the nerve cell until it reaches the end of the axon. Here, the nerve impulse triggers the release of neurotransmitters. These chemicals carry messages from the axons across synapses (gaps between nerve cells) to the dendrites or the cell bodies of other neurons. Scientists estimate that the typical neuron has up to 15,000 synapses. Neurotransmitters carrying messages bind to specific receptor sites on the receiving end of dendrites of adjacent nerve cells. Receptors are proteins (molecules that determine the physical and chemical traits of cells and organisms) that recognize and bind to chemical messengers from other cells.

When the above receptors are activated, they open channels into the receiving nerve cell's interior or start other processes that determine what the receiving nerve cell will do. Some neurotransmitters inhibit nerve cell function; that is, they make a neuron less likely to act. Other neurotransmitters stimulate nerve cells; they prime the receiving cell to become active or send a message.

In this way, signals travel back and forth across the brain in a fraction of a second. Millions of signals flash through the brain all the time.

Groups of neurons in the brain have specific jobs. For example, the brain's cerebral cortex is a large collection of neurons all over the surface of the brain. Some of these nerve cells are involved in thinking, learning, remembering, and planning.

The survival of nerve cells in the brain depends on the healthy functioning of three dynamic mechanisms all working in harmony. These mechanisms control nerve cell activities related to communicating information, using energy, and repairing cells and tissues. The first mechanism, communication between nerve cells, is described in the preceding paragraphs. The loss or absence of any one of several chemical messengers or receptors disrupts cell-to-cell communication and interferes with normal brain function.

In the second mechanism, metabolism, cells and molecules break down chemicals and nutrients into energy. Efficient metabolism in nerve cells requires adequate blood circulation to supply the cells with important nutrients, such as oxygen and glucose (a sugar). Glucose is the only source of energy available to the brain under normal circumstances. Depriving the brain of oxygen or glucose causes nerve cells to die within minutes.

The third mechanism repairs injured nerve cells. Unlike most other body cells, neurons live a long time. Brain neurons are built to last more than 100 years. In the adult, when neurons die (due to disease or injury), they are not replaced. To prevent their own death, living neurons constantly must maintain and remodel themselves. If cell cleanup and repair slow down or stop for any reason, the nerve cell cannot function properly. It is not clear when and why some neurons start to die and some synapses stop working.

Research shows that the damage seen in Alzheimer's Disease involves changes in all three mechanisms: nerve cell communication, metabolism, and repair.

Changes in the Brain in Alzheimer's Disease

In AD, communication between some nerve cells breaks down. The destruction from AD ultimately causes these nerve cells to stop functioning, lose connections with other nerve cells, and die. Death of many neurons in key parts of the brain harms memory, thinking, and behavior.

AD destroys neurons in parts of the brain controlling memory, especially the hippocampus (a structure deep in the brain that helps code memories). As nerve cells in the hippocampus stop functioning properly, short-term memory fails, and often, the person's ability to do familiar tasks begins to decline. AD also attacks the cerebral cortex. The greatest damage occurs in areas of the cerebral cortex responsible for functions such as language and reasoning. Here, AD begins to take away language skills and change a person's judgment. Personality changes also occur; emotional outbursts and disturbing behavior, such as wandering and agitation, appear and can happen more and more often as the disease runs its course.

Two abnormal structures are found in the AD brain: amyloid plaques and neurofibrillary tangles. Plaques are dense deposits of an amyloid protein, other associated proteins, and non-nerve cells that gradually accumulate (build up) outside and around neurons. Amyloid is a generic name for protein fragments that aggregate (collect or mass together) in a specific way to form insoluble deposits. The fragments can arise from different processes. Neurofibrillary tangles are insoluble twisted fibers that build up inside neurons. Much progress has been made in determining the makeup of amyloid plaques and neurofibrillary tangles and in proposing mechanisms that could account for their buildup in AD.

Amyloid Plaques

In AD, plaques develop in areas of the brain used for memory. These plaques consist of beta-amyloid intermingled with neurites from neurons and with non-nerve cells. These non-nerve cells include glial cells and microglia (cells that surround and digest damaged cells or foreign substances).

In plaques, beta-amyloid is a protein fragment snipped from a larger protein—called amyloid precursor protein (APP)—during metabolism. Researchers do not know yet whether amyloid plaques cause AD or result from it. APP is a member of a large family of proteins that are associated with cell membranes. The cell membrane encloses the cell and acts as a barrier that selects which substances can go in and out of the cell. During metabolism, APP becomes embedded in the membrane of the nerve cell, partly inside and partly outside of the cell, like a needle poking partway through a piece of fabric. While APP is embedded in the cell membrane, proteases cleave APP apart. Proteases are enzymes (substances that speed up or cause chemical reactions in the body) that snip proteins into smaller pieces. Beta-amyloid is produced only when the cleavage happens at the wrong place in APP.

After beta-amyloid is formed, scientists do not yet know exactly how it moves through or around nerve cells. In the final stages of its journey, it joins with other beta-amyloid filaments and fragments of dead and dying neurites to form the dense, insoluble plaques that are a hallmark for identifying AD in brain tissue. Researchers believe that beta-amyloid sets off the AD process and/or is an early byproduct in the slow, many-step process that ultimately leads to nerve cell damage and death in the brain.

Many studies have centered on how beta-amyloid is processed and how enzymes break down APP. Investigators are looking for clues in beta-amyloid's environment. For example, normally, substances may bind to beta-amyloid and keep it in solution. But in AD, according to one theory, something causes beta-amyloid fragments to aggregate together, just as fluid proteins in eggs become hard after being cooked. Beta-amyloid aggregates gradually build up to form dense, insoluble plaques that the body cannot dispose of or recycle.

Other areas of research focus on how beta-amyloid affects neurons. In one laboratory study, neurons from the hippocampal area of the brain died when aggregated beta-amyloid was added to the cell culture, suggesting that the protein fragment is deadly to neurons. Results of a recent study suggest that beta-amyloid causes the release of free radicals, which then attack neurons.

Similar laboratory studies conducted by researchers at NIA's Gerontology Research Center (GRC) in Baltimore, Maryland, are looking at the effects of beta-amyloid on nerve cells from the cerebral cortex. So far, they have found that the cells try to defend themselves against attack from beta-amyloid by making cell stress proteins and other proteins that help prevent cell death. These scientists continue to study why these defense mechanisms fail to fully protect the cells.

Still, the way that beta-amyloid may cause nerve cells to die remains a mystery. Some studies indicate that beta-amyloid disrupts potassium channels, which in turn can affect calcium levels inside the cell. Potassium (an element or electrolyte) helps control the normal activity of nerves and muscles. Among other things, potassium channels (tunnel-like structures in cell membranes) help balance the amount of calcium that the cell takes in and removes. Calcium (another element or electrolyte) helps cells do many things, such as carry nerve signals. The correct amount of electrolytes, such as potassium and calcium, also helps the body use energy. However, too much calcium inside the cell leads to cell death.

A recent finding suggests that beta-amyloid itself is able to form small channels in the nerve cell membrane. These channels may allow too much calcium to enter a nerve cell, killing the cell.

Yet another study links beta-amyloid to lower choline levels in nerve cells. Since choline is a basic part of acetylcholine (a neurotransmitter), this finding suggests a link between beta-amyloid and decreases in acetylcholine levels found in the brains of people with AD.

Following a different line of reasoning, NIA researchers at the GRC in Baltimore suggest that APP may help repair injured brain cells. Scientists do not yet know how APP acts, but these researchers think that it may help keep brain tissue healthy and boost brain repair activities. According to these NIA investigators, someday, a form of APP may be used as a therapy to help reverse or even prevent further destruction due to AD.

More research is needed to determine the exact mechanism of selective nerve cell damage in the AD brain and the roles that beta-amyloid and APP play in this process.

Neurofibrillary Tangles

Neurofibrillary tangles are abnormal collections of twisted threads found inside nerve cells. The chief component of tangles is one form of the protein, tau. In the central nervous system, tau proteins are best known for their ability to bind and help stabilize microtubules (the cell's internal support structure or skeleton).

In healthy neurons, microtubules form structures like train tracks, which guide nutrients and molecules from the bodies of the cells down to the ends of the axons. In cells affected by AD, these structures collapse. Tau normally forms the "railroad ties" or connector pieces of the microtubule train tracks. However, in AD tau is changed chemically, and this altered tau can no longer hold the railroad ties together, causing the microtubule train tracks to fall apart. This collapse of the transport system first may result in malfunctions in communication between nerve cells and later may lead to neuron death.

In AD, chemically altered tau twists into paired helical filaments (two threads wound around each other). These filaments are the major substance found in neurofibrillary tangles.

Chapter 20

Advances in Identifying Risk Factors for Alzheimer's Disease

Researchers believe that Alzheimer's Disease (AD) is caused not by a single factor, but by a number of factors that interact differently in different people. Age remains the strongest risk factor identified for AD so far. In addition, having both apoE4 (a form of a certain protein called apolipoprotein E that is now recognized as a genetic risk factor for the common late-onset form of Alzheimer's disease) and a severe head injury that leads to even a brief loss of consciousness may increase a person's risk of developing AD later in life.

In most cases, genetic risk factors alone, as noted for apoE4, are not enough to trigger AD. Other risk factors may combine with a person's genetic makeup to increase his or her chances of developing AD.

Researchers looking at the frequency of AD and related dementias in people over age 65 seek to identify additional risk factors for AD and to show how and why AD develops. By studying various ethnic, racial, and social groups of people, scientists may discover new risk factors for AD. These risk factors, in turn, may suggest new theories about mechanisms involved in setting up and/or triggering the disease process.

Last year, researchers funded by the National Institute on Aging (NIA) made advances in many areas, including understanding the role of presenilin proteins 1 and 2 in AD, the possible relation between oxidative damage and AD, and how cultural or environmental changes

Excerpted from *Progress Report on Alzheimer's Disease, 1997,* National Institute on Aging, NIH Pub. No. 97-4014, November 1997.

may affect Japanese Americans' likelihood of developing AD. Findings from these and other investigations eventually may lead to new treatments and strategies for prevention.

Presenilins

In 1992, investigators supported by the NIA and the National Institute on Neurological Disorders and Stroke (NINDS) identified a defective gene (called presenilin 1) on chromosome 14 in people with AD in some inherited, early-onset AD families. Although researchers believe that presenilin 1 accounts for close to 50 percent of all cases of FAD (the most aggressive form), they do not know the function of this gene.

Scientists at several ADCs have found almost 30 mutations of presenilin 1 in approximately 50 early-onset AD families. These defects are scattered across the protein encoded by the mutated gene. Some of these mutations may lead to AD earlier than others. Rather than cause protein products to stop working, mutations may produce altered, harmful protein products.

Scientists do not know the normal function of presenilins or how mutations of these genes affect the onset of FAD. They also do not know whether presenilins play any role in the more common, sporadic or non-familial form of late-onset AD.

Much evidence suggests that neurons are a major source of the beta-amyloid that forms plaques in AD. Thus, it is important to study how presenilins function in neurons. Researchers are looking at how presenilins 1 and 2 interact with APP processing, plaques, tangles, and beta-amyloid. A recent study showed that people with early-onset AD and presenilin 1 and 2 mutations have more of a longer form of beta-amyloid in their brains than do those with the sporadic form of AD. This finding suggests that mutations in the presenilins may drive the production of amyloid in AD.

Oxidative Damage and Alzheimer's Disease

One long-standing theory of aging suggests that the buildup of damage from oxidation in the body causes nerve cells to gradually decay. Scientists believe that free radicals produced through oxidative mechanisms play a role in several diseases, including cancer and AD.

A free radical is a molecule with one unpaired (leftover) electron in its outer shell. Healthy metabolism can produce free radicals of oxygen with unpaired electrons. The body produces free radicals to help cells in certain ways, such as in fighting infections. However, having too many free radicals is bad for cells. Free radicals are highly reactive; they readily latch onto other molecules available nearby, such as part of the cell membrane or a piece of DNA. The resulting, newly combined molecule then can set off a chain reaction, releasing unwanted chemicals that can damage cells.

Free radicals are suspected to play a role in the development of AD for several reasons. They attach to molecules of fat in nerve cell membranes and thus may upset the delicate membrane machinery that regulates substances that go into and out of a cell, for example, calcium. As mentioned before, too much calcium can kill cells. Further, oxidation due to free radicals may alter proteins; these new forms of proteins may be associated with the development of AD. Some of these oxidative changes are found in amyloid plaques in AD, where beta-amyloid causes the release of free radicals. Reactions like these also produce several free radicals of oxygen that may target the internal support structures of nerve cells.

Scientists at Columbia University in New York City are studying a receptor on microglia (very small non-neuron cells found in the brain). They recently found that this receptor helps microglia bind to beta-amyloid. This binding leads to the release of reactive oxygen molecules and causes cells to become immobilized. Further studies are needed to understand the relation of oxidation to nerve cell damage in AD.

In 1996, investigators also at Columbia University identified a protein that binds to synthetic beta-amyloid. This protein is identical to the central receptor for advanced glycation end products (AGEs), which are the results of certain molecular processes within the body. This receptor for AGE may define how beta-amyloid interacts with nerve cells and surrounding cells. Interactions between beta-amyloid and this receptor may contribute directly to nerve cell damage that leads to dementia.

In another study, scientists at NIA's Laboratory of Biological Chemistry in Baltimore exposed nerve cell lines to the APP gene and the presenilin 2 gene, which each had mutations like those found in people with early-onset AD. These nerve cells were killed by the mutant products of the genes through programmed cell death. Nerve cells with extra mutated APP appeared to produce more free radicals. By adding anti-oxidants, such as vitamin E, that may intercept or latch onto free radicals before they have a chance to damage cells, researchers were able to prevent nerve cell damage related to beta-amyloid and caused by free radicals. These findings suggest that in AD, cell damage related to free radicals may cause nerve cells to die, and that anti-oxidants may help prevent nerve cell death. Anti-oxidants are found in common foods, especially those rich in vitamins A, C, and E.

Cultural or Environmental Changes, Japanese Americans, and Alzheimer's Disease

Looking at findings from the Honolulu-Asia Aging Study, NIA-supported researchers found that older Japanese American men have a higher rate of AD than their counterparts living in Japan. Analysts looked at data describing Japanese American men born between 1900 and 1919 who were living on Oahu, Hawaii, in 1965, when the study began.

Based on data collected between 1991 and 1993 for 3,734 survivors, 9.3 percent had dementia (from all causes) and 5.4 percent had AD. The scientists compared these findings to those from studies of similar men living in Japan.

In one such study, Japanese researchers recently found AD in 1.5 percent of 887 residents of Hisayama who were 65 years of age and older. Other Japanese studies also suggest lower rates of AD in the Japanese population.

The same NIA study looked at the frequency of vascular dementia-mental decline caused by reduced blood flow to the brain and small strokes. Researchers found that 4.2 percent of the Oahu participants had vascular dementia, compared to 3.2 percent of the Hisayama residents.

These comparisons suggest that AD is almost as common among older Japanese American men in Hawaii as it is in Americans of European ancestry, but it is less frequent in Japanese men living in Japan. Vascular dementia is only slightly less frequent among these Japanese Americans than among the Japanese. Researchers believe that environmental and lifestyle changes associated with migrating from Japan to Hawaii may have influenced the development of AD, while risk factors affecting the development of vascular dementia may have remained the same. Based on the results of the Oahu study, researchers will do more population studies to see if lifestyle changes after migration influence the occurrence of AD.

Brain Infarction and Alzheimer's Disease

NIA-funded researchers at the University of Kentucky's Sanders-Brown Research Center on Aging in Lexington studied the relationship between brain infarction and clinical signs of AD in a group of nuns. A brain infarction is an area of injury in brain tissue that occurs when the blood supply to that area is interrupted, or, less often, when a vein that carries blood away from the area is blocked in some way. Infarcts can be a sign of blood vessel disease and are thought to play a role in some strokes.

Scientists studied 102 members of the School Sisters of Notre Dame religious order who took part in the Nun Study, a long-term study of aging and AD. While in this study, the nuns completed regularly scheduled cognitive tests. Clinical signs of AD include impairments in the following skills: memory, concentration, language, visuospatial ability, orientation to time and place, and social and daily function. Autopsies were performed when the nuns died. During autopsies, researchers identified infarcts, amyloid plaques, and neurofibrillary tangles in the brains of these nuns.

Among 61 deceased participants who met the criteria for AD (had many amyloid plaques and neurofibrillary tangles in the brain), those with infarcts in particular brain regions previously had shown poorer cognitive function and more dementia than those without infarcts. Among 41 participants who did not meet the criteria for AD, brain infarcts were only weakly associated with previous poor cognitive function and dementia.

These findings suggest that at least some brain infarcts do not themselves cause dementia, but may play an important role in increasing the severity of the clinical signs of AD. In addition, other signs of disease related to the brain's blood vessels or blood supply, such as atherosclerosis, may be involved in the development of AD. Atherosclerosis (often called "hardening of the arteries") is a common disorder of the arteries in which yellowish plaques of cholesterol, fat, and other remains are deposited in the walls of some arteries (blood vessels that carry blood with oxygen away from the heart to the rest of the body). Further research is needed to understand whether preventing these types of blood vessel diseases in the brain can help reduce the clinical signs of AD.

Chapter 21

Genetic Factors in Alzheimer's Disease

Every healthy person has 46 chromosomes in 23 pairs. Usually, people receive one chromosome in each pair from each parent. Chromosomes are rod-like structures in the cell nucleus. In each chromosome, DNA forms two long, intertwined, thread-like strands that carry inherited information in the form of genes.

Genes are basic units of heredity that can direct almost every aspect of the construction, operation, and repair of living organisms. Each gene is a set of chemical instructions that tells a cell how to make one of the many unique proteins in the body. Every human cell has from 50,000 to 100,000 genes arranged on the chromosomes like beads on a string.

Genes are made up of four chemicals (bases) arranged in various patterns along the strands of DNA. In each gene, the bases are lined up in a different order, and each sequence of bases directs the production of a different protein. Even slight changes in a gene's DNA code can make a faulty protein, and a faulty protein can lead to cell malfunction and possibly disease.

Two types of Alzheimer's disease (AD) exist: familial Alzheimer's disease (FAD), which is found in families where AD follows a certain inheritance pattern; and sporadic (seemingly random) AD, where no obvious inheritance pattern is seen. Because of differences in age at onset, AD is further described as either early-onset (younger than 65

Excerpted from *Progress Report on Alzheimer's Disease, 1997*, National Institute on Aging, NIH Pub. No. 97-4014, November 1997.

years old) or late-onset (65 years and older). Early-onset AD is rare and generally affects people aged 30 to 60. Early-onset AD progresses faster than the more common, late-onset forms of AD.

Almost all FAD known so far is early-onset, and many cases involve defects in three genes located on three different chromosomes (chromosomes 1, 14, and 21). Until recently, AD genetic research was dominated by the discovery that an unidentified defective gene on a particular region of chromosome 21 was the cause of AD in a few early-onset families. This finding was followed by the identification of gene mutations in the APP gene on chromosome 21 as the cause of AD in these families. (In affected people, the gene on chromosome 21 carries the code for an abnormal form of APP.)

This emphasis shifted in 1992, when researchers at the University of Washington Alzheimer's Disease Center (ADC) in Seattle—supported by the NIA and the National Institute of Neurological Disorders and Stroke (NINDS)—discovered a link between other FAD cases and genes in a particular region of chromosome 14. They subsequently identified the defective gene and named it presenilin 1.

More recently, these same scientists also found a link between FAD in families descended from a group of Germans living in the Volga Valley of the former Soviet Union (called the Volga Germans) and a gene in a particular region of chromosome 1. These families have a higher than average occurrence of AD and show no link to AD through genes on either chromosome 21 or 14. These investigators and others funded by the NIA and the NINDS at the Massachusetts ADC in Boston and in Toronto, Canada, identified the defective gene on chromosome 1 and called it presenilin 2. In these inherited forms of the disease, inheriting the mutation almost always results in the person getting AD. Only a very small fraction of early-onset FAD is caused by mutations in the presenilin 2 gene.

Together, these mutations (presenilins 1 and 2) account for approximately 50 percent of early-onset FAD. The other genes have yet to be identified. (For additional information about these "presenilin" genes, see Presenilins.)

Pursuing another avenue, researchers at the NIA are looking at Down's syndrome because it shares some traits with AD. Down's syndrome is caused by a birth defect in which the person has three, rather than the normal two, copies of chromosome 21. Down's syndrome is associated with mental retardation and the development of AD pathology. Because the gene for APP has been mapped to chromosome 21, researchers believe that AD is related to the "overexpression" of APP.

Some gene changes occur more often in AD patients than among people in general. In 1992, researchers at the Duke University ADC in Durham, North Carolina, found an increased risk for late-onset AD with inheritance of the apoE4 (apolipoprotein E4) allele on chromosome 19. An allele is one of two or more alternate forms of the same gene. This finding helped scientists explain variations in age at onset, based on whether people had zero, one, or two copies of apoE4.

Every person has two apoE genes, one inherited from each parent. AD researchers are interested in three common alleles of apoE: apoE2, apoE3, and apoE4. They are studying people who inherit different forms of this gene to learn more about risk factors for AD. A simple blood test can be used to determine which alleles a person has inherited.

ApoE is a protein that sits on the surface of the cholesterol molecule and helps carry blood cholesterol throughout the body. ApoE is found in neurons of healthy brains, but also is associated with the plaques and neurofibrillary tangles found in AD brains.

The relatively rare apoE2 may protect some people against the disease; it seems to be associated with a lower risk for AD and later age of onset. ApoE2 also appears to protect people with Down's syndrome from developing AD. ApoE3 is the most common version found in the general population; researchers believe it plays a neutral role in AD.

AD scientists are most interested in apoE4 because it is linked to an increased risk of the disease. The apoE4 form in AD patients is not limited to those with a family history of AD. In addition, people who carry two copies of apoE4 are more likely to get AD than those with one copy of apoE4. How apoE4 increases a person's susceptibility to AD (likelihood of developing AD) is not yet known. ApoE4 may contribute to beta-amyloid buildup and APP regulation. ApoE4 also appears to lower the age of onset of AD, perhaps because apoE4 speeds up the AD process in some unknown way. Researchers believe that AD risk related to apoE4 may increase because the age of onset decreases.

A flurry of activity has followed the apoE findings to discover the molecular mechanisms that underlie the effects of the different forms of apoE on the development of AD. Scientists are looking at how the different forms of apoE interact with both beta-amyloid and tau. Researchers also are studying how forms of apoE affect the way that cells remodel themselves and grow after being damaged.

Whatever its role in AD, the mere inheritance of an apoE4 gene does not predict AD with certainty; that is, apoE4 is a risk factor gene.

A person can have an apoE4 gene and not get the disease, and a person with AD may not have any apoE4 genes. As of now, no predictive test for AD exists. Even with the current knowledge about apoE, scientists cannot predict whether or when any person might develop AD, no more than a doctor can predict whether a person with high cholesterol will have a stroke. However, many researchers believe that inheriting an apoE4 gene, in association with lower memory performance in older people that gradually worsens with time, may be a predictor for who is going to develop AD.

Genetic analysis someday could help scientists find people with probable AD to include in clinical trials of promising treatments. Because of the increased risk associated with apoE4, people with clinical signs of AD who have this allele may be among the first volunteers to be studied in clinical trials of experimental drugs.

It may follow that having multiple risk-factor genes may increase a person's likelihood of developing AD. With each new finding, researchers gain more clues about basic mechanisms in AD and move closer to understanding the disease and designing treatments that slow its progression, delay its onset, or even prevent it.

Transgenic Mouse Model for Alzheimer's Disease

A team of researchers at the University of Minnesota in Rochester; Veterans Administration Medical Center in Sepulveda, California; Mayo Clinic in Jacksonville, Florida; and other institutions have developed a new mouse model for AD. The National Institutes on Aging (NIA), the National Institute of Neurological Disorders and Stroke (NINDS), and the Alzheimer's Association supported this research.

This research team has used the gene coding for APP to breed mice that make the mutated version of the APP protein in brain cells. The mice are double mutants of a human APP form in which two parts of the protein are changed. These changes mimic those in APP found in a large human family with early-onset FAD. This genetically-engineered (transgenic) mouse is the first to show cognitive signs of AD as well as protein-derived plaques like those found in the brain tissue of AD patients.

Early in life, at 2 to 3 months of age, these transgenic mice appear normal. But later, at 9 to 10 months and older, the mice have problems doing several memory and spatial learning tasks that a group of healthy, similarly trained mice can do without difficulty. These deficits were correlated with a greater buildup of both amyloid and the mutant APP. In 1-year-old transgenic mice, plaques and amyloid deposits outside nerve cells were observed in the cerebral cortex. These deposits were not found in younger mice and controls. The oldest transgenic mice had between 5 and 14 times more beta-amyloid peptides (small protein fragments) associated with amyloid plaques than did younger, healthy mice. Thus, there was an association between the amounts of mutant APP and the onset of problems in learning and memory in the oldest transgenic mice.

These mice give scientists the opportunity to study the relationship among certain mutations related to AD, abnormal behaviors, and changes in the brain, for example, the evolution and control of plaque development. This animal model will increase researchers' understanding of how AD progresses and ultimately make it possible for them to test promising therapies in mice showing some AD symptoms.

For years, scientists have debated whether amyloid plaques cause AD or result from some process in the development of AD. The transgenic mouse model is the first animal model to show that amyloid is associated with deficits in learning and memory. However, researchers do not yet know whether the deficits are caused by, or merely correlate with, the buildup of amyloid. The mouse model can be used to study this question.

Chapter 22

Advances in Diagnosing Alzheimer's Disease

Alzheimer's disease (AD) is diagnosed conclusively only by an autopsy after death. Its telltale signs during life, such as dementia symptoms, also may be caused by other problems. To confirm AD, pathologists look for the presence of characteristic plaques and tangles in brain tissue during an autopsy.

Through the work of many researchers, the diagnosis of AD in living people has become more and more accurate. In specialized research facilities, neurologists now can diagnose AD with up to 90 percent accuracy, as confirmed later at autopsy. The diagnosis includes taking a personal history from patients and their families, doing a physical exam and tests, and administering memory and psychological tests to patients. Nonetheless, important questions and knowledge gaps remain.

Now, tests of mental status are needed that can pinpoint the gradual loss of cognitive ability in AD patients and identify people who are at a very early stage in the course of the disease. The search continues for reliable biological markers for diagnosing AD. The sooner an accurate diagnosis of AD is made, the greater the gain in managing symptoms, determining the natural history of AD, and defining subtypes of patients. An early, accurate diagnosis of AD is especially important to patients and their families because it helps them plan for the future and pursue care options, while the patient still can take part in decisions.

Excerpted from *Progress Report on Alzheimer's Disease, 1997*, National Institute on Aging, NIH Pub. No. 97-4014, November 1997.

The National Institute on Aging (NIA) supports research aimed at developing and testing reliable, valid diagnostic tools for AD and other dementias in older people. One possible advance in AD diagnosis was the discovery of apoE4 by NIA-funded researchers at the Duke University ADC in 1992. Before 1992, scientists studied people who were said to have probable or possible AD based on a clinical diagnosis alone. A later Duke University study asked whether obtaining a person's apoE4 status would increase diagnostic accuracy while the person still was alive.

In this study, each study participant's clinical diagnosis was confirmed after death with an autopsy, and each participant's apoE status was determined. The findings show that every participant with at least one apoE4 allele and a clinical diagnosis of probable or possible AD was confirmed to have AD according to the autopsy criteria. These initial results need to be verified in a larger sample. Currently, all of the ADCs are taking part in a further cooperative study to determine if these preliminary results can be confirmed.

Another promising new finding could contribute to the identification of patients at risk for AD. Collaborating scientists at the NIA, the National Cancer Institute, and the Howard University College of Medicine in Washington, District of Columbia, studied fibroblasts (cells from tissue that supports and joins collections of cells or parts of the body) and lymphocytes (one of two types of small white blood cells that play a role in fighting disease). They exposed the cells to fluorescent light and used agents to block the cells' natural tendency to repair strands of DNA. Cells from study participants with Down's syndrome or AD showed flaws in how the cells tried to repair the damage to DNA caused by fluorescent light. These results suggest that scientists might be able to use such techniques to develop a test that identifies people at higher and lower risk for losing cognitive skills due to AD. Further research is needed to confirm these initial findings.

Other research by NIA scientists indicates that autopsied brain tissue from AD patients shows a marked decrease in messenger ribonucleic acid (RNA) and protein needed for enzymes involved in a body process related to metabolism, especially in neurons containing high levels of tangles. This decrease may be a marker for the loss in the ability of cells to communicate with each other in affected regions of the AD brain. Within a cell, messenger RNA is a substance that carries genetic information from DNA in the nucleus to the rest of the cell where proteins are made. When levels of messenger RNA and proteins needed for certain metabolic processes fall, nerve cells may be less able to communicate between themselves and tangles may develop within cells. Additional work will aim to distinguish whether the molecular changes are the cause or the result of decreased neuron activity, and whether it might be possible to reverse the changes, thus making the neurons more active again.

In addition, many researchers are working to develop a better way to picture metabolism in the living brain using positron emission tomography (PET) scanning. NIA's Laboratory of Neurosciences (LNS) in Bethesda, Maryland, has begun to use certain fatty acids as one agent in imaging studies. Fatty acids may help scientists evaluate metabolic processes in the brain related to how the body breaks down and uses important energy-producing substances, including fatty acids and nitrogen. Some scientists believe that this type of metabolism in the brain is a better indicator of brain activity than just blood flow, which is routinely measured in PET scans.

In continuing the search for ways to diagnose AD, other NIA researchers studying brain function in people with Down's syndrome have shown a gradual decline in cerebral blood flow that seems to mimic that in AD. The difference in metabolic activity in certain brain regions at rest versus stimulation may be an early indicator of disease. The failure of certain areas to show an increase in metabolic activity when the patient performs a memory task is a sign that the brain is not functioning properly. This finding could lead to an early diagnosis of AD in patients in high risk groups based on their family history or apoE4 status.

Scientists at NIA's LNS have developed a passive test of memory that does not require patients to actively take part in a study. To complete standard memory tests, patients must be able to think, hear, see, speak, and write well enough to do memory tasks on demand. Most patients in the later stages of AD and dementia are unable to take part in research studies or to complete tests because they have lost so many of these abilities or they forget the instructions.

LNS's researchers have developed tests to get around this major obstacle. Instead of using standard memory tests, they show a particular visual pattern of dots to AD patients. Viewing dots that are arranged in even or balanced patterns causes activity in the cerebral cortex of the brain that mimics what happens when a patient is asked to remember something. After repeated exposure to the even patterns, stimulation of the hippocampus can be seen, even in patients who are in the later stages of AD and cannot take part in standard learning and memory tests. This test may enable scientists to study patients with severe dementia and to look for ways to improve their cortical

239

function. It may lead to a way for scientists to measure how treatments that might improve cognition affect pathways in the brain activated by passive stimulation.

Ongoing work by NIA researchers has shown that at least part of the low performance of AD patients on memory tasks is due to their poor visual attention span. Being able to maintain visuospatial attention leads to better performance on memory tests. In 1996, scientists showed that one subgroup of possible AD patients with visual disturbances had lower metabolic activity mainly toward the back of the brain, in regions associated with vision. The common form of AD has low metabolic activity in other areas of the brain. Autopsy confirmation of the clinical diagnosis in these patients will show whether they had a form of AD or a different disease.

In addition, investigators at NIA's Laboratory of Personality and Cognition at the Gerontology Research Center in Baltimore are evaluating other tests as early indicators of AD. They found that an exam called the Trail-Making Test can tell the difference between normal and abnormal changes in cognition with age. This test may help identify patients with early AD who might be candidates for treatment. However, before this test can be used outside of a research setting, further studies are needed to confirm these findings.

Diagnostic Criteria for Alzheimer's Disease

Criteria for diagnosing AD at autopsy were developed in 1983. Now, researchers are trying to refine diagnostic methods using new knowledge about the locations of plaques and tangles in the brain.

An international panel of 17 neuroscientists—the National Institute on Aging and Reagan Institute Working Group on Diagnostic Criteria for the Neuropathological Assessment of Alzheimer's Disease—met in November of 1996 to revise the guidelines for diagnosing AD at autopsy. The Working Group examined recent research concerning changes in plaques and tangles, synapses, dendrites, and molecular events that may lead to the formation of plaques and tangles. They discussed how these findings eventually might improve AD diagnosis.

Earlier guidelines called for evaluating plaque density as a diagnostic marker for AD. The Working Group called for definitions of low, moderate, and high probability of AD based on the numbers of neuritic plaques as well as neurofibrillary tangles in brain tissue after death. The Working Group recommended that pathologists record the number of amyloid plaques and neurofibrillary tangles that they find during an autopsy, along with other signs of damage, such as Lewy bodies and vascular lesions, that are likely to cause loss of mental function. (In Lewy body dementia, round, abnormal structures called Lewy bodies develop in cells within the midbrain and cerebral cortex, and significant plaques and tangles are absent.)

New Guidelines for Early Recognition and Assessment of Alzheimer's Disease Symptoms

The Agency for Health Care Policy and Research (AHCPR), part of the Federal Government's Public Health Service, brought together a panel of experts from the private sector to develop a Clinical Practice Guideline (AHCPR Guideline 19) for identifying AD and related dementias. The NIA provided some staff as leaders for the panel.

The panel focused on identifying early dementia in people showing certain symptoms that signal the need for further assessment. The panel's primary goal was to increase the early recognition and assessment of a potential dementing illness to: eliminate concern when it is not warranted, identify and address treatable conditions, and diagnose non-reversible conditions early enough so patients and their families might plan for the future. The panel also sought to improve the early detection of AD and related dementias in people showing certain signs and behaviors; educate health professionals, patients, and their families about symptoms that suggest the need for an initial assessment for a dementing disorder; and identify areas for further research on early recognition of dementia.

In 1996, the AHCPR reported the following major findings of the panel:

- certain triggers should prompt a doctor to perform an initial assessment for dementia, rather than attribute apparent signs of mental decline to aging

- an initial clinical assessment should combine information from a focused history and physical exam, an evaluation of mental and functional status, reliable informant reports, as well as assessments for delirium and depression

- the Functional Activities Questionnaire is useful in the initial assessment for functional impairment

- the Mini-Mental State Examination, the Blessed Information-Memory-Concentration Test, the Blessed Orientation-Memory-Concentration Test, and the Short Test of Mental Status are

241

effective mental status tests that discriminate early-stage dementia equally well

- doctors should assess and consider factors such as sensory impairment and physical disability in selecting mental and functional status tests, and other confounding factors such as older age, educational level, and cultural influence in interpreting test results

In people who have possible risk factors for AD (e.g., family history and Down's syndrome) but do not show obvious symptoms, the panel recommends that the doctor's judgment and knowledge of the patient's current condition, history, and social situation should guide the decision to initiate an assessment for dementia.

In summary, AHCPR Guideline 19 outlines methods for assessing people for dementia and interpreting results; the role of neuropsychological testing; the importance of followup; key points about AD for health care providers and patients; and symptoms that might indicate dementia.

Chapter 23

New Research Suggests Method for Pre-symptomatic Diagnosis of Dementias

A research study at the National Institute on Aging (NIA) suggests that a new method using brain scans may detect brain changes predictive of dementia before memory loss begins. If this or other methods prove effective in larger scale testing, then research could be directed at developing drugs to help arrest or slow the disease process before significant damage is done to the brain.

The research is reported in the August, 1997 issue of *The American Journal of Psychiatry* (Pietrini P et al., "Low Glucose Metabolism During Brain Stimulation in Older Down's Syndrome Subjects at Risk for Alzheimer's Disease Prior to Dementia", *Am J. Psychiatry*, 154:8, 1997), and was conducted by a team of NIA scientists headed by Pietro Pietrini, M.D. Ph.D., and Mark B. Schapiro, M.D. The researchers studied volunteers with Down's syndrome because most patients exhibit neuropathology similar to that of Alzheimer's disease after middle age and develop many cognitive defects similar to those in Alzheimer's disease later in life.

In order to test whether development of an Alzheimer's-like dementia could be predicted well before the onset of any outward mental or physical signs, the researchers chose 16 healthy Down's syndrome adults. They divided the patients into a younger group between the ages of 32 to 38 and an older group between the ages 43 to 61 which might be expected to be developing early Alzheimer's-like pathology. By using positron emission tomography (PET), the scientists were able

National Institute on Aging, Press Release, August 1, 1997.

to observe brain activity while the subjects were at rest (wearing earplugs and blindfolds) or while their brains were stimulated by viewing a movie. In order to assure their comfort and ease, we monitored these patients' anxiety levels during PET testing. Variations in activity in specific regions of brain in the PET scans showed researchers where there were low activity levels, which are associated with early Alzheimer's disease.

According to Dr. Pietrini, "although persons with Down's do not develop dementia at the same ages as persons who develop Alzheimer's disease, they comprise an excellent group for study because of the high incidence rate for Alzheimer's-like dementia in this population. I believe we have identified evidence of dementia at a much earlier stage than previously described by other investigators. We saw no difference in resting brain activity but when we looked at stimulated brain activity, we were able to see decreases in our older group of patients in areas of the brain that we know show Alzheimer's-like tissue changes."

Dr. Schapiro adds, "The subjects in the present study were all healthy and exhibited no outward signs of dementia. The inability of this group to respond normally to visual stimulation indicates that the disease process leads to changes in brain function even sooner than we expected. We also found that in this older group, during stimulation, the left side of the brain seemed to be more impaired than the right, suggesting that the left side of the brain may be preferentially affected early in the disease process. As an interesting unexpected observation, cognitive function that was not related to memory was not impaired, suggesting some plasticity, which is the ability of the brain to compensate for metabolic impairments during the stimulation activity."

According to Dr. Pietrini, "It must be pointed out, however, that this study was done on a small group of persons with Down's and must be replicated on a much larger scale and in other people at risk for Alzheimer's before actual testing of interventions using this procedure could be advised or planned. Studies that specifically identified persons in the pre-symptomatic stages of Alzheimer's would give us early clues as to the promise of actual interventions that could be put into practice in years to come."

Alzheimer's disease affects 4 million Americans and that number is expected to increase several-fold as more people live longer. Prevention or treatment of the disease is thus of great practical importance, and as has been learned in many human diseases, the earlier one can intervene in the disease process, the greater the likelihood for a positive long-term outcome.

Other investigators who took part in the study from the NIA are Alessio Dani, M.D., Maura Furey, Ph.D., Gene E. Alexander, Ph.D., Ulderico Freo, M.D., Cheryl L. Grady, Ph.D., Marc J. Mentis, M.D., David Mangot, B.S., Elliot W. Simon, Ph.D., Barry Horwitz, Ph.D., and James V. Haxby, Ph.D.

The National Institute on Aging, one of the 18 Institutes which make up the National Institutes of Health, leads the Federal effort supporting basic, clinical, epidemiological and social research on Alzheimer's disease and the special needs of older people.

For more information on the NIA and aging in general, please visit our web site at http://www.nih.gov/nia. For general information on Alzheimer's disease and for information on participation in NIA clinical studies, contact NIA's Alzheimer's Disease Education and Referral (ADEAR) Center, toll-free, at 1-800-438-4380.

For more information on the NIA and aging in general, please visit our web site at http://www.nih.gov/nia. General information is also available from our resource center by calling, toll-free, 1-800-222-2225.

Chapter 24

Advances in Treating and Preventing Alzheimer's Disease

Immediate goals in treating and managing the dementia symptoms of Alzheimer's disease are to slow, reduce, and/or reverse its mental and behavioral signs. The eventual goal is to stop the disease process altogether. Scientists are pursuing many leads to accomplish these goals, but the current focus is on the patient's symptoms and unusual behaviors.

Researchers, including those supported by the NIA, have begun to test the effectiveness of drugs on the mental and behavioral aspects of AD. Several clinical trials are testing a variety of compounds. Scientists are looking for treatments that work on many patients, stay effective for a long time, ease a broad range of symptoms, improve patients' activities of daily living and cognitive function, and have no serious side effects.

Treatments also are needed for managing unusual behaviors, such as verbal and physical aggression, agitation, wandering, depression, sleep disturbances, and delusions that occur in AD. Preliminary studies suggest that these types of behaviors greatly influence families' decisions to move loved ones to care outside the home. Improving these behaviors could delay or even prevent placement in long-term care facilities, maintain patients' dignity, reduce caregiver stress, and lower overall costs to families and to society.

Excerpted from *Progress Report on Alzheimer's Disease, 1997*, National Institute on Aging, NIH Pub. No. 97-4014, 1997.

247

In 1996, the Food and Drug Administration (FDA) approved donepezil hydrochloride (Aricept) to help treat some mild to moderate symptoms of AD. Aricept (also known as E2020) is the second drug approved by the FDA to treat AD. The first drug, tacrine (Cognex), has been marketed since 1993.

Both Aricept and Cognex slow the breakdown of acetylcholine, a key neurotransmitter in cognitive functioning. However, neither drug stops nor reverses the progression of AD. Occasional side effects of Aricept include diarrhea and nausea. The drug also can cause an irregular heartbeat, especially in patients with heart conditions. Fainting spells have been reported in some patients. However, Aricept seems not to affect liver enzymes, an effect that prevented many patients from taking Cognex. Most researchers agree that neither Aricept nor Cognex works for all, or even most, patients so that the drugs' effects and duration of usefulness are limited.

In studies on animals, scientists at the NIA have preliminary evidence suggesting that a new drug, phenserine (a cholinesterase inhibitor), may be useful in treating AD patients. In animal models of cognitive decline, phenserine was significantly more effective in enhancing performance and learning in a maze test than drugs currently marketed to treat AD. Phenserine is undergoing toxicology testing (studies to find safe doses and any potentially problematic side effects). Similarly, NIA scientists recently found that a drug called arecoline seems to improve cognitive function and the process whereby chemical messages are sent across synapses in animals. Researchers now are studying the effects of arecoline in people.

Still other NIA investigators have found that physostigmine helps improve working memory in healthy people by shortening the amount of time needed to react to study tasks and enhancing activity in a certain part of the brain. Physostigmine is a drug that also blocks the breakdown of acetylcholine and improves the way that acetylcholine sends messages at synapses. Scientists now are studying this drug in AD patients.

These drugs (Aricept, Cognex, and physostigmine) only temporarily halt or reverse cognitive losses from AD, and do not prevent AD from continuing to kill the nerve cells that normally produce acetylcholine. Therefore, researchers are looking for other drugs to slow or prevent AD and to help vital acetylcholine-producing cells survive longer.

The search for more effective ways to treat and prevent AD includes studying the use of estrogen, anti-inflammatory drugs, and other compounds in AD patients; determining which groups of people develop AD; and conducting several initiatives related to caregiving.

Estrogen Replacement Therapy and Alzheimer's Disease

In looking for factors associated with earlier or later onset of AD, the NIA and the National Center for Research Resources funded researchers at Columbia University. These investigators found that estrogen replacement therapy (ERT) was associated with a reduced incidence of AD in a group of older women. Incidence is the rate at which new cases of a disease occur. Study volunteers, initially free of AD, were taking part in a long-term study of aging and health. This 5-year investigation was unique because all of the women were examined and interviewed about their estrogen use before they developed AD symptoms; and it was the first AD study group with similar numbers of older women of African American, European, and Hispanic American ancestry. Previous studies depended on the review of death certificates and patients' and/or caregivers' memories of using estrogen.

Researchers compared the self-reported history of estrogen use, medical history, apoE4 status, ethnic group, age, and education of 1,124 women. In this study, only 9 of the 156 women age 70 and older who had used estrogen for from 2 months to 49 years developed AD. Among 968 participants who never had used estrogen, 158 developed AD during the study. The estimated annual incidence rate for AD among women in the study who took estrogen was 2.7 percent, compared to 8.4 percent among those who did not take estrogen.

These results suggest that estrogen use during and after menopause may significantly lower the risk of AD and delay the onset of AD symptoms. The duration of estrogen use also seemed important in reducing risk. Women with a history of long-term use (more than 10 years) had the lowest risk. But, even women who took estrogen for a short time and then stopped also benefited. From this study, researchers conclude, for example, that a woman who takes estrogen for 10 years at and after menopause may reduce her risk of developing AD by 30 to 40 percent, compared to other women her age.

Scientists at Johns Hopkins University in Baltimore reported similar results related to estrogen use among women in the Baltimore Longitudinal Study of Aging (BLSA). A long-term NIA study, the BLSA includes a physical and mental assessment of 2,283 men and women who were healthy at the start of the study. In a retrospective study (looking at what occurred in the past) of one group of BLSA women, a history of ERT was associated with a reduction in AD risk by about half, also suggesting that estrogen helps protect women from AD. This beneficial effect is added to the lower incidence of heart disease and osteoporosis (a disorder in which normal bone tissue is lost) for women who take estrogen after menopause.

Estrogen is a hormone, a body chemical that starts or runs the activity of an organ or a group of cells. Some scientists believe that estrogen's role is in helping brain cells survive, which in turn delays the onset of AD. Other researchers think that estrogen aids the metabolism of APP, preventing it from forming beta-amyloid fibers. Still others propose that estrogen may work as an anti-oxidant to protect nerve cells. Additional laboratory research is needed to learn exactly how estrogen may protect women from AD. In turn, this research will help scientists develop new treatments for the disease.

While these findings are encouraging, clinical trials are needed before doctors can recommend estrogen to women for delaying or preventing AD. Clinical trials will determine whether estrogen therapy can delay or prevent the onset of AD as well as the safety, dose, and duration of estrogen treatment needed to produce these effects. One such clinical trial, the Alzheimer's disease Cooperative Study (ADCS) trial of estrogen, is assessing the effect of ERT on the progression of AD in postmenopausal women who have the disease.

Anti-Inflammatory Drugs and Alzheimer's Disease

A growing body of evidence suggests a link between inflammation and some changes that occur in the brains of AD patients. However, scientists do not know yet whether inflammation is a cause or an effect of the disease.

Researchers in NIA's 40-year BLSA believe they have found a link between anti-inflammatory drugs and a lowered risk of AD. Scientists surveyed 1,417 men and 648 women enrolled in the BLSA between 1955 and 1994 about their use of medications. A total of 110 participants eventually were diagnosed with AD. Those who regularly used non-steroidal anti-inflammatory drugs (NSAIDs) other than aspirin had a lower risk of developing AD than those who took acetaminophen (Tylenol) or no painkillers at all. For men and women in the BLSA study who took NSAIDs regularly for even as little as 2 years, researchers found a lower risk of AD by as much as 60 percent. NSAIDs include ibuprofen (Advil, Motrin), naproxen sodium (Aleve), indomethacin (Indocin), and many other painkillers. Tylenol has no anti-inflammatory properties. Aspirin users had a slightly decreased risk of AD, but this drop was not statistically significant in this particular study.

Scientists advise against taking NSAIDs to prevent AD based on these results alone. The BLSA survey neither distinguished among the various NSAIDs nor compared specific doses. Further, it relied on the self-reports of those interviewed. Moreover, NSAIDs have potentially serious side effects, particularly stomach irritation and ulcers. Further research is needed to determine whether NSAIDs decrease a person's risk of developing AD and, if decreased risk is established, to develop anti-inflammatory drugs with less severe side effects.

Another NIA-supported study suggests that older people who regularly take aspirin or other anti-inflammatory drugs may be at lower risk of age-related cognitive decline, including AD. Scientists studied changes in mental ability over 3 years among 7,671 older volunteers who are taking part in the Established Populations for Epidemiologic Studies of the Elderly. Twenty-one percent of the participants took NSAIDs regularly at the beginning of the study.

After 3 years, participants who regularly used NSAIDs had significantly better cognitive function than those who had not taken NSAIDs. On average, the cognitive ability of a volunteer taking NSAIDs was equal to that of a person 3.5 years younger. Using NSAIDs was associated with a reduced risk of significant cognitive decline by about 20 percent. Mental decline was more likely to occur in female, older, and less-educated volunteers and in participants who had survived a previous stroke.

Researchers previously had noted that AD is less common in arthritis patients. Now it appears that this finding may be associated with the high rate of NSAID use by arthritis patients. The way NSAIDs might reduce the risk of cognitive decline is unclear. However, some scientists think that NSAIDs may help prevent the inflammation found in the brains of people with AD.

These findings do not confirm that taking NSAIDs can prevent cognitive decline. As with estrogen, the only way to prove a cause-and-effect relationship is through careful studies (clinical trials) in which older participants are assigned randomly to take NSAIDs or not and then reexamined several times over a long period. Until these studies are performed and the results carefully evaluated, taking NSAIDs to preserve cognitive function is not advised unless recommended by a doctor. Information gleaned from these and other studies (such as the ADCS's investigation of the steroidal anti-inflammatory drug, prednisone) brings scientists closer to being able to treat AD patients.

Use of Selegiline and Vitamin E to Treat Alzheimer's Disease

Oxidative changes are seen in the brains of AD patients. Studies of compounds that fight oxidation put researchers one step closer to understanding processes that damage cells and finding ways to treat and possibly prevent AD. The NIA-supported ADCS trial of selegiline (l-deprenyl or Eldepryl) and alpha-tocopherol (vitamin E) is one such study.

Both selegiline and vitamin E act as anti-oxidants. Selegiline, which has been used to treat patients with Parkinson's disease, works by inhibiting an enzyme in the brain that impairs certain neurotransmitter systems.

For 2 years, researchers studied 341 moderately impaired patients with probable AD who were recruited from 23 centers taking part in the ADCS. Participants were divided into four groups that received different treatments: selegiline, vitamin E, both selegiline and vitamin E, or a placebo (an inactive substance). Scientists compared the amount of time it took patients in each group to reach one of the following outcomes: death, institutionalization, loss of the ability to do basic activities of daily living (such as handling money, bathing, dressing, and eating), and severe dementia. They looked at the signs of AD that can worsen over time.

The results suggest that compared to those who took a placebo, the estimated average time to reach any one of the four outcomes increased by 230 days for participants who took vitamin E, 215 days for those who took selegiline, and 145 days for those took both selegiline and vitamin E combined. Also compared to those who took a placebo, members of the treatment groups showed some improvements related to their level of independence and behavioral symptoms. No effect was found on cognitive measures.

Overall, this study shows that treatment with selegiline or vitamin E reduced moderately impaired AD patients' risk of reaching one of the four primary outcomes, with an estimated average delay of 6.5 months. In addition, these findings support the idea that damage due to oxidation plays a role in AD.

Scientists caution that further research is needed to confirm these preliminary findings. Researchers need to find out if these types of drugs actually can delay the development of symptoms much earlier in the course of the disease and learn how these drugs might affect patients at different stages of AD. They also need to study if the positive findings related to function occurred because the anti-oxidants improved other aspects of the patients' health, such as heart-related effects, rather than specifically fighting oxidation in the brain.

Investigators further warn that selegiline may have potential side effects and interactions with other drugs. In addition, the dosage of vitamin E used in this study was much higher than that typically found in daily supplements. Vitamin E may be associated with an increased risk of bleeding in some people. AD patients and their families should consult their doctors to see whether these drugs or others approved by the FDA may be appropriate for a particular AD patient.

Alzheimer's Disease Cooperative Study

The ADCS was established in 1991 to build the organizational structure needed for many centers to cooperate in testing promising drugs in AD and to develop and improve tests for evaluating AD patients in clinical trials.

The following six studies began in the first 5-year grant period (some were completed by June 1996 and others still are ongoing): safety and effectiveness of selegiline and vitamin E (results published); tests in English that measure treatment efficacy (results in press); tests in Spanish that measure treatment efficacy (results in analysis); use of haloperidol, trazodone, and behavioral management techniques in patients with disruptive agitated behavior (results in analysis); use of ERT in women with mild to moderate AD (still recruiting participants); and use of the anti-inflammatory drug prednisone (results in analysis).

Five more proposed studies have been approved for the next 5-year grant period: development of improved measures of treatment efficacy; an anti-inflammatory study; AIT-082 (a molecule derived from hypoxanthine and procaine) in AD (in a Phase I study, which means the drug is being given to a small number of volunteers to determine toxic levels and safe doses); melatonin and sleep disorders in AD; and divalproex sodium (Depakote), an anti-seizure drug, as therapy for agitation and dementia in nursing home residents.

Alzheimer's Disease Centers

The NIA funds 27 ADCs across the United States. Each ADC supports four common functions: clinical practice, neuropathology, education and information transfer, and administration. The comprehensive ADCs also receive funding to perform specific research studies on AD. ADCs also perform other functions, such as neuroimaging. The primary goals of the ADC Program are to promote research, training and education, technology transfer, and multicenter and cooperative studies in the diagnosis and treatment of AD.

Much of the success in AD research in this country since 1985 can be attributed to resources provided by the NIA to the ADCs. Recent advances include linking genes on chromosomes 1, 14, and 21 to FAD and identifying inherited risk factors related to apoE. In addition, researchers at the ADCs helped lay the groundwork for studying how proteins associated with amyloid plaques and neurofibrillary tangles are processed.

Other programs funded by the NIA depend on research activities at the ADCs, including regular, investigator-initiated studies; the Consortium To Establish a Registry for Alzheimer's Disease (CERAD); and the ADCS. In addition to conducting research and pilot research projects, the ADCs contribute resources such as patient data, brain and other tissue samples, and molecular probes to other scientific programs. The ADCs also serve as a resource for many types of studies testing new AD treatments.

In 1990, NIA began a program to link satellite diagnostic and treatment clinics to the ADCs. The satellite clinics offer diagnostic and treatment services to minority, rural, and other underserved people; and help increase diversity among research volunteers, so that answers to research questions apply to a wider group of people. This program makes it easier for diverse populations to take part in research studies and clinical drug trials through the parent ADC.

Twenty-seven satellite clinics serve communities with broad ethnic and cultural diversity, including African Americans, Asian Americans, Hispanic Americans, and Native Americans. Eleven clinics serve rural areas, 12 serve urban areas, and 4 serve a combination of urban and rural areas.

Consortium to Establish a Registry for Alzheimer's Disease

In 1986, the NIA established CERAD to bring uniformity to clinical and pathological studies of AD patients by standardizing clinical, neuropsychological, neuroimaging, and neuropathological assessments. Members of the Consortium conduct followup, observation, and autopsies of patients; review data for consistency, accuracy, and completeness; and promote use of this unique data resource for publications by both CERAD and non-CERAD investigators. In fiscal year 1995, CERAD received funding from the NIA to maintain data on the current group of more than 1,200 AD patients and controls.

Special Care Units Initiative

Throughout 1996, researchers reported preliminary findings from the NIA-supported Special Care Unit (SCU) Initiative. SCUs are separate sections in nursing homes for residents with dementia. The idea behind SCUs is that people with dementia might benefit from specially designed programs or environments different from those provided in a traditional nursing home. The SCU Initiative is a study at several sites, including researchers at some ADCs, to evaluate the effectiveness and costs of special care for AD patients at nursing homes. Participating scientists already have contributed to what is known about nursing home care for people with dementia.

Ten sites take part in this research consortium, funded for 5 years to:

- identify key elements of care
- specify appropriate outcomes
- evaluate the effects of key elements of care

Study designs among the sites range from case studies to multi-State evaluations to a national assessment. Most of these collaborative investigations use large data sets to compare care and outcomes in SCUs with those in traditional nursing home care units. Researchers also seek to standardize a definition of units that provide special care.

NIA-funded scientists compared national survey data on nursing homes for 1991 and 1995. Compared to 1,497 SCUs in 1991, there were more than 3,746 SCUs in 1995. Of these, 3,263 were units, wings, or clusters within units; and 483 were programs. In 1995, among the nation's 16,827 nursing facilities, more than 22 percent offered specialized care in some form for people with dementia and the total SCU capacity was 122,479 patients.

The national study also showed several differences between residents in SCUs and those in traditional care. Compared with residents in traditional care, those in service-rich, specialized care settings are less likely to fall even though they are more likely to be up and about; less likely to be restrained, and when restrained, are restrained for fewer days; and more likely to be prescribed psychotropic medications (drugs that are designed to ease their negative behaviors). However, prescription use by the SCU goes down during the initial 6 month period of placement, suggesting a tailoring of medication to suit patients' changing needs. Moreover, residence in an SCU environment is associated with less agitated behavior, after controlling for gender and other baseline factors such as initial levels of agitation and cognitive impairment.

The data also suggest that using strategies that match the needs of residents with dementia can have positive effects on behavior and emotional states of both patients and staff. Even within a broadly defined SCU, placement in an SCU environment lowers aggressive and agitated behaviors after 6 months. Not only are patients' aggressive behaviors decreased, but their positive behaviors and social interactions are increased.

The final research year of the SCU Initiative, 1997, is devoted to comparing the data among the different nursing homes. Investigators hope to translate this research into practical guidelines for nursing home administrators and policy makers.

Enhancing Family Caregiving

In 1995, the NIH established a major initiative to develop and test new ways for families and friends to manage the daily activities and stresses of caregiving for people with AD. Called REACH—Resources for Enhancing Alzheimer's Caregiver Health—the studies are sponsored by the NIA and the National Institute of Nursing Research. This 5-year effort is a critical part of NIA's support for research on AD patients receiving care at home.

Participating researchers are from the Center for Aging at the University of Alabama in Birmingham; Veterans Affairs Medical Center and the University of Tennessee at Memphis; the Center on Adult Development and Aging at the University of Miami, Florida; Veterans Affairs Palo Alto Health Care System and Stanford University, California; the Center for Collaborative Research at Thomas Jefferson University in Philadelphia, Pennsylvania; the Medical Information Systems Unit at the Boston University Medical Center, Massachusetts; and the University Center for Social and Urban Research at the University of Pittsburgh, Pennsylvania. They are studying the effects of educational support groups, behavioral skills training, family-based interventions, environmental redesign, and computer-based information services for African American, Caucasian, and Hispanic American families.

The NIA has funded a Coordinating Center to develop and maintain a common database. Data from this initiative will enable researchers to study the feasibility and outcomes of different interventions at the participating sites.

REACH is designed to stimulate research on home- and community-based interventions to help families provide care for loved ones with mild and moderate dementia. For example, NIA-supported researchers at the Center for Collaborative Research at Thomas Jefferson University are looking at the role of adjustments in the home environment (design changes and ways of managing tasks) in supporting family caregivers and enhancing their well-being. Both types of adjustments reflect adaptive strategies that caregivers may use to simplify the environment, make tasks easier, and increase patient safety.

Stress Reduction for Family Caregivers: Effects of Using Day Care

NIA-supported researchers at Pennsylvania State University in University Park and Kent State University in Kent, Ohio, studied the mental health benefits of adult day care use by 326 family caregivers of dementia patients. The participants were divided into a treatment group (122 people) and a control group (204 people). The treatment group used day care at least 2 days a week for 3 months. The control group used neither adult day care nor any other respite services during the study.

During the time the treatment group of caregivers enrolled their loved ones in day care, researchers measured changes in caregivers' attitudes about their own primary stressors and well-being. Scientists compared the results of the treatment and control groups on rating scales that assess overload, worry and strain, caregiver role, lack of emotional control, distress, depression, well-being, anger, and positive feelings.

Preliminary results suggest that 3 months of use of adult day care services by caregivers of dementia patients helped improve their well-being and greatly reduced stress within a relatively brief time. Using adult day care decreased participants' feelings of overload, depression, worry, and strain. Further study is needed to confirm this initial research.

Exploratory Centers on Demography of Aging: Alzheimer's Disease

The NIA supports research at nine collaborating Exploratory Centers on the Demography of Aging. Demography refers to the study of certain health factors—in this case, aging—in human populations.

The goal of these centers is to provide innovative and public policy-relevant research on health, long-term care, and the economic aspects of aging. Each center brings experts from different backgrounds together to conduct research in several areas of interest.

In the second year of this program, four new pilot projects are under way studying aspects of AD along with other demographic factors. As part of two of these, researchers at Duke University are studying the development of AD and the effects of different apoE gene statuses on AD. In other areas, the Duke University team is trying to forecast the life expectancy of older people and health service needs, studying how life expectancy can be extended, and measuring the rate of disease and disability in the U.S. population. Researchers in one of these studies are examining the costs and benefits of different medical treatments for older people.

In another exploratory center study, scientists at the University of Chicago, Illinois, are investigating the well-being of spouses of institutionalized AD patients. University of Chicago researchers also are studying the economics of aging from a historical perspective, retirement prospects and minority issues for Hispanic Americans, and differences in family care and social supports between African Americans and Caucasians.

Lastly, exploratory center researchers at the University of Pennsylvania are studying AD and life in nursing homes. These scientists are working to develop new measures of AD progression for use in projecting population and disability rates. They also are examining relationships between members of different generations, measuring death rates for African Americans from 1930 to the present, comparing English and Spanish versions of the Dementia Severity Measure, and looking for ways to encourage minority researchers.

By collecting and analyzing data about health and economic trends in the older population, exploratory centers foster a better understanding of aging and its effects on both individuals and society.

Chapter 25

Biomedical Research That Will Carry Us into the 21st Century

We are engaged in a remarkable period of Alzheimer's disease discovery. Not long ago, "senility" was thought to be an inevitable consequence of aging, but research has since proved that, without disease, the human brain continues to function well throughout life.

Dementia, or the loss of intellectual function, results from disease, and Alzheimer's disease is the most common cause of dementia in older people. Tragically, an estimated four million people now suffer from Alzheimer's disease, a progressive brain disorder marked by an irreversible decline in intellectual abilities and by changes in behavior and personality. Alzheimer's disease devastates its victims. Although the early signs involve mild forgetfulness, the dementia ultimately leaves patients incapable of caring for themselves. Behavior changes may cause patients to become agitated, sometimes to the point of causing harm to themselves or others. As a result, Alzheimer's disease has a profound effect on the millions of family members and other loved ones who provide most of the care for people with this disease.

Because the prevalence of Alzheimer's disease doubles every five years beyond age 65, the rapid growth of the oldest old population is expected to place a significantly greater number of people at risk for the disease. Some scientists have projected a tripling of Alzheimer's

Statement of Richard J. Hodes, M.D. Director, National Institute on Aging, Hearing of the U.S. Senate Labor and Human Resources Committee, Subcommittee on Aging, June 5, 1997.

disease patients by the year 2050 to 14 million individuals. It is urgent that we define the causes and features of Alzheimer's disease and find ways to combat it.

Fortunately, as understanding of the disease grows, so do the opportunities for developing interventions to halt or slow its progress. The National Institute on Aging (NIA) leads a national effort, in collaboration with several components of the National Institutes of Health and other agencies, to conquer this devastating disease by working to understand the biological mechanisms underlying Alzheimer's disease, to develop treatments and cures based on research findings, and eventually to discover ways to prevent the disease.

Pathological Signs

When Dr. Alois Alzheimer studied the pathology of this dementia in 1907, he described two distinctive features in the brain that still characterize the disease. The first feature is the plaque, composed largely of a protein fragment called beta-amyloid, normally secreted by brain cells. Plaques gradually accumulate in the spaces between nerve cells in the brains of patients with Alzheimer's disease. Many scientists believe that beta-amyloid contributes to the nerve cell death that leads to dementia in Alzheimer's disease.

The other feature is the neurofibrillary tangle, which is composed mainly of an abnormal form of a protein called tau. Normally, tau supports the microtubular structure that transports molecules within nerve cells. In Alzheimer's disease, however, abnormal tau accumulates to form tangles inside nerve cells, disrupting cell functions. Scientists also believe that tangles could cause cell injury and death as they build up inside cells.

While some plaques and tangles occur with normal aging, they are much more numerous in persons with Alzheimer's disease. A significant amount of research is devoted to understanding the origin of plaques and tangles in Alzheimer's disease and to learning how they relate to nerve cell death, loss of neuronal connections, and other features, such as inflammation, also seen in the brains of Alzheimer's disease patients. Scientists hope to translate this knowledge into therapies that will slow or prevent the progress of Alzheimer's disease.

For many decades after Dr. Alzheimer described plaques and tangles, these features were not commonly associated with the dementia of old age, which was widely believed to be an inevitable consequence of aging. This belief has largely been dispelled by a broad scientific initiative to understand the disease. Researchers have recognized different forms of Alzheimer's disease. In some individuals, symptoms occur in persons as young as 30 years. This rare, early-onset form of Alzheimer's disease occurs in a small number of individuals and accounts for approximately 10 percent of cases of Alzheimer's disease. The common, late-onset form of Alzheimer's disease, in which symptoms appear after age 65, accounts for approximately 90 percent of cases.

Genetic Links

Beginning in 1990, research has produced a remarkable series of genetic discoveries. Researchers identified mutations in three genes that cause the familial, early-onset form of the disease, and identified a fourth gene that is a risk factor for the common, late-onset form of the disease. The first early-onset gene mutation discovered, on chromosome 21, is in the gene that codes for the parent protein of the beta-amyloid peptide found in plaques. Mutations were soon found in genes on chromosomes 14 and 1, associated with early-onset Alzheimer's disease. Mutations in the chromosome 14 gene are the most common, being responsible for 40 to 50 percent of early-onset cases inherited in families. In these early onset cases, inheritance of just one copy of the mutated gene causes the disease. In addition, there remain some familial, early-onset Alzheimer's disease cases not caused by mutations in any of the known genes, making it likely that there are more genes still to be identified.

The fourth gene, associated with the more common form of Alzheimer's disease in which symptoms occur in later years, was found on chromosome 19. Knowing that there were families in which many members developed Alzheimer's disease late in life, researchers looked for a genetic link. The search led to a gene that codes for forms (alleles) of the protein apolipoprotein E (ApoE). One of the forms, ApoE4, is now recognized as the first genetic risk factor identified for the common, late-onset form of Alzheimer's disease. Epidemiologic studies have suggested that the age of onset of Alzheimer's disease can vary by as much as 20 years depending on whether a person inherits no copies, one copy, or two copies of ApoE4. Recent research findings support the possibility that development of at least some cases of late-onset Alzheimer's disease involves other risk factor genes, and investigators are pursuing the location of these genes on other chromosomes, as well as their identification.

To aid in analyzing the disease process in the different forms of Alzheimer's disease, researchers last year genetically engineered a transgenic mouse. The mouse carries mutated human genes associated with Alzheimer's disease. This is the first animal model to exhibit some of the cognitive as well as the neuropathological features of Alzheimer's disease. This model provides an important research tool for understanding Alzheimer's disease and for expediting the testing of potential Alzheimer's disease drug therapies.

Ethical Issues

A degenerative disease such as Alzheimer's disease raises important ethical questions regarding care, genetic testing, and research. Considerable attention has been given to the ethics of elective genetic testing for Alzheimer's disease, apart from research purposes. Predictive testing is possible in the autosomal dominant genes linked to early-onset families. The ApoE allele, however, is not absolutely predictive of Alzheimer's disease in asymptomatic individuals. To date, there is a consensus among most researchers, policy experts, ethicists, and others, that except for autosomal dominant early-onset families, Alzheimer's disease genetic testing should not be used for screening or diagnosis in asymptomatic individuals. Genetic testing is currently a particular concern given the potential for employment and insurance discrimination.

Issues of informed consent, both for health care and for participation in research, are of particular concern for Alzheimer's disease patients and others with diminished cognitive abilities. Special efforts are being made to improve the consent process for care, to encourage advance care planning while the patient is able, and to make the consent process meaningful to potential participants in Alzheimer's disease intervention studies.

Potential for Early Detection

The genetic involvement of Alzheimer's disease offers a number of opportunities for discovering disease mechanisms, improving diagnostic tests, and identifying targets for treatment. For example, scientists recently studied the cognitive and brain function of volunteers aged 50 to 64 years to compare those having two copies of the ApoE4 allele (who are at high risk for developing Alzheimer's disease) with controls having no ApoE4 allele. Although neuropsychological tests found all volunteers to be cognitively normal, brain imaging technology showed that an increased proportion of individuals with two ApoE4 alleles had reduced glucose metabolism in the same areas of the brain as patients with probable Alzheimer's disease. These findings indicate that it may be possible to identify brain function abnormalities in persons with no clinical symptoms who are at high risk for Alzheimer's disease many years before they would be expected to develop such symptoms. This provides opportunities for the development of early interventions that would delay or prevent the brain damage seen in fully developed Alzheimer's disease. Stopping or delaying the progression of the disease prior to onset of noticeable symptoms would make a major contribution to quality of life and continued function.

Early recognition and appropriate assessment of Alzheimer's disease are critical goals. Family members, especially spouses, can be instrumental in interpreting early signs and symptoms and seeking evaluation and treatment. A study of Japanese-American men and their families in Hawaii, however, found that many wives and other family members had not recognized or reported memory problems in individuals with mild to more severe dementia. Further, more than half of the individuals with recognized memory problems had not received a dementia evaluation. These results highlight the importance of public education efforts to improve recognition and reporting of symptoms very early in the illness in order to take advantage of interventions for individuals with potentially treatable dementias and to help patients and families plan for the future.

Epidemiologic Research

While determining the prevalence of Alzheimer's disease in the United States is important for health policy formulation and research planning, differing Alzheimer's disease prevalence estimates generated by studies in various populations provide key evidence suggesting potential risk factors (both genetic and environmental) as well as protective factors. Epidemiologic studies, particularly those comparing different populations, provide crucial clues to these factors, as well as to the causes of and potential treatments for Alzheimer's disease. Triggered by clues from basic research, epidemiologic studies have been very effective, for example, in helping to identify genetic and environmental risk and protective factors for Alzheimer's disease. As a result of epidemiologic research, age, a history of severe head trauma, and coexisting medical conditions, such as vascular disease, are now viewed as potential Alzheimer's disease risk factors. In contrast, high levels of education and cognitive ability have been linked to lower risk for developing Alzheimer s disease in late life.

Epidemiologic studies have also suggested that estrogen replacement therapy, use of non-steroidal anti-inflammatory drugs, and use of anti-oxidants are protective against Alzheimer's disease. One such study provided the strongest evidence to date that taking estrogen after menopause may delay the onset and reduce the risk of Alzheimer's disease in postmenopausal women. In this study, 16.3 percent of the women who had not used estrogen developed Alzheimer's disease, while only 5.8 percent of the women who had taken estrogen developed the disorder. Recent results of a 15-year study found that anti-inflammatory drugs such as ibuprofen, taken for as little as two years, also appear to reduce the risk of Alzheimer's disease. In most forms of Alzheimer's disease, therefore, disease progress may be influenced by multiple factors.

Coexisting Vascular Disease

We are also learning more about the relationship of AD to other conditions affecting older persons. In a recent finding that described the coexistence of Alzheimer's disease with vascular disease in elderly U.S. nuns, the presence of small strokes in parts of the brain below the cortex resulted in more severe dementia than expected on the basis of Alzheimer's disease neuropathology alone. In comparison, people with such small strokes in any brain region in the absence of Alzheimer's disease neuropathology generally had no significant changes in cognitive function when compared with controls. Approximately half of the demented patients in this autopsy study had these small strokes. These results strongly suggest that prevention or treatment of vascular disease could delay or reduce the development of symptoms in many Alzheimer's disease patients.

Clinical Studies

In order to speed the discovery, development, and testing of new compounds to treat Alzheimer's disease, the NIA complements its broad basic research efforts with strategies that encourage the translation of basic research findings to the development of interventions to be tested in clinical studies. NIA's Drug Discovery Groups represent an innovative approach to fostering this process. These research teams are expanding the range of pharmacologic and behavioral approaches to the treatment of Alzheimer's disease and exploring the development of novel delivery systems to the brain.

NIA's Alzheimer's Disease Cooperative Study (ADCS) coordinates the efforts of 35 institutions to rapidly respond to ideas for potential treatments by conducting clinical studies for the treatment of cognitive impairment and behavioral disorders associated with Alzheimer's disease. The design of this consortium makes it possible to conduct multiple clinical studies simultaneously in response to rapidly-emerging scientific opportunities. Evidence from basic and epidemiologic research has stimulated clinical studies of antioxidants, anti-inflammatory agents, and estrogen to explore ways of slowing the degenerative progress of Alzheimer's disease. A recently completed clinical trial, conducted by the ADCS, assessed the effectiveness of selegiline (an anti-oxidant drug used in Parkinson's disease) and vitamin E (an antioxidant vitamin), both separately and in combination, in delaying the progression of Alzheimer's disease. This trial showed that selegiline and vitamin E may slow development of functional signs and symptoms of Alzheimer's disease by about seven months. Each of the two drugs delayed important milestones for people with moderately severe Alzheimer's disease, such as entry into nursing homes and loss of ability to perform activities of daily living. Delays in the onset of ever more troubling symptoms are viewed by caregivers as an important step.

The ADCS is now studying the effects of other promising therapies, including the steroidal anti-inflammatory agent prednisone, the efficacy of estrogen replacement therapy in women with mild to moderate Alzheimer's disease; and the impact of psychoactive drugs and behavior management techniques on reducing disruptive, agitated behavior in Alzheimer's disease patients.

In addition, a large NIH randomized trial of hormonal replacement, the Women's Health Initiative, is being used to test the ability of hormonal replacement to prevent cognitive decline.

Caregiving

The prolonged and intense caregiving of Alzheimer's disease patients affects the physical, mental, and social health of the caregiver. Fatigue, insomnia, and other physical symptoms are frequent. Depression is not uncommon. Cardiovascular risk factors, such as high blood pressure, may be affected. In response, scientists are testing various methods to help family members who care for people with Alzheimer's disease. Strategies are being developed to increase the caregiver's emotional support, improve services that ease the burden for caregivers, and provide knowledge and skills training useful for coping with the symptoms of Alzheimer's disease.

Families find decisions surrounding placement in a nursing home extremely difficult. Research is helping to define whether and when to turn to a nursing home, and to evaluate what type of care is best for the patient. Additional studies are identifying the strategies that promote the most effective, highest quality institutional care.

Future Research

Alzheimer's disease is a devastating condition that ruins the lives of those who have the disease and disrupts the lives of their caregivers. Over the last five years, research has resulted in major advances in our understanding of the disease, including the discovery of genetic components, detection of risk factors, and identification of potential protective interventions. As the pace of research accelerates, new findings will make possible better understanding of factors contributing to nerve cell death and will improve our ability to predict who is at risk for developing Alzheimer's disease. We are at the threshold of further discoveries that will lead to more accurate methods of diagnosis, and to the development of more effective treatments and preventive interventions to reduce the scourge of Alzheimer's disease.

Chapter 26

Alzheimer's Disease Drug Research

Patients, families, and caregivers all seek treatments to ease the symptoms of Alzheimer's disease (AD). For most of them, it is an immediate concern. They want treatments to relieve their loved ones' suffering right now. To meet this pressing need, researchers across the country are working to develop drugs to treat AD.

Drug Development

Drug development generally consists of the following basic steps: drug discovery, pre-clinical testing, investigational new drug (IND) application to the U.S. Food and Drug Administration (FDA), clinical trials, and review and approval by the FDA.

The search for AD treatments begins with basic laboratory research and animal studies. This early research does not predict how a new drug will work in people. Therefore, the most promising drugs are studied in patients, hopefully leading to treatments that may help many people.

Drug Discovery

Using sophisticated techniques and equipment, chemists work with known molecules and develop new ones. A molecule is a very small piece of matter that is a combination of two or more atoms that form a specific chemical. A molecule is the smallest amount of a chemical

National Institute on Aging, *Connections*, Vol. 6 (1), Spring 1997.

that can exist alone. Biologists test the molecules in living cells taken from various animal and human organs to discover if the molecules have a beneficial action against AD.

Federal Government's Role

The National Institute on Aging (NIA) and other parts of the National Institutes of Health (NIH) play an important role in AD drug discovery. The NIA and NIH fund and conduct basic research on healthy brain functioning and disease processes. The goal is to identify abnormal activities in cells and molecules that may suggest ways to treat AD.

The NIA established the following research programs to advance AD drug research:

- Alzheimer's Disease Centers (ADCs)—Research facilities at major medical institutions across the country conduct clinical studies on AD.

- Alzheimer's Disease Cooperative Study (ADCS)—A consortium of 31 research centers tests the safety and efficacy of potential treatments.

- Drug Discovery Groups for Alzheimer's Disease—Research facilities work to discover promising compounds to treat or prevent AD.

- Drug Toxicity Testing—In this NIH contract for animal testing of compounds, studies are done to determine if potential therapeutic compounds have any toxic properties.

- Satellite Diagnostic and Treatment Clinics—These ADC-affiliated research facilities recruit minority, rural, and other underserved patients to increase the diversity of study volunteers.

The Drug Discovery Groups and ADCS sometimes work in tandem with drug company efforts. Drug Discovery Groups focus on the early stages of developing innovative treatments. These groups seek to produce new compounds and to find better ways of delivering drugs through the blood-brain barrier into the brain. By taking the first practical steps to apply new theories, NIA's AD drug discovery efforts may lay the groundwork for further drug development by pharmaceutical manufacturers.

The ADCS evaluates three kinds of potential treatments: medications that lack commercial appeal because their patents have expired; treatments that are on the market for other conditions; and new classes of drugs developed by small companies without the financial resources to test them. In contrast, drugs based on more established theories of action and use (i.e., cholinergic drugs), which carry relatively less financial risk, are being tested widely by pharmaceutical companies.

Private Industry's Role

Drug innovation is an expensive, high-risk venture. The Pharmaceutical Research and Manufacturers of America (PhRMA) estimates that it takes an average of 12 years, nearly $500 million, and thousands of people to move a drug from the laboratory to the pharmacy. Every step along the way is critical and builds on previous ones. According to the PhRMA, only 1 drug out of 5,000 tested will make it to pharmacy shelves.

Of the estimated $16 billion that drug companies spent on research and development (R&D) in 1995, about $3 billion went to products acting on the central nervous system and sense organs, such as those for AD and Parkinson's disease. According to the PhRMA, drug companies developed over 90 percent of new medicines approved in the United States between 1981 and 1991.

Nearly 60 percent of drug companies' expenditures for R&D are for development—technical activities that translate research findings into products. About 40 percent of the pharmaceutical industry's R&D expenses are for research, mostly applied research. The industry often uses basic research findings from the NIH and academia as the foundation for drug research.

Pre-Clinical Testing

A compound that has a desirable effect in laboratory studies goes on to toxicity studies. These inquiries provide information about toxic side effects and safety at different doses in animals. Scientists study how much of the drug's active ingredients are absorbed by the blood and tissues, how body chemicals break down the drug, how toxic the drug is, and how quickly the body excretes it.

Toxicity studies are important because they enable researchers to study the actions and effects of a variety of compounds in large, readily-accessible groups of subjects. Many experimental drugs never go beyond pre-clinical testing because they do not work well enough, are poorly absorbed, or are unsafe.

Investigational New Drug (IND) Application

Researchers with promising results from animal testing submit an IND application to the FDA proposing that they start clinical trials in people. The IND application describes the study plan and the drug, including its formula, animal test results, and manufacturing information. The FDA has only 30 days to review the application, and allows initial clinical trials to proceed only if the information provided in the application shows that participants in the research will not be at undue risk. The FDA estimates that for every 100 drugs for which an IND application has been submitted about 20 will be approved for marketing.

Clinical Trials

Laboratory, including animal, studies lack the means to fully predict or measure the effects of a new drug in humans. Clinical trials, studies of a drug's effects in humans, link basic research and patients. The goal of these trials is to translate the best of that research into treatments that help patients. With any new treatment, risks and benefits are possible. Clinical trials are the primary basis for researchers to find out if a promising treatment is safe and effective for patients. Clinical trials also tell researchers which treatments are more effective than others.

Sponsors of drug development programs may conduct or support clinical trials at private research facilities, teaching hospitals, specialized AD research clinics, or doctors' offices. Some studies involve hospitalized patients; others are done on an outpatient basis. Participants commonly have to follow strict dosing schedules, keep detailed records of symptoms, periodically give blood samples, and undergo several evaluations over time to assess the effects of the test drug and how the disease is progressing. All participants in clinical trials are monitored carefully during a trial and followed up afterwards.

In some clinical trials, not all participants will receive the drug being studied. In controlled clinical trials, participants are divided into a test group and a control group for comparison. Members of test and control groups generally are similar in age, health status, and other factors that may affect treatment outcome. The test group may receive varying doses of one or more test compounds. The control group may receive no treatment, treatment with a drug already known to be effective, a combination of test drugs or other interventions, or a placebo. A placebo is an inactive substance that looks like the test drug.

Legitimate clinical research is federally regulated, with safeguards built in to protect patients. Risks and discomforts are fully disclosed to each participant, along with information about his or her rights as a volunteer to leave the study at any time. Participants also must be advised of any significant new findings from the study that might relate to their willingness to continue to take part in the study, such as recently noted toxic effects.

An Institutional Review Board (IRB) monitors the study. An IRB is a panel of five or more scientists, ethicists, and non-scientists at the facility that is doing the research. IRB's make sure studies are well-designed and present only minimal risks to participants; evaluate each participant's informed consent form; maintain fairness in selection, safety, and privacy of participants; keep data confidential; and review the study at least annually. IRB's are designed to protect patients and to see that risks are reasonable in relation to benefits. Well-run clinical trials are reviewed carefully by the research institution for medical ethics, patient safety, and scientific merit.

If the treatment in a trial is not helping patients or if one treatment is found to be clearly superior to another treatment in the trial, the researchers often will choose to halt the trial before it has been completed, particularly if significant adverse events have been reported.

Patients take part in clinical trials for many reasons. Usually, they hope for benefits for themselves. They also may hope for a cure, a longer time to live, or a way to feel better. Often, they want to contribute to research that may help others.

Advances in medicine and science are the results of new ideas and approaches developed through research. By participating in clinical trials, both healthy volunteers and people with AD enable researchers to gain more information about potential treatments, risks, and how well treatments may or may not work. If people did not take part in clinical trials, scientists could not find new and better ways to help those with AD.

Phases of Clinical Drug Trials

Phase I. A new research treatment is given to 20 to 100 volunteers to study how it is absorbed, distributed, metabolized, and excreted;

how long it works; and its safe dosage range. Researchers look for the best way to give a new treatment and test how much of it can be given safely. They watch closely for harmful side effects. While the research treatment has been well tested in laboratory studies of animals, no one knows yet how humans will react. For this reason, these studies may involve significant risks. This phase usually lasts less than 1 year. Once a treatment and its effects have been characterized and if a treatment has not been shown to be unsafe in Phase I, it moves to Phase II.

Phase II. Between 100 and 300 patients take part in controlled studies to evaluate the research treatment's effectiveness. Phase II generally lasts from several months up to 2 years. If a treatment has shown activity against disease and has not been shown to be unsafe in Phase II, it moves to Phase III.

Phase III. The research treatment is given to between 1,000 and 3,000 patients in hospitals, doctor's offices, and clinics to confirm Phase II results and identify infrequent adverse reactions. This phase usually lasts 1 to 4 years. If research data show safety and effectiveness, the FDA reviews the data and issues approval for doctors to begin prescribing the new treatment to patients.

Phase IV. Once approved by the FDA, some drugs may continue to be studied for long-term effects while in general use by doctors for their patients. These are Phase IV or post-marketing studies.

Preventing Research Bias

Researchers use two methods to make sure a clinical trial is conducted without bias:

Blinding. Volunteers who agree to take part in a single-blind study do not know if they are taking the test drug or a placebo (an inactive substance). In a double-blind study, neither volunteers, investigators, nor data analysts know who is getting the test drug. Blinding helps eliminate bias for and against the test drug.

Randomization. Patients agree to be randomly assigned (selected by chance) to one group or another: those in the treatment group receive the research treatment(s), and those in the control group either do not receive the research treatment(s) or receive standard accepted treatment. Randomization helps protect the results from being slanted, because it keeps researchers from giving the test drug only to certain people they select intentionally or unintentionally.

Recruiting and Retaining Research Volunteers

In addition to the general challenges of drug research, AD presents a unique set of problems in recruiting patients and retaining them in clinical trials:

Assessment. Problems include the lack of tests that can detect changes in patients with severe AD; difficulty in conducting cognitive assessments of people who have problems hearing or seeing; and use of measures that do not take into account patients' cultural or ethnic backgrounds.

Dr. Mary Sano is the Director of Clinical Trials in Alzheimer's Disease, an Associate Professor of Neuropsychology, and an Irving Scholar at Columbia University in New York City. "To increase cultural or ethnic sensitivity, we have found that it helps if the research center includes staff members and doctors from the same ethnic groups as patients taking part in a clinical trial," says Dr. Sano. "This may help increase the patients' comfort level and improve the staff's ability to serve them." In addition, many researchers are working to develop more effective measurement tools for use with AD patients.

Ethical Concerns. One of the most important ethical issues is that AD patients lose their ability to think and make decisions. These skills are needed for volunteers to give informed consent to take part in research. To protect this vulnerable population, those involved must resolve the question of who can provide informed proxy consent for AD patients. To address these issues, researchers in most studies ask that families review and fill out informed proxy consent forms for their loved ones to make sure they understand what it means to participate in research. This usually is done as part of the process whereby researchers determine whether or not patients are eligible to take part in a study.

Fairness to patients is another concern that researchers in all clinical trials share. The following considerations are at the heart of the issue of fairness: giving placebos to people with AD, who will continually get worse during the period of drug evaluation; and exposing vulnerable patients to experimental drugs that may have dangerous side effects or make other conditions worse. To help deal with these concerns, many studies are structured so that at some point all participants get the drug. In addition, scientists conduct animal studies to detect harmful side effects before administering an experimental drug to patients.

Geographic Distribution. The distance from AD patients' homes to clinical trial sites may make study participation difficult, expensive, and time consuming. According to Dr. Sano, whose program is a member of the ADCS, "One way to address these problems is to design clinical trials so that some of the research can be conducted in the patients' communities (i.e., in churches or senior centers). Another way is to provide patients and their caregivers with affordable and reasonable transportation to and from the research center."

Patient Selection. Most researchers recruit early-stage patients, because patients with more severe forms of AD usually are too cognitively impaired to take part in research. Recruiting early-stage patients limits scientists' ability to generalize research results and excludes many people whose more pronounced symptoms may be the reason why their families are interested in taking part in a clinical trial.

Unrealistic Expectations. Research on treatments for AD and other illnesses offers great promise. However, discoveries of drugs that reverse symptoms or make diseases disappear are rare, and claims of such cures must be viewed with skepticism.

Scientific conferences, scholarly journals, and the mainstream media often report encouraging but preliminary results from clinical studies. Frequently, information targeted to medical professionals and researchers, who are trained to interpret the data, reaches the general public in a brief form, where some meanings may be lost. In some cases, test results may be misinterpreted as being more conclusive, dramatic, or promising than they are.

It is important for research participants and their families to know beforehand that clinical trials usually do not have miraculous or definitive outcomes. Researchers may find that a drug relieves one or more AD symptoms, changes a clinical measurement, or reduces the risk of death. Although these important outcomes may not have practical benefits for the family, they eventually may help others.

Some people may drop out of trials because of unrealistic expectations, trouble going in for testing, low tolerance for the treatment, or other study-related problems. Others may elect not to participate because they know beforehand that the study is unlikely to cure the disease, or the treatment may cause only a slight improvement.

According to Dr. Sano, "A strategy that has worked for the Columbia University program is the development of support groups for both the AD patients who volunteer and their caregivers. These support groups enable patients and families to discuss their needs. Another way to keep patients in a clinical study is to involve caregivers in the study." Caregivers are essential to an accurate and thorough patient history. In addition to tracking changes in patients and making sure they comply with study requirements, caregivers can make participation easier for patients, for instance, by helping them get to and from research centers. "Interestingly, some researchers have found that the increased scrutiny that patients receive during clinical trials often helps both patients and their caregivers adjust to the disease," says Dr. Sano.

Drug Review and Approval

Once the key controlled clinical trials are completed, the sponsor submits a New Drug Application (NDA) to the FDA. An NDA is a request for approval to market a new drug. It provides detailed information about the drug. FDA approval depends largely on well-controlled clinical studies that provide substantial evidence of effectiveness and safety, that is, demonstration that the drug's benefits outweigh its risks.

To determine a drug's effectiveness and safety, scientists and other staff at the FDA's Center for Drug Evaluation and Research (CDER) evaluate the study design and validity of analyses; the drug's therapeutic and adverse effects; and the product's chemical stability, packaging, and labeling. In many cases, the FDA will discuss the NDA during a public meeting with an advisory panel of research and medical experts, with this panel issuing recommendations for FDA action.

After reviewing the NDA, the FDA notifies the drug sponsor that the drug has been approved for marketing, may be approved with minor changes, or cannot be approved because of major problems. If a drug is not approved, the drug's sponsor may amend or withdraw the NDA, or request a hearing to discuss the matter further.

Once the FDA has approved an NDA, the sponsoring company produces and distributes the drug to pharmacies and doctors, and the CDER periodically inspects the company's production processes for consistency and quality. Thereafter, the FDA requires periodic reports from the drug company about adverse reactions and quality control.

For some medications, the FDA requires post-marketing studies. After a drug is in use by the public, medical practitioners report its long-term effects to the FDA.

References

Pharmaceutical Research and Manufacturers of America. *Pharmaceutical News*: The Case for FDA Reform. Washington, DC: Pharmaceutical Research and Manufacturers of America. March 11, 1996.

Pharmaceutical Research and Manufacturers of America. *PhRMA Industry Profile*, 1996. Washington, DC: Pharmaceutical Research and Manufacturers of America. 1996.

U.S. Food and Drug Administration. *From Test Tube to Patient: New Drug Development in the United States, 2nd ed*. Pittsburgh, PA: U.S. Government Printing Office. January 1995. Stock Number 017-012-00371-1.

Chapter 27

Estrogen, Anti-Inflammatories, and Other Promising Drugs

The road to discovering and developing new drugs to treat Alzheimer's disease (AD) is long and difficult. Ideally, an effective AD drug will do several things: benefit many patients for a long time, slow down or stop the disease, improve patients' mental abilities and functioning in activities of daily living, and have few serious side effects.

Tacrine (trade name Cognex) and donepezil (trade name Aricept) are the only drugs that the Food and Drug Administration (FDA) has approved so far to treat some symptoms of AD.

An important first step in developing these drugs was the discovery that the brains of AD patients have a shortage of acetylcholine. Acetylcholine is a chemical messenger or neurotransmitter that aids communication between neurons in the brain, especially those responsible for learning and memory. Drugs like tacrine and donepezil increase the brain's supply of acetylcholine, allaying some symptoms and helping brain cells function more efficiently in some patients.

Researchers now believe that the brain deficit of acetylcholine may not be a central event in AD, but only one of a cascade of biochemical events, some of which cause brain cells to die. Several other medications that enhance or mimic the action of acetylcholine in the brain are in the later stages of the FDA drug-approval process. These other cholinergic drugs may prove to be more effective or have fewer side effects than either tacrine or donepezil. However, many researchers believe that any cholinergic drug will offer only moderate and temporary

---

National Institute on Aging, *Connections*, Vol. 6 (1), Spring 1997.

benefits. Therefore, they are searching for new treatments that prevent cell death; neither tacrine nor donepezil does this.

Current Research

Scientists are looking at estrogen, estrogen-like molecules, anti-inflammatory drugs, and anti-oxidants. Some researchers believe that one or the other of these drugs may help nerve cells survive by preventing damage from oxidation and inflammation.

Estrogen and Anti-Inflammatory Drugs

Through epidemiologic research, scientists have identified two kinds of drugs that may slow or stop AD: estrogen and anti-inflammatory drugs. Epidemiologists study AD incidence, prevalence, and various risk factors in culturally-diverse populations. Incidence is the rate at which new cases of a disease occur. Prevalence is the percentage of the entire population with the disease at a given time.

When epidemiologic studies showed some potential benefits of estrogen and anti-inflammatory drugs in treating AD, the National Institute on Aging's (NIA's) Alzheimer's Disease Cooperative Study (ADCS) launched pilot studies to assess their effectiveness. The ADCS is part of the Federal Government's AD research effort. Dr. Leon Thal directs the ADCS and the Alzheimer's Disease Center (ADC) at the University of California in San Diego. According to Dr. Thal, these are the first attempts to gauge the therapeutic potential of these drugs in AD in controlled research studies.

"The epidemiologic research is not completely reliable because it is based partly on the recall of people with AD. Further, it does not show whether the medications actually benefit those who have the disease," says Dr. Thal. "Only one small-scale controlled study of an anti-inflammatory drug—indomethacin—has been done, and no adequately sized and properly controlled studies have involved estrogen," he adds. Controlled clinical studies are needed to confirm and add to these epidemiologic findings.

Biological evidence suggests that both estrogen and anti-inflammatory drugs may help treat and possibly prevent AD. Estrogen is a hormone, a chemical with important roles in the brain and other parts of the body such as the female reproductive system. Scientists have found that estrogen has positive effects on motor and cognitive abilities, mood, and behavior. Researchers now believe that cells in brain areas severely affected by AD (including the limbic system, cerebral cortex, and hippocampus) use estrogen. The cerebral cortex is the part of the brain most involved in learning, language, and reasoning. The hippocampus is a structure deep in the brain involved in memory storage.

Estrogen appears to interact with nerve growth factor (NGF) to help brain cells—particularly those that use acetylcholine—develop and survive. NGF is a substance that helps promote the repair of cholinergic neurons (nerve cells that contain or are stimulated by acetylcholine).

Estrogen may work as an anti-oxidant, stopping the harmful action of oxygen molecules. Oxygen molecules combine readily with other molecules and, in doing so, sometimes damage cells (see Other Anti-Oxidants below).

The current ADCS trial of prednisone (a steroidal anti-inflammatory drug) is for "proof of the concept," Dr. Thal notes. Evidence shows that an inflammatory response by the body's immune system may be associated with the production of beta-amyloid. Beta-amyloid is an abnormal protein fragment that makes up the neuritic plaques (deposits of amyloid mixed with pieces of dead and dying neurons) found in the brains of AD patients. Beta-amyloid is cut out from the larger amyloid precursor protein (APP).

"Prednisone has proven useful in another inflammatory central nervous system disorder—lupus. It also has more general effects in the central nervous system than other anti-inflammatory drugs. Therefore, tests of prednisone provide the best chance of identifying a positive effect, if there is one.

If the pilot study with prednisone is encouraging, then researchers may begin to home in on a better long-term therapy, perhaps one of the nonsteroidal, anti-inflammatory drugs (NSAIDs)," says Dr. Thal. NSAIDs are a drug class that includes ibuprofen and aspirin. In general, NSAIDs have less serious side effects than prednisone. And, recent findings using data from the Baltimore Longitudinal Study of Aging (BLSA) suggest that regular use of NSAIDs may lower the risk of AD by as much as 60 percent. These results are from a study of 1,686 BLSA participants (older people) who were followed for 1 or more years between 1980 and 1995.

Even if results from the ADCS's pilot studies of estrogen and prednisone are promising, much work still must be done before medical experts will recommend these drugs for everyday use in battling AD. For example, researchers will need to find safe and effective anti-inflammatory drugs with reasonably few side effects after extended use.

Estrogen-Like Molecules

In addition to pursuing today's strongest prospects in their search for effective AD therapies, NIA's Drug Discovery Groups open new lines of inquiry and reexamine areas of research that others may assume are closed. Dr. James Simpkins, who directs a Drug Discovery Group at the University of Florida in Gainesville, says that the progress of his own career in AD research proves the value of exploring a range of theories—unpopular as well as popular. "My colleagues and I first became interested in estrogen in the mid-1980's. At that time, most researchers dismissed the idea that it had any role in AD. Today, estrogen has taken center stage."

Currently, Dr. Simpkins's team is working to transform the estrogen molecule into a safe and beneficial compound for people who have or are at risk for AD. Describing the group's efforts, he says, "Based on the substantial evidence that estrogen protects neurons, we set out to build models that explain how it works." Studying animals and tissue cultures, this team eventually linked estrogen's benefits to its antioxidant function. "With estrogen, we drastically reduced oxidation damage in tissue cultures and correlated that activity with less cell death," notes Dr. Simpkins. In addition, the group found that estrogen's neuron-protecting activities are not related to its "feminizing" properties, and that activating estrogen receptors is unnecessary to protect neurons. Receptors are proteins that recognize and bind to chemical messengers, such as neurotransmitters.

Building on these discoveries, Dr. Simpkins's team made a series of minor changes at various places in the structure of the estrogen molecule. The team sought to produce new substances that kept estrogen's anti-oxidant potential, but lost its feminizing qualities. They developed 10 molecules that may help protect neurons but do not act like sex hormones. Dr. Simpkins speculates that hundreds of similar, estrogen-like molecules may be found.

The University of Florida team also found that normal levels of estrogen help protect neurons. This finding suggests that estrogen-like therapies may be administered effectively at relatively low doses over many years. Dr. Simpkins notes that estrogen may help with other diseases of the central nervous system, including Parkinson's disease, and strokes.

In an agreement with a pharmaceutical company, Dr. Simpkins and his colleagues will further develop 3 of the 10 modified estrogen molecules prepared at the University of Florida. Paving the way for clinical trials, the drug company will test these substances in mice

280

genetically engineered to produce abnormally high levels of APP. The company seeks to find out if the substances protect brain cells from the possibly toxic effects of amyloid.

Other Anti-Oxidants

Results are due soon from a trial completed by the ADCSs to test the drug selegiline, vitamin E, and their combination for AD. Selegiline, or deprenyl, is an FDA-approved therapy for Parkinson's disease that increases the supply of dopamine. Another neurotransmitter, dopamine is decreased in AD, although not to the same extent as acetylcholine. Like vitamin E, selegiline is an anti-oxidant.

One long-standing theory of aging suggests that the buildup of damage due to oxidation causes nerve cells to degenerate. Scientists believe that free radicals generated through oxidative mechanisms play a role in AD, cancer, and many other diseases.

A free radical is a molecule with an unpaired electron in its outer shell. Normal metabolism produces free radicals of oxygen with unpaired electrons. The body produces free radicals to help cells in certain ways, such as in fighting infections. But, having too many free radicals is bad for cells. Free radicals are extremely reactive; they will latch readily onto other molecules, such as a part of the cell membrane or a piece of deoxyribonucleic acid (DNA). This can set off a chain reaction, releasing chemicals that can harm cells.

In AD, free radicals are suspects for several reasons. They attack molecules of fat in nerve cell membranes and may upset the delicate membrane machinery that regulates what goes into and out of a cell, such as calcium. In addition, oxidation may alter proteins, and these alterations may be associated with the development of AD. Some of these oxidative changes are found in amyloid plaques in AD. Researchers have shown that in neuritic plaques, beta-amyloid causes the release of free radicals. All of the above are changes that cannot be reversed. Reactions like those mentioned also produce several free radical oxidation molecules that may target the internal support structures of nerve cells.

Studies of compounds that fight oxidation—such as the ADCS trial of selegiline and vitamin E—put researchers one step closer to understanding processes that damage cells in AD and finding ways to treat and possibly prevent AD.

Future Directions

The final proof that estrogen, anti-oxidants, and anti-inflammatory drugs are valuable in treating AD will come from prospective research, that is, studies to see if people who take these drugs for an extended period do not develop AD. Because such long-term research is expensive, Dr. Thal emphasizes the importance of designing the study so that it clarifies all issues involved.

Dr. Thal believes that this long-term research is economical when "piggy-backed" on other studies. This research can capitalize on the fact that estrogen and anti-inflammatory drugs also are effective in other diseases of aging. For example, the Women's Health Initiative— a long-term study sponsored by the National Institutes of Health— will examine the effectiveness of estrogen in preventing both memory impairment and osteoporosis.

Nerve Growth Factor

In the near future, NIA's ADCS plans to test several other therapies for AD. In addition to estrogen, drugs that interact with or increase the supply of NGF are promising. However, because NGF is a relatively large molecule, it cannot go through the protective blood-brain barrier, and thus, cannot be used in drug form. The blood-brain barrier is a system of tightly knit cells that form a boundary around the blood vessels of the brain and permit only certain substances to cross from the blood into the brain. "Many drugs may never get a fair shot," says Dr. Simpkins. "One issue that repeatedly derails promising compounds is that with no effective transport system, many good drugs do not get into the brain. Often, enormous therapeutic opportunities are lost."

In looking for ways to enhance the benefits of drugs in the brain, a small biotechnology company has developed a drug that stimulates the release of NGF and other neurotrophins (substances that help neurons grow and regenerate). The ADCS is considering a clinical trial to evaluate this drug.

Protease Inhibitors

Other promising classes of substances need more refinement before they are safe for testing in people. One class, called protease inhibitors, may stop the production of beta-amyloid. A protease is an enzyme that cuts a protein into smaller sections. Protease inhibitors stop the faulty protein-breaking process that produces beta-amyloid in AD.

"Several readily-available protease inhibitors may act on APP," according to Dr. Thal. "The problem is that they also work on a wide variety of other proteins, so they could disturb and interfere with critical brain functions." Therefore, researchers are working to develop highly-specific protease inhibitors that only stop APP splitting.

New Drug Delivery Systems

Perhaps as important as the University of Florida Drug Discovery Group's development of new compounds is its work to find better ways to deliver drugs to the brain. The expensive and fierce competition in commercial drug development often means that if a drug does not yield immediate results, it is abandoned quickly, even when ineffective delivery is the reason.

Nicholas Bodor, a chemist with the University of Florida Drug Discovery Group, is working to develop effective chemical delivery systems. These systems combine substances with drugs to assist entry into the brain. The University of Florida group has developed a chemical delivery system that consists of cholesterol and several other proteins. This system seems to disguise the appearance of a neuropeptide called thyrotropin releasing hormone (TRH) so that it can pass through the blood-brain barrier. Once TRH enters the brain, enzymes break down the chemical delivery system in a way that locks TRH in the brain, thereby strengthening its effects.

"Enhancing the effects of drugs in the brain with chemical delivery systems may lead to new treatments for AD and increase the effectiveness of some drugs as much as 50 times," says Dr. Simpkins. He believes that delivery systems could significantly enhance cholinergic therapy.

Drugs like tacrine increase the availability of acetylcholine to neurons by inhibiting cholinesterase, an enzyme that breaks down acetylcholine. Cholinergic therapy also includes drugs called cholinergic agonists that act in place of acetylcholine. Cholinergic agonists directly stimulate neuron receptors. Because high doses can damage vital organs such as the heart and liver, both types of cholinergic drugs must be used sparingly. But, the right chemical delivery system may raise the effectiveness of safe doses of cholinergic therapy.

Other Areas of Research

The ADCS plans additional effectiveness studies on drugs used to treat the behavioral symptoms of AD. Early in 1996, the consortium finished enrolling volunteers for a clinical trial to measure the effectiveness of trazodone and haldol in preventing or reducing agitation.

References

Aisen, P.S.; Davis, K.L. Inflammatory Mechanisms in Alzheimer's Disease: Implications for Therapy. *American Journal of Psychiatry.* 151(8): 1105-1113. August 1994.

Paganini-Hill, A.; Henderson, V.W. Estrogen Deficiency and Risk of Alzheimer's Disease in Women. *American Journal of Epidemiology.* 140(3): 256-261. August 1, 1994.

Rogers, J.; et al. Clinical Trial of Indomethacin in Alzheimer's Disease. *Neurology.* 43(8): 1609-1611. August 1993.

Simpkins, J.W.; Singh, M.; Bishop, J. The Potential Role for Estrogen Replacement Therapy in the Treatment of the Cognitive Decline and Neurodegeneration Associated With Alzheimer's Disease. *Neurobiology of Aging.* 15(Suppl 2): S195-S197. 1994.

Stewart, W.F.; et al. Risk of Alzheimer's Disease and Duration of NSAID Use. *Neurology.* 48(3): 626-632. March 1997.

Tang, M.X.; et al. Effect of Oestrogen During Menopause on Risk and Age at Onset of Alzheimer's Disease. *The Lancet.* 348(9025): 429-432. August 17, 1996.

Thal, L. Future Directions for Research in Alzheimer's Disease. *Neurobiology of Aging.* 15(Suppl 2): S71-S72. 1994.

Whitehouse, P.J. Cholinergic Therapy in Dementia. *ACTA Neurology Scandinavia.* Suppl 149: 42-45. 1993.

Chapter 28

Autopsy Assistance Network

The Network was established because families were increasingly aware that diagnosis of Alzheimer's disease or a related disorder can be confirmed only through brain autopsy after death. Planning ahead helps families in making the difficult decision for autopsy; families need support and guidance in making the decision and planning for autopsy.

Obviously, there is an ongoing need for tissue for research. But equally important is the listing of Alzheimer's disease or a related disorder on the death certificate. If the autopsy diagnosis shows a type of dementing illness other than Alzheimer's disease, death certificates should be corrected through the attending physician. This will eventually provide the basis for more reliable studies and statistics on the prevalence of dementia.

The primary purposes of the Autopsy Assistance Network are:

- To provide families with information regarding autopsy.
- To assist in obtaining a confirmed diagnosis.

Additional benefits of the Autopsy Assistance Network include:

- Providing tissue for Alzheimer's disease research.

- Establishing diagnosis for purpose of clinical and epidemiological studies.

NOTE: The Alzheimer's Association Medical and Scientific Advisory Board recommends that the body organs of the patient with Alzheimer's disease *not* be donated for transplant purposes.

Procedure for Prearranging a Brain Autopsy

1. Meet with the entire family to make the autopsy decision and preplan for the autopsy.

2. If the patient is in a hospital, nursing home or Veteran's Administration Medical Center, contact the doctor in charge and state your intention that an autopsy be performed.

3. State your intentions for autopsy to the nursing home, care center and/or attending physician, along with a written statement requesting an autopsy to be placed in the patient's medical record.

4. If the family wishes to donate brain tissue for research, contact your regional Autopsy Assistance Network Representative for further details.

5. It is advisable to plan in advance with the funeral director for the autopsy procedure. Inform the funeral director that an autopsy is to take place. Work with the funeral director to make the autopsy arrangements.

6. There may be costs associated with the autopsy. For information concerning those costs, contact your local Alzheimer's Association Network Representative (your local Chapter or the national office can give you the telephone number).

Procedure At the Time of Death

1. All states require a signed autopsy permit. In some states, it is possible to pre-sign an autopsy permit, but the decision for brain autopsy must be confirmed verbally at the time of death. Autopsy permit forms are available from your pathologist or hospital.

2. The pathologist will arrange the details of the autopsy.

3. Families can expect a written autopsy report from the pathologist, neuropathologist, or research center within a reasonable time after the death of the patient.

Questions and Answers about Autopsy

Q. Who may request an autopsy?

A. Legally, the next-of-kin or guardian is the person to make that decision. If the spouse is deceased, the oldest child is considered next-of-kin.

Q. Is a complete autopsy performed?

A. No. In instances where Alzheimer's disease is suspected, only the brain tissue need be examined for diagnosis; however, a complete autopsy is recommended.

Q. Where is the autopsy performed?

A. If death occurs in a hospital, the autopsy may be performed in that facility; if death takes place in a nursing home, other arrangements will have to be made with a pathologist.

Q. Can I have an open casket?

A. Yes. Brain tissue removal leaves no apparent disfigurement.

Q. Will my relatives know the brain has been removed?

A. Only on close inspection would anyone know an autopsy had been performed, because tissue is removed from a non-visible area.

Q. Hasn't the patient suffered enough? Why put him/her through anything more?

A. It may appear callous to discuss a need for autopsy when dealing with those emotionally burdened, but a refusal based on "they have suffered enough" is the result of an emotional state of mind. Only through autopsy can the diagnosis be certain.

Q. Is it important for children of Alzheimer's disease patients to have confirmed diagnosis through autopsy?

287

A. Yes. As our knowledge increases, it becomes more important for families to have complete medical records. If other family members develop dementia, an autopsy-confirmed diagnosis of previous cases will be essential for any early treatment the future may bring.

About Alzheimer's Disease

Alzheimer's disease is a progressive, degenerative disease that attacks the brain and results in impaired memory, thinking and behavior. Approximately 4 million Americans are affected. Its symptoms include loss of recent memory, decline in ability to perform on the job or at home, difficulty in learning, impairment of judgment, personality change, and difficulty with movement and speech. The disease eventually renders its victims totally incapable of caring for themselves.

Alzheimer's disease is the leading cause of dementia among the elderly and the fourth leading cause of death among American adults. At this time, there is no known cause or cure for Alzheimer's disease.

About the Alzheimer's Association and Its Mission

The Alzheimer's Association is the national voluntary health organization dedicated to research for the prevention, cure and treatment of Alzheimer's disease and related disorders, and to providing support and assistance to the afflicted patients and their families.

The Alzheimer's Association's mission is carried out through:

- Research into the cause, prevention, treatment and cure for Alzheimer's disease and related disorders.

- Education of the public and information for health care professionals.

- Chapter formation for a nationwide family support network and to implement programs at the local level.

- Advocacy for improved public policy and needed legislation.

- Patient and family services to aid present and future victims and caregivers.

Part Four

Long-Term Care Issues

Chapter 29

Information for Families of Alzheimer's Patients

Someone to Stand by You

Coping with Alzheimer's disease (AD) or a related disorder does not have to be a lonely experience, although it is common to feel alone, to think that no one can understand what is happening in your life. Participating in a family group can help, by giving you a chance to share your feelings with others who do understand because they too have a loved one with dementia.

If you are a caregiver, you probably are aware that you will need help and support as the disease progresses. However, caregivers can easily become isolated with their patients because of the demands of caregiving, the forced changes in lifestyle, the loss of friends or the lack of family assistance. A family support group can help, by giving you a chance to meet others who also are facing the caregiving struggle. Support groups were established so that those who care for someone with dementia do not become "victims" of the disease themselves.

Text in this chapter was taken from "Standing by You: Family Support Groups," © 1990 The Alzheimer's Disease and Related Disorders Association, Inc., 919 North Michigan Ave., Chicago, Il 60611-1676. This information was reprinted with permission from the Alzheimer's Association. For more information about Alzheimer's disease, call (800) 272-3900. The Alzheimer's Association regrets that the original document from which this text was taken is no longer available to the public.

What Is a Support Group?

A family support group is made up of caregivers, family members and friends of those with AD or a related disorder. Although these people begin as strangers, they quickly become friends and, in a sense, a family.

The support group leader(s) may be a family member and/or a health care professional. The meeting may focus on emotional support and sharing experiences, or it may focus on education, with experts speaking on topics such as legal issues, nutrition, caregiving techniques and community resources.

The number of participants will vary, in some cases depending on the format. For instance, educational groups are usually larger. However, the ideal size for a support group is 6 to 12 members.

Meetings are usually held monthly or bi-monthly at members' homes, a hospital, church, library, nursing home or senior center.

The purpose of an Alzheimer's Association support group is to offer families support and information that is specific to dementia. Some Alzheimer's Association Chapters have support groups especially for adolescents, male spouses, adult children caring for a parent, family members of nursing home residents, or widows and widowers. Some Chapters also have a special orientation for family members of a newly-diagnosed patient.

Family support groups that are sponsored by an Alzheimer's Association Chapter are open to the public and free of charge. These support groups depend on the Chapters they are affiliated with to provide resources such as literature, updates on legislation and research, and newsletters. Alzheimer's Association Chapters serve larger areas than the support groups and they provide resources to the community as well.

Alzheimer's Association support groups encourage members to share information, give and receive mutual support and exchange coping skills with one another. Support group members share practical suggestions for caring based on their caregiving experiences. Caring for a dementia patient requires different techniques than those needed to care for a patient who is not cognitively impaired. Experienced caregivers have found that some methods of providing care, ideas that may not be found in books or articles, can make caregiving easier. Sharing those ideas in a support group can prevent caregivers from having to "re-invent the wheel."

The support group setting also assists families in learning about and locating community resources, such as adult day care and transportation services. Through sharing common experiences, families can obtain consumer information, such as listings of physicians who are familiar with dementia or nursing homes in the area that accept dementia patients.

Perhaps what is most important about a support group is the atmosphere of caring, frankness and confidentiality it provides. Family members need the freedom to express their emotions without feeling guilt, and caregivers need the positive reinforcement that can be given by others who know the hard work involved in providing care. A support group gives its members the chance to vent their frustrations, anger and disappointments, as well as share their successes in a safe, non-judgmental environment. In the process, members take a first step in restructuring their lives by forming new relationships with each other.

Why Do I Need a Support Group?

Attending a support group is often difficult at first. It takes time to feel comfortable sharing your problems with people you do not know. However, the experience of many family members is that once they opened up, they found that their problems were not so different from those of other support group members. Suddenly, the people they were sharing with were not strangers at all, and by sharing with others in the same situation they felt less alone.

If you are having difficulty talking to family or friends about your feelings, you may find that it is easier to express yourself in a support group, where you can be honest with others who are facing similar problems.

A support group also can help you feel more in control of your life, by helping you understand more about the disease. Because you will have heard how others have coped or are coping with similar situations, you will know what to expect. By sharing with those people and learning from their experiences, you may find it easier to solve problems and make difficult decisions.

Through participation in a support group, you will be better prepared and perhaps feel less devastated as your loved one's condition becomes worse. You also may be able to find some hope, from seeing that others who have been caring longer have survived the caregiving experience.

Finally, a support group can give you encouragement and moral support. The group's members can help you rebuild the self-esteem that may have been damaged in the caregiving process. In many cases, the support group members can become a second family, especially if you are not receiving help from family members or friends.

What If

What if you cannot attend the support group meeting at the time it is normally scheduled?

If you work during the day or you have difficulty with transportation at night, ask the Alzheimer's Association Chapter if there are others in your area who would like to meet at a different time and who may be interested in starting another group.

What if you do not drive?

Ask the Chapter if a support group member lives in your area and could pick you up, or if there are transportation services you could use.

What if you cannot leave your patient?

Ask the Chapter if respite services are available. Sometimes the support group will have a care provider(s) available during the meeting so family caregivers can attend while someone looks after their patients.

What if you already have too many demands on your time?

Try attending a support group meeting at least once. For many caregivers, attending their support group meeting becomes the single best hour-and-a-half they spend each week. It is the one time and place where they can relax and be themselves.

What if your circumstances make it impossible to attend?

Ask the Chapter if it has a telephone support network established for housebound caregivers.

What if you are not the primary caregiver?

If you live miles away from your loved ones, a local support group still can be useful by helping you understand what the caregiver is facing so you can offer assistance. It can be the source of caregiving suggestions and research updates that you can share with your loved one's caregiver. A support group also will give you the opportunity to share your emotions and fears with other family members. Their understanding and experience can help you cope with your situation.

How Do I Find a Support Group?

Check your local phone book for the listing of the nearest Alzheimer's Association Chapter, or call the Alzheimer's Association toll-free telephone number for a Chapter referral: 1-800-272-3900.

If there is not an Alzheimer's Association Chapter in your area, the nearest Area Agency on Aging (AAA) office should be able to provide you with information on support groups. If you are interested in starting a support group, call, toll-free, the nearest Alzheimer's Association Chapter or the Association's national office.

Chapter 30

Communicating with People with Alzheimer's Disease

Talking with people with Alzheimer's disease represents a special challenge, as Alzheimer's patients often exhibit the following behaviors and speech patterns:

- May substitute or make up words that sound like or mean something like the word they are trying to find.

- May repeat favorite words, even tactless curses.

- May have trouble organizing words into thoughts or lose their train of thought.

- May become angry or frustrated if misunderstood or may stop talking to avoid making mistakes.

- May misunderstand directions.

Nevertheless, people with Alzheimer's are very sensitive to tone and expression of voice, and generally understand more than they can express.

Excerpted from *You Are One of Us: Successful Clergy/Church Connections to Alzheimer's Families* by Lisa P. Gwyther, Center for Aging, Alzheimer's Family Support Program, The Joseph and Kathleen Bryan Alzheimer's Disease Research Center, © 1995 Duke University Medical Center; reprinted with permission.

297

Tips on Talking to People with Alzheimer's

- Never talk about her as if she were not there.

- Use non-verbal cues—pointing, touch, smiles, humor, demonstration or start the motion for him.

- Get her attention: approach from the front and maintain a distance that is comfortable; reduce confusing background noise.

- Be calm and supportive; make eye contact, hold hands.

- If you don't understand, ask her to point, gesture, or describe again.

- Help her find a missing word by guessing and asking if you are on the right track.

- Begin by identifying yourself and calling the person by name.

- Speak slowly and distinctly in a low pitch or into the person's good ear if hearing is impaired.

- Use familiar words and short sentences, but watch the tone of your voice—no talking down.

- Give simple one-step directions.

- Ask one question at a time and give her a chance to respond.

- Talk in positive terms; e.g., "Let's go," not "Don't do that."

- Avoid expressions she may no longer understand, like "Hop into the car."

- Don't correct, confront, explain or rationalize.

- Move slowly, touch gently and avoid startling her.

Responding to Changes in Behavior

- Rethink: Is the behavior harmful to her or others? Can you accept it or not take it personally?

- Redirect: Can she pace or work off her restlessness in some safer, more productive way?

- Distract: Snacks, treats, a walk, or a cup of tea may divert or calm someone down.

- Reassure: Let her know you understand she is scared and you will protect her from embarrassment or danger.

- Routines, rituals, repetition: Limit changes or need to make decisions.

- Slow down: avoid crowds, noise, demands, confrontations.

- Celebrate retained skills: e.g., remind her that she is still a great singer.

- Help her do it or do it for her to avoid failure.

Chapter 31

Dementia and Depression

Common concerns of primary care physicians working with geriatric patients include management of depression and dementia.[1] These disorders are major causes of morbidity and mortality in the elderly and present significant diagnostic challenges.

Dementia is a common geriatric disorder, affecting one in five persons over the age of 85 years. This disorder, which has many etiologies, represents a global impairment of intellect that interferes with all aspects of life, including social, cognitive and behavioral spheres. Alzheimer's disease accounts for 75 percent of dementias, but all patients presenting with symptoms of a dementing illness require a thorough investigation to rule out reversible causes.

Depression affects approximately 15 percent of the geriatric population.[2,3] Recognition of depression in this age group is important because suicide rates are higher in the elderly, especially in white men and persons with debilitating chronic illnesses.[4] Although rare, suicide in patients with Alzheimer's disease has been reported, and its risk should not be overlooked.[5] Depression is a disorder of mood that, like dementia, affects multiple spheres of functioning.[6]

Depression may be difficult to diagnose in elderly patients, for a variety of reasons. Sociocultural differences in beliefs about the meaning of dysphoria in the elderly may affect the willingness of patients

"Comorbid Disease in Geriatric Patients: Dementia and Depression," by Rebecca S. Lundquist, Anthony Bernens, and Cynthia G. Olsen, *American Family Physician*, June 1997, v55 n8 p2687(9), © 1997 American Academy of Family Physicians; reprinted with permission.

to report symptoms to their physician. In addition, the higher prevalence of disabling and painful physical disorders in the elderly may make the somatic signs and symptoms of depression more difficult to elucidate and separate from those of medical illness. These somatic symptoms may include fatigue, sleep disturbance, weight change or constipation.

Comorbidity

Memory loss, disinterest in surroundings and cognitive impairment are problems that need to be addressed because they are not signs of the normal aging process. Patients with mild dementia and patients with depression commonly complain about memory deficits, whereas patients with moderate to severe dementia may overestimate their memory.[6]

Coexistence of depression and dementing illness (especially mild to moderate dementia) is common, with an incidence ranging from 19 to 86 percent in some studies.[7,8] In some patients, depression can be mistaken for dementia when changes in cognition result directly from changes in mood. This reversible condition is referred to as "pseudodementia."

Elderly patients with Alzheimer's disease who are admitted to a nursing facility or who experience some other change in their environment, such as a change in caregiver status, frequently respond negatively to the disruption. The resultant behavior problems are easily attributed to the dementing illness, and the diagnosis of depression can be missed. When depression is not recognized, these patients may not receive treatment and symptomatic relief.

Finally, and perhaps most intriguingly, late-onset depression may be a harbinger of dementia. In one study,[9] Alzheimer's disease developed within two years in 39 percent of patients with late-onset depression. Studies that followed a group of patients with pseudodementia for three years[10] and eight years[11] found that Alzheimer's disease developed in 89 percent of these patients. The exact relationship between depression and the progression toward dementia is unclear.

Diagnosis

Since memory loss, cognitive deficit and lack of interest in surroundings are not part of the normal aging process, geriatric patients should be screened for both depression and dementia. In this context, the particular strengths of the primary care physician include a continuing relationship with the patient and the family, as well as a sense of the community in which the patient resides. These are extraordinary assets when working with elderly patients, particularly those with depression and dementia. Both dementia and depression affect not only cognition and behavior but also the activities of daily living. The physician's knowledge of the patient, combined with data from the patient's history, physical examination and laboratory studies, are invaluable in assessing both the presence and degree of depression and dementia.

It can be difficult to distinguish between depression with cognitive impairment and early Alzheimer's disease with depressive symptoms.[12] Memory deficits in major depression include problems with attention, concentration and speed of processing. Marked and profound memory deficits, visuospatial disorientation and wandering behavior are uncommon in primary depression. Likewise, neurologic signs of aphasia (speech impairment), apraxia (inability to use tools or execute purposeful movements) and acalculia (inability to perform simple calculations) are features of Alzheimer's disease and are not seen in patients who have depression without dementing illness.[13]

Depression may have an atypical presentation in moderately to severely depressed patients with Alzheimer's disease. In such patients, a significant underlying depressive disorder may be manifested by the new onset of aggressive behavior, agitation, wandering, crying out or shouting, angry outbursts, apathy, insomnia, resistiveness, cursing, picking, or the refusal of food or medication.[14]

The new onset of agitation in patients with Alzheimer's disease has a broad differential diagnosis, and other causes must be considered before a diagnosis of depression is made. These causes may include infectious illness, any pain syndrome, medication effects, cardiac ischemia and hypoxia. Furthermore, many patients with Alzheimer's disease who have a change in environment or caregiver may demonstrate a brief period of agitation.

A change in the functional status of patients with Alzheimer's disease may be the sign of a new illness, including depression. Caregivers of patients with Alzheimer's disease need to be interviewed regularly for evidence of deterioration in the functions of feeding, dressing, grooming, toileting and ambulation.

Screening Instruments

A number of screening instruments for dementia and depression can be used in the office setting. While screening tools are not diagnostic, they may assist in confirming the diagnostic impression. When used in combination with information from family members about a patient's level of functioning at home, screening tools can be extremely helpful in unmasking dementia and depression.

Because of its ease of administration and proven validity, the Mini-Mental State Examination (MMSE) is perhaps the best dementia screening tool available to primary care physicians.[15,16] The MMSE has been criticized for being less useful in patients with low levels of education and for being based more on language skills than on visuospatial skills. Some of the bias of the MMSE toward language deficit can be overcome by adding a simple test in which the patient is asked to draw a clock and then number the clock face. The clock test helps to identify patients with the visuospatial deficits of dementia.[17] With periodic administration every three to six months, the MMSE (or a comparable screening test) may also be used to evaluate disease progression.

While a number of depression scales are available, many are too lengthy and time-consuming to be used in the office. The Geriatric Depression Scale (GDS) does have an easily administered short form that has been well validated in geriatric populations.[18,19] Furthermore, the GDS relies less on somatic symptoms, such as constipation and insomnia, that may also be present in elderly patients who do not have depression. Disagreement exists concerning the use of the GDS in demented patients. However, mild to moderate dementia (a MMSE score higher than 15/30) does not seem to affect the usefulness of the GDS, especially when the test is orally administered, rather than self-administered.[20,21]

Screening for depression often can be accomplished by asking the patient one simple question: "Do you often feel sad or depressed?"[22]

Interviewing the family is important in uncovering information and often adds clarity to the evaluation. In one study,[23] researchers interviewed 36 patients with Alzheimer's disease and their caregivers. Based on information given by the patients alone, only 4.3 percent met the criteria for major depression as given in the Diagnostic and Statistical Manual of Mental Disorders (DSM-III-R).[24] When information from caregivers was used, 30.6 percent of patients met the criteria for depression. Other investigators have found similar discrepancies between patient and caregiver reports, underscoring the importance of involving caregivers and family members in the diagnostic process.[25]

Laboratory and Imaging Studies

The role of laboratory and imaging studies in the diagnosis of dementia and depression varies from patient to patient. Reversible causes for both disorders must be sought through the history and the physical examination, as well as through laboratory and imaging studies.[26] Among the reversible causes of dementia are drug toxicity, metabolic disorders, endocrine disorders, sensory deficits, nutritional disorders, intracranial pathology, infection and inflammatory complications. Many of these conditions can also produce an organic affective disorder with depressed mood (i.e., depression with an identifiable organic cause).

Laboratory tests are used in the medical evaluation of depressed and demented elderly persons. Patients who are both demented and depressed may have a vascular lesion, such as subdural hematoma, cortical cerebrovascular accident, arteriosclerosis, lacunar infarction, or periventricular small-vessel disease from hypertension (Binswanger's disease).

Although it is not possible to diagnose dementia or depression with any currently available imaging study, many physicians believe that mass lesions, intracranial bleeding and hydrocephalus should be ruled out with either computed tomographic scanning or magnetic resonance imaging. It would be unusual, however, for a patient to be diagnosed with any of these conditions in the absence of localizing signs or other clues in the history or the physical examination.[27]

Management

A variety of pharmacologic and nonpharmacologic treatments are used to manage Alzheimer's disease, depression and related behavior problems. Although no currently available drug can reverse the dementia of Alzheimer's disease, concurrent depression is amenable to treatment.

Nonpharmacologic Treatment

Once the diagnosis of depression is established in the patient with dementia, possible therapies should be discussed with family members and other caregivers, and a treatment plan should be formulated. Providing environmental stability and maintaining a structured daily routine can help reduce the patient's fear and agitation.[28] Having familiar persons and mementos in the environment can help reduce the anxiety often experienced by a patient with Alzheimer's disease and depression.

Caregivers must be educated about the dementing process, and they need to be instructed to change their expectations of the patient's ability to perform tasks and respond to situations. Depression is often caused by the patient's realization of his or her progressive functional impairment. Caregivers can help reduce the resulting despair and frustration by structuring the patient's tasks and activities in ways that reduce the likelihood of failure and increase opportunities for success and satisfaction.[29,30]

Adult day care and outpatient psychiatric care can increase patient functioning and help relieve depression, as well as decrease caregiver burden. Cognitive behavior therapy has been shown to be useful in the patient with early-stage Alzheimer's disease and concomitant depression. Caregivers must be monitored for burnout and depression, with support and referrals given when necessary.[30]

Pharmacotherapy

Antidepressant therapy is extremely beneficial in patients with concomitant dementia and depression. Drug treatment may actually be diagnostic of depression by improving depressed mood, decreasing agitation and sometimes lessening memory symptoms.[31] However, cognitive function improves only minimally and remains in the dementia range.[32] The correlation between the presence and severity of depression in patients with Alzheimer's disease and a resulting decline in cognitive function has been recognized. Whether functional improvement can occur with antidepressant therapy has yet to be established.[33]

Drug therapy for Alzheimer's disease has consisted of attempts to treat the dementing illness as well as accompanying disruptive behavior symptoms. The U.S. Food and Drug Administration has approved the use of tacrine (Cognex), a long-acting cholinesterase inhibitor, for the treatment of Alzheimer's disease, even though some doubts exist about the drug's efficacy for this indication.

One double-blind, placebo-controlled study[34] of tacrine in mildly to moderately impaired patients with Alzheimer's disease found that treated patients had a smaller decline in both cognitive function and activities of daily living. However, physicians who independently evaluated these patients detected no global difference between the treated group and the control group.

Alzheimer's disease appears to be a heterogeneous disorder in which the response to cholinesterase inhibition varies considerably. In patients who benefit from tacrine, clinically significant findings (recognized by both physician and caregiver) usually occur within 12 weeks of gradually increasing doses. Liver toxicity may occur, but it is reversible and is easily detected by monitoring alanine amino-transferase levels every other week for 16 weeks, monthly for two months and then quarterly. Tacrine does not appear to improve depressive symptoms in patients with Alzheimer's disease. The length of time that this drug is useful for the individual patient has yet to be determined.[35]

Other classes of psychoactive drugs are often used to control the behavior effects of Alzheimer's disease. The drug classes most commonly used for this purpose are the antipsychotics and the anxiolytics. While a full discussion of these drugs is beyond the scope of this chapter, it is important to note that antipsychotic and anxiolytic agents can have significant side effects, especially when they are used in large doses over long periods. These drugs do not alleviate depression in patients with Alzheimer's disease.[36]

While antidepressant therapy is efficacious in patients with Alzheimer's disease and concomitant depression, elderly patients are more susceptible to the most common and dangerous side effects of these medications, including central and peripheral anticholinergic effects (which can result in delirium), cardiovascular effects and sedative effects. Thus, in treating a geriatic patient with depression, it is very important to choose a drug that has a favorable side effect profile.

Lower doses of most antidepressants are effective in the elderly. Treatment is generally initiated at one half the recommended dose, and the patient is monitored for side effects as the dosage is titrated upward. Some physicians obtain an electrocardiogram and orthostatic blood pressures soon after a patient is started on an antidepressant medication.[37]

Antidepressants with greater anticholinergic effects, such as amitriptyline (Elavil, Endep), doxepin (Sinequan) and imipramine (Tofranil), generally are not favorable choices for elderly patients with dementia. Of the tricyclic antidepressants, nortriptyline (Pamelor) and desipramine (Norpramin) are considered to be more appropriate choices because of their decreased anticholinergic and sedative properties. Trazodone (Desyrel) is useful for its sedating effects, and it has been shown to reduce agitation.[37]

Tricyclic antidepressants do not change cognitive function in patients with Alzheimer's disease. Furthermore, the beneficial effects of these drugs may not become apparent until patients have been receiving an effective dose for at least four weeks.

In recent years, a number of drugs with novel structures and mechanisms of action have become available.[38] Selective serotonin reuptake inhibitors (SSRIs), including fluoxetine (Prozac), sertraline

307

(Zoloft), paroxetine (Paxil) and others, have been marketed heavily for use in geriatric populations. Although the SSRIs appear to have fewer anticholinergic and cardiac side effects, more work needs to be done to determine whether these agents are appropriate for patients with cognitive impairment and dementia. Preliminary studies in these patients tend to show equivalent efficacy for the various SSRIs. However, these agents may cause agitation, insomnia, gastrointestinal disturbance and weight loss. Other recently introduced drugs, such as nefazodone (Serzone) and venlafaxine (Effexor), show promise as alternative antidepressants with low side effect profiles.[39]

Referral to a psychiatrist should be considered for patients with intolerance of an antidepressant or nonresponse at six to eight weeks after the initiation of antidepressant drug therapy.

Final Comment

Numerous resources are available to primary care physicians who are managing patients with Alzheimer's disease and depression. Local chapters of the Alzheimer's Association can provide information on resources for patients and caregivers. Psychiatric consultation can be helpful when a patient is difficult to manage or has exhausted the resources and knowledge of the physician.

References

1. Williams ME, Connolly NK. What practicing physicians in North Carolina rate as their most challenging geriatric medicine concerns. *J Am Geriatr Soc* 1990;38:1230-4.

2. Gurland B, Dean L, Cross B. The epidemiology of depression and dementia in the elderly: the use of multiple indicators of these conditions. In: Cole JO, Barrett JE, eds. *Psychopathology in the aged*. New York: Raven Press, 1980.

3. Murrell SA, Himmelfarb S, Wright K. Prevalence of depression and its correlates in older adults. *Am J Epidemiol* 1983;117:173-85.

4. Carney SS, Rich CL, Burke PA, Fowler RC. Suicide over 60: the San Diego study. *J Am Geriatr Soc* 1994;42:174-80.

5. Koenig HG, Cohen HJ, Blazer DG, Krishnan KR, Sibert TE. Profile of depressive symptoms in younger and older medical

inpatients with major depression. *J Am Geriatr Soc* 1993;41:1169-76.

6. Grut M, Jorm AF, Fratiglioni L, Forsell Y, Viitanen M, Winblad B. Memory complaints of elderly people in a population survey: variation according to dementia stage and depression. *J Am Geriatr Soc* 1993;41:1295-300.

7. Reifler BV, Larson E, Hanley R. Coexistence of cognitive impairment and depression in geriatric outpatients. *Am J Psychiatry* 1982;139:623-6.

8. Merriam AE, Aronson MK, Gaston P, Wey SL, Katz I. The psychiatric symptoms of Alzheimer's disease. *J Am Geriatr Soc* 1988;36:7-12.

9. Alexopolous GS, Young RC, Meyers BS, Abrams RC, Shamoian CA. Late-onset depression. *Psychiatr Clin North Am* 1988;11:101-15.

10. Reding M, Haycox J, Blass J. Depression in patients referred to a dementia clinic. A three-year prospective study. *Arch Neurol* 1985;42:894-6.

11. Kral VA, Emery OB. Long-term follow-up of depressive pseudodementia of the aged. *Can J Psychiatry* 1989;34:445-6.

12. Wells CE. Pseudodementia. *Am J Psychiatry* 1979;136:895-900.

13. Reuben DB, Yoshikawa TT, Besdine RW, eds. *Geriatrics review syllabus; a core curriculum in geriatric medicine*. New York: American Geriatrics Society, 1993:11005-25.

14. Volicer BL, Hurley AC, Mahoney E. Management of behavioral symptoms of dementia. *Nursing Home Med* 1995;3:300-6.

15. Folstein MF, Folstein SE, McHugh PR. "Mini-mental state." A practical method for grading the cognitive state of patients for the clinician. *J Psychiatr Res* 1975;12:189-98.

16. Cockrell JR, Folstein MF. Mini-Mental State Examination (MMSE). *Psychopharmacol Bull* 1988;24:689-92.

17. Wolf-Klein GP, Silverstone FA, Levy AP, Brod MS. Screening for Alzheimer's disease by clock drawing. *J Am Geriatr Soc* 1989;37:730-4.

18. Sunderland T, Alterman IS, Yount D, Hill JL, Tariot PN, Newhouse PA, et al. A new scale for the assessment of depressed mood in demented patients. *Am J Psychiatry* 1988;145:955-9.

19. Yesavage JA, Brink TL, Rose TL, Lum O, Huang V, Adey M, et al. Development and validation of a geriatric depression screening scale: a preliminary report. *J Psychiatr Res* 1982-83;17:37-49.

20. Yesavage JA. Geriatric Depression Scale. *Psychopharmacol Bull* 1988;24:709-11.

21. McGivney SA, Mulvihill M, Taylor B. Validating the GDS depression screen in the nursing home. *J Am Geriatr Soc* 1994;42:490-2.

22. Mahoney J, Drinka TJ, Abler R, Gunter-Hunt G, Matthews C, Gravenstein S, et al. Screening for depression: single question versus GDS. *J Am Geriatr Soc* 1994;42:1006-8.

23. Mackenzie TB, Robiner WN, Knopman DS. Differences between patient and family assessments of depression in Alzheimer's disease. *Am J Psychiatry* 1989;146:1174-8.

24. *Diagnostic and statistical manual of mental disorders. 3d ed rev.* Washington, D.C.: American Psychiatric Association, 1987.

25. Teri L, Wagner AW. Assessment of depression in patients with Alzheimer's disease: concordance among informants. *Psychol Aging* 1991;6:280-5.

26. Larson EB, Reifler BV, Sumi SM, Canfield CG, Chinn NM. Diagnostic tests in the evaluation of dementia. A prospective study of 200 elderly outpatients. *Arch Intern Med* 1986;146:1917-22.

27. Katzman R. Should a major imaging procedure (CT or MRI) be required in the workup of dementia? An affirmative view. *J Fam Pract* 1990;31:401-5.

28. Mahusay N, Mahusay AJ. Depression in the agitated, demented elderly. *Nursing Home Medicine*. 1995;3:243-7.

29. Banazak DA. Difficult dementia: six steps to control problem behaviors. *Geriatrics* 1996;51:36-42.

30. Carlson DL, Fleming KC, Smith GE, Evans JM. Management of dementia-related behavioral disturbances: a nonpharmacologic approach. *Mayo Clin Proc* 1995;70:1108-15.

31. Teri L, Reifler BV, Veith RC, Barnes R, White E, McLean P, et al. Imipramine in the treatment of depressed Alzheimer's patients: impact on cognition. *J Gerontol* 1991;46:372-7.

32. Stoudemire A, Hill CD, Morris R, Martino-Saltzman D, Markwalter H, Lewison B. Cognitive outcome following tricyclic and electroconvulsive treatment of major depression in the elderly. *Am J Psychiatry* 1991;148:1336-40.

33. Fitz AG, Teri L. Depression, cognition, and functional ability in patients with Alzheimer's disease. *J Am Geriatr Soc* 1994;42:186-91.

34. Farlow M, Gracon SI, Hershey LA, Lewis KW, Sadowsky CH, Dolan-Ureno J. A controlled trial of tacrine in Alzheimer's disease. The Tacrine Study Group. *JAMA* 1992;268:2523-9.

35. Freeman SE, Dawson RM. Tacrine: a pharmacological review. *Prog Neurobiol* 1991;36:257-77.

36. Fleming KC, Evans JM. Pharmacologic therapies in dementia. *Mayo Clin Proc* 1995;70:1116-23.

37. Jenike MA. Treatment of affective illness in the elderly with drugs and electroconvulsive therapy *J Geriatr Psychiatry* 1989;22:77-112.

38. Sussman N. New approaches to the pharmacologic management of anxiety and depression in the elderly. *Clin Geriatrics* 1996;4:54-72.

39. Goldberg RJ. Nefazodone and venlafaxine: two new agents for the treatment of depression. *J Fam Pract* 1995;41:591-4.

Rebecca S. Lundquist, M.D. is a fourth-year resident in the Harvard Longwood psychiatry residency program and the Department of Psychiatry at Harvard Medical School, Boston. Dr. Lundquist received her medical degree from Wright State University School of Medicine, Dayton, Ohio.

Anthony Bernens, M.D. is a fourth-year resident in the Department of Internal Medicine at the University of California, Davis, Medical Center, Sacramento. He graduated from Wright State University School of Medicine.

Cynthia G. Olsen, M.D. is executive vice chair and associate professor in the Department of Family Medicine at Wright State University School of Medicine, where she earned her medical degree. Dr. Olsen completed a family practice residency at Good Samaritan Hospital, Dayton, and also earned a certificate of added qualifications in geriatric medicine.

Chapter 32

Exploring Care Options for a Relative with Alzheimer's Disease

When to Consider Getting Help for a Relative with Alzheimer's Disease

There is no standard answer to the question of when to seek help. Each family must examine its unique situation, considering both the needs of the person who is ill and the needs of the caregivers.

Family members who try to manage at home often far surpass their own endurance levels. They become physically and mentally exhausted long before they are willing to acknowledge that home and community-based services, assisted living or nursing home care may be a viable consideration.

"Home and community-based services" refers to the whole array of supportive services that help older persons continue to live in their homes and communities. Adult day care and companion services are just some of the services that may benefit persons with Alzheimer's disease and their families.

Assisted living residences offer a resident help with daily living activities such as bathing, dressing and eating. Many assisted living residences also provide some health care. Assisted living bridges the gap between living on one's own and living in a nursing home.

When a person with Alzheimer's disease reaches the point at which he or she needs round-the-clock, skilled health care, nursing home care may be the appropriate care option.

In spite of the confusion and mixed feelings you may be having as a caregiver, you probably should begin to familiarize yourself with home and community-based services, assisted living residences and nursing homes in your community and their requirements for admission. Do this as soon as possible after Alzheimer's disease is diagnosed. When you are faced with long-term care decisions, this information will help you make informed choices.

Financial Assistance Available for Home and Community-based Services

Financial assistance that is available depends on the type of service, the area in which you live and the type of insurance you have. Meals and transportation are often available through local senior programs for a suggested contribution.

Medicaid is the joint federal and state program that helps older people and those with disabilities pay for nursing home care and health care at home after they can no longer afford the expenses themselves. Medicaid pays for some community services, usually limited home health, hospice and personal care, depending on the state in which you live.

Medicare, the federal program that underwrites health insurance for persons 65 and older and some persons with disability, also covers limited home health and hospice care. Other federal assistance, such as the Older Americans Act and social services block grant funds, pays for some supportive services.

Adult day care and respite care are often available through community groups, sometimes on a sliding fee schedule. Insurance policies are beginning to cover some community services, such as day care and care management.

Financial Assistance for Assisted Living

Costs in assisted living residences range from less than $1,000 a month to $3,000 or more a month, depending on the services and accommodations offered. The facility's charges will reflect the number of services to which you have access. In addition to basic charges, there may be extra charges for some services. The cost may also vary according to the size of the room or apartment.

In some states, funds are available for those who cannot afford assisted living. In those states, the service component of assisted living may be paid for by Medicaid if the state has applied for and been approved under a home and community-based waiver. The waiver is for persons who are determined to be eligible for nursing home care. The resident may then use Supplemental Security Income (SSI) to pay for the room and board costs. In most cases, however, the resident or family pays for the majority of assisted living services.

Financial Assistance for Nursing Homes

Nursing home care, like all good health care, is costly. Before you enter into a contract, understand completely all the financial arrangements of the home you have selected. Nursing homes charge a basic daily or monthly rate.

Many residents or their families pay for nursing home care out of their own private funds. One way to help defray nursing home expenses is to purchase private long-term care insurance. Others whose finances are depleted rely on Medicaid to cover the costs of their nursing home care.

Ask the admissions staff at the nursing home of your choice what the basic monthly fee is and what it includes. Ask if the home charges extra for physician's fees, medications, laundry, special feeding, frequent linen changes or special supplies such as wheelchairs and walkers. Are therapies included in the basic charge? Is a deposit required?

To find out whether a resident is financially eligible for Medicaid, call the Department of Social Services in your area. Contact your Social Security office about Medicare, but be aware that Medicare pays for very little nursing home care, and never for a long-term stay.

In addition, if your relative is a veteran of the U.S. armed forces, it will be to your advantage to investigate services available through the Veterans Administration.

The nursing home may ask for financial disclosure to determine the appropriate payment mechanism. Admissions personnel will assist you in determining what information is necessary and what forms need to be filed to expedite placement.

Because some nursing homes have waiting lists, you might want to have paperwork done in advance in the event that an emergency placement is necessary.

Making the Transition

You, your family and close friends provide a special link between your relative and his or her past. You are familiar and are likely to have a calming effect. Frequent visits will help make the transition to an assisted living residence or nursing home care easier. Visiting is also important because it gives you the opportunity to get to know the facility staff and to help the staff get to know your relative. Visits also can help reassure you that your relative is getting the proper care. It is important that you stay involved in the resident's care.

Rituals can help ensure a smooth adjustment. For example, if your relative always reads the newspaper after lunch, then the act of reading or having a newspaper in hand—whether or not it can be read or understood—may be a comforting activity.

Creating a home-like atmosphere by personalizing his or her room with family photos, a favorite chair or a special blanket also can contribute to feeling secure. Because memories of earlier years remain accessible to persons with Alzheimer's disease much longer than events from the recent past, tapping the past can help create a familiar and safe situation in the present.

As a caregiver, you are dealing with feelings, pressures, and concerns that leave you under a tremendous amount of stress. Although it seems impossible now, you must take time for your own needs in addition to the needs of your relative. Joining an Alzheimer's family support group offers the opportunity to meet and gain strength from others with similar concerns. Your local area agency on aging, primary care physician, or an assisted living or nursing home staff member can provide information on support group meetings in your area.

Additionally, the Alzheimer's Disease and Related Disorders Association has a toll-free hot-line you can call for information about group meetings in your area. (Telephone 1-800-272-3900.)

Where to Write for Help

The American Association of Homes and Services for the Aging (AAHSA) has published a guidebook for relatives of persons with Alzheimer's disease. The authors are experienced long-term care providers who not only have cared for persons with Alzheimer's disease but also have provided counseling and services for their families.

The guidebook, titled *The Nursing Home and You: Partners in Caring for a Relative With Alzheimer's Disease*, offers insights and answers to common questions and concerns.

Topics include:

• Loneliness and Depression
• Working with Nursing Home Staff
• Solving the Lack of Privacy Problem

- Deciding about Home Visits
- How Often to Visit and What to Do
- Dating and Companionship
- Dealing with Behavior Changes
- Financial and Legal Concerns
- Confidentiality in Medical Care
- Recommended Readings

To order the guidebook or other AAHSA publications, call AAHSA publications at 1-800-508-9442 or, in the Washington, D.C. area, call 301-490-0677. You may also visit www.aahsa.org.

About the American Association of Homes and Services for the Aging

The American Association of Homes and Services for the Aging (AAHSA) is a national nonprofit organization representing nearly 5,000 not-for-profit nursing homes, continuing care retirement communities, assisted living and senior housing facilities and community service organizations for the elderly. AAHSA's mission is to represent the interest of its members and promote the association's vision through ethical leadership, advocacy, education, information and other services. AAHSA's vision is a world in which every community offers a continuum of high-quality, affordable and innovative health care, housing and community services and in which self-determination, compassion, benevolence, individual dignity, diversity and social responsibility are valued.

Chapter 33

Learning about Home and Community-Based Services

Most older people prefer to live independently in their own homes for as long as possible. "Home and community-based services" refers to the whole array of supportive services that help older persons live independently in their homes and communities.

Home and community-based services can help persons with daily living activities such as shopping, transportation, bathing and dressing. Many community services also create opportunities for social interaction. This is especially important to those who may be isolated. Often community services are provided by not-for-profit organizations sponsored by religious or fraternal groups or other community organizations.

Who Can Benefit from Home and Community-based Services?

Many older persons and their caregivers can benefit from some type of home or community-based service. One person may need only a little help with shopping to be able to stay at home. Another person may need a mix of services such as help with housekeeping, transportation and preparing meals. Others may seek social contacts through senior centers or volunteer activities, such as the foster grandparent or senior companion program.

Caregivers of older people who have chronic illnesses or disabilities often benefit from home and community-based services. For example, adult day care and respite care enable caregivers to work or take time off from caregiving responsibilities, knowing their loved ones are getting the care they need.

Just as everyone is different, so are individuals' needs different as they grow older. A variety of community service options can be put together in many combinations to meet an older person's needs.

What Types of Home and Community-based Services are Readily Available?

While many different community services exist for older people, not all are available in every community. The most commonly available services are described below.

- Adult day care services provide a variety of health, social and related support services in a protective setting during the day. Some day care programs are designed especially for those with Alzheimer's disease.

- Care coordination or case management helps older persons and their families gain access to needed services. A care manager works with the older person and family members to determine which services are most appropriate for their needs. The manager then puts together a plan of care and arranges for services.

- Congregate meal programs offer free or low-cost, nutritious meals in group settings, often in a senior center or senior housing facility.

- Financial counseling programs help older people balance their checkbooks, file income and property taxes and pay bills. They also help the elderly complete Medicaid, Medicare or insurance forms.

- Friendly visiting or companionship services provide socialization, supervision and support services to older persons in their own homes.

- Health maintenance services usually are provided in a congregate setting, such as a senior center. They include such services as blood pressure checks.

- Home health care services are provided in a person's own home. They can include part-time nursing services; personal care and homemaker or chore services provided under the supervision of a licensed nurse; medical supplies or equipment, and physical, occupational and speech therapies provided by licensed professionals.

- Homemaker or chore services help with general household activities, such as meal preparation and routine household care. They also help with heavy household chores such as washing floors, windows and walls and shoveling snow.

- Hospice care provides comfort, nursing care and other supportive services, such as counseling and homemaker services, to terminally ill persons and their families. Hospice care is provided in the client's home, in a nursing facility or in a community-based hospice.

- Home-delivered meals, often called meals-on-wheels, bring nutritionally balanced meals to those who are unable to prepare their own meals.

- Information and assistance referral services provide older persons and their families with information about available public and voluntary services and resources. Referrals to services often include contact and follow-up with the provider and/or client.

- Personal care services assist persons with daily living activities, such as eating, bathing, dressing and grooming.

- Respite care gives families temporary relief from the responsibility of caring for older persons who are unable to care for themselves. Respite care is offered in a variety of settings including the older person's home, the caregiver's home or a nursing facility.

- Rehabilitation services provide restorative care to an older person. These services try to reduce a person's physical or mental disability.

- Senior centers offer a variety of social and recreational services. Senior centers enable older adults to maintain social contacts, reduce social isolation and improve satisfaction with one's own life.

- Telephone reassurance is a service that maintains regular telephone contact. It ensures that people living alone have continued contact with the outside world.

- Transportation services help older people get to and from shopping centers, keep appointments and, generally, access a variety of community services and resources.

Is Any Financial Assistance Available for Home and Community-based Services?

The availability of financial assistance depends on the type of service, the area in which you live and the type of insurance you have. Meals and transportation are often available through local senior programs for a suggested contribution.

Medicaid is the joint federal and state program that helps older people and those with disabilities pay for nursing home care and health care at home after they can no longer afford the expenses themselves. Medicaid pays for some community services, usually limited home health, hospice and personal care, depending on the state in which you live.

Medicare, the federal program that underwrites health insurance for persons 65 and older and some persons with disability, also covers limited home health and hospice care. Other federal assistance, such as the Older Americans Act and social services block grant funds, pays for some supportive services.

Adult day care and respite care are often available through community groups, sometimes on a sliding fee schedule. Insurance policies are beginning to cover some community services, such as day care and care management.

The Continuing Care Retirement Community: A Guidebook for Consumers examines a variety of contractual agreements offered by continuing care retirement communities (CCRCs). A consumer checklist and financial worksheet help you make a decision before signing a continuing care contract. *The Consumers' Directory of Continuing Care Retirement Communities* will help you choose the CCRC that's right for you. It profiles over 500 CCRCs. (AAHSA publications can be ordered by calling 1-800-508-9442 or by visiting www.aahsa.org.)

Where Can I Get Further Information?

When contacting any organizations, be sure to state your need. For example, tell them you need daily help in preparing meals or that you need help getting to places. The agency you contact needs specific information in order to recommend the best support.

The best place to start is your local telephone directory. Check under county government or aged/aging services for a listing of the area agency on aging. If you have trouble locating your area agency on aging, call the toll-free Eldercare Locator at 1-800-677-1116 for referral to the agency near you.

About the American Association of Homes and Services for the Aging

The American Association of Homes and Services for the Aging (AAHSA) is a national nonprofit organization representing nearly 5,000 not-for-profit nursing homes, continuing care retirement communities, assisted living and senior housing facilities and community service organizations for the elderly. AAHSA's mission is to represent the interest of its members and promote the association's vision through ethical leadership, advocacy, education, information and other services. AAHSA's vision is a world in which every community offers a continuum of high-quality, affordable and innovative health care, housing and community services and in which self-determination, compassion, benevolence, individual dignity, diversity and social responsibility are valued.

323

Chapter 34

Choosing a Nursing Home

This publication discusses how to select a nursing home. It is not a legal document. The official provisions of the Medicare and Medicaid programs are contained in the relevant laws, regulations, and rulings.

Introduction

Selecting a nursing home is one of the most important and difficult decisions that you may be asked to make. Though it may be difficult to admit, you may spend several years in a nursing home. So it is important that you make the best decision possible, and base your decision on the most complete and timely information available.

The Health Care Financing Administration (HCFA) wants you to make a good choice when choosing a nursing home. This text is designed to help you choose a nursing home. It provides you with a step-by-step process that will assist you. It also provides you with some key resources that will help you conduct a wise search for the nursing home or long-term care facility that best fits your needs.

Step 1: Building a Network

Before you begin searching for a nursing home, it is a good idea to put together a network of people who can help you make the right choice. This team should include the family and friends who are im-

Health Care and Financing Administration, Pub. No. HCFA 02174, last updated December 10, 1996.

portant to you. It should also include the doctors and health professionals who understand your needs. Clergy and social workers may also be valuable network members.

Consult with your network. Family and friends may be willing to share responsibilities and should be treated as partners. Remember that two heads are better than one, and many heads are better than two.

If you are helping to select a nursing home for a relative, make every effort to involve your relative in the selection process. If your relative is mentally alert, it is essential that his or her wishes be respected. People who are involved in the selection process are better prepared when the time comes to move into a nursing home.

Finding a nursing home that provides the right services for you in a pleasant, comfortable environment often requires research. Ideally, you will have ample time to plan ahead, examine several nursing homes, and make the appropriate financial plans. By planning ahead, you will have more control over the selection process, more time to gather good information, and more time to make certain that everyone in your network is comfortable with the ultimate choice. Planning ahead is the best way to ease the stress that accompanies choosing a nursing home, and helps assure that you will make a good choice.

Unfortunately, a great many people must select a nursing home with little notice—frequently during a family crisis or right after a serious illness or operation. If you are in this situation, this chapter should still be helpful. Though you may not be able to follow all of the steps in the upcoming pages, by reading this chapter you will gain valuable information about nursing homes, learn about the people who might be able to help you, and pick up some tips about what to look for in a nursing home.

Step 2: Long-Term Care Options

Until recently, few alternatives to nursing homes existed for people who could no longer take care of themselves. Even today, some people are placed in nursing homes simply because neither they nor their family know about the alternatives to nursing homes. Today, people who cannot live completely independently may choose from a variety of living arrangements that offer different levels of care. For many, these alternatives are preferable to nursing homes.

Home and Community Care

Most people want to remain at home as long as possible. A person who is ill or disabled and needs help may be able to get a variety of home services that might make moving into a nursing home unnecessary. Home services include meals on wheels programs, friendly visiting and shopper services, and adult day care. In addition, there are a variety of programs that help care for people in their homes. Some nursing homes offer respite care—when they admit a person for a short period of time to give the home caregivers a break. Depending on the case, Medicare, private insurance, and Medicaid may pay some home care costs.

Subsidized Senior Housing

There are Federal and State programs that subsidize housing for older people with low to moderate incomes. A number of these facilities offer assistance to residents who need help with certain tasks, such as shopping and laundry, but residents generally live independently in an apartment within the senior housing complex. In this way, subsidized senior housing serves as a lower cost alternative to assisted living—though assisted living communities are frequently newer and more luxurious.

Assisted Living (Non-Medical Senior Housing)

Some people need help with only a small number of tasks, such as cooking and laundry. Some may only need to be reminded to take their medications. For those people who need only a small amount of help, assisted living facilities may be worth considering. Assisted living is a general term for living arrangements in which some services are available to residents (meals, laundry, medication reminders), but residents still live independently within the assisted living complex. In most cases, assisted living residents pay a regular monthly rent, and then pay additional fees for the services that they require.

Board and Care Homes

These are group living arrangements (sometimes called group or domiciliary homes) that are designed to meet the needs of people who cannot live independently, but do not require nursing home services. These homes offer a wider range of services than independent living options. Most provide help with some of the activities of daily living, including eating, walking, bathing, and toileting. In some cases, private long-term care insurance and medical assistance programs will help pay for this type of living.

327

Continuing Care Retirement Communities (CCRCs)

CCRCs are housing communities that provide different levels of care based on the needs of their residents—from independent living apartments to skilled nursing in an affiliated nursing home. Residents move from one setting to another based on their needs, but continue to remain a part of their CCRC's community. Many CCRCs require a large payment prior to admission, then charge monthly fees above that. For this reason, many CCRCs are too expensive for older people with modest incomes.

What Is a Nursing Home?

A nursing home is a residence that provides room, meals, recreational activities, help with daily living, and protective supervision to residents. Generally, nursing home residents have physical or mental impairments which keep them from living independently. Nursing homes are certified to provide different levels of care, from custodial to skilled nursing (services that can only be administered by a trained professional).

Before deciding which care setting is most appropriate for you or your relative, talk to your doctor or a social worker and get a realistic assessment of care needs. If you are considering home care, be sure you understand all the work that comes with caring for a chronically ill person. If you are considering independent living, consider the risks associated with an unsupervised environment.

Be sure to discuss long-term care options with family members who will be the main home care givers and/or visitors to your new home. Consider how you will pay for your own long-term care.

Remember that caring for someone who is very sick requires a lot of work. Nursing homes are designed to meet the needs of the acutely or chronically ill. The options discussed above may work for people who require less than skilled care, or who require skilled care for only brief periods of time, but many people with long-term skilled care needs require a level and amount of care that cannot be easily handled outside of a nursing home.

Step 3: Gathering Information

Once you have decided that a nursing home is the right choice for you, it is time to gather information about the nursing homes in your area. A good first step in this process is finding out exactly how many nursing homes there are in your area (because nursing homes are frequently located in out of the way areas, there might be more than you think).

There are a number of ways that you can learn about the nursing homes in your area. The easiest ways to find out about local nursing homes begin with the phone book. Your yellow pages list many of the nursing homes in your area. In addition, your local Office on Aging (in the Blue Pages of your Phone Book) should have a listing of nursing homes in your area and will be able to refer you to your local Long-Term Care Ombudsman.

You can get information on the nursing homes in your area from a variety of sources. Word of mouth can be a good source of information. Ask your friends and neighbors if they know people who have stayed in local nursing homes. Learn all you can from these different sources.

Some Facts about Nursing Homes

On any given day, nursing homes are caring for about one in twenty Americans over the age of 65. Almost half of all Americans turning 65 this year will be admitted into a nursing home at least once. One fifth of those people admitted into nursing homes stay at least one year—one tenth stay three years or more.

The Long-Term Care Ombudsman

One of the best sources of information is your local long-term care ombudsman. Nationwide, there are more than 500 local ombudsman programs. Ombudsman visit nursing homes on a regular basis—their job is to investigate complaints, advocate for residents, and mediate disputes. Ombudsman often have very good knowledge about the quality of life and care inside each nursing home in their area.

Ombudsman are not allowed to recommend one nursing home over another. But when asked about specific nursing homes they can provide information on these important subjects:

- the results of the latest survey,
- the number of outstanding complaints,
- the number and nature of complaints lodged in the last year,
- the results and conclusions of recent complaint investigations.

In addition, the ombudsman may provide general advice on what to look for when visiting the various area nursing homes. The phone

329

number of your State Long-Term Care Ombudsman is provided in the "Additional Help and Information" section.

Other Community Resources

In addition to the Long-Term Care Ombudsman, there are many other resources that you should consult before selecting a nursing home. Some other people who might be helpful are:

- hospital discharge planners or social workers,
- physicians who serve the elderly,
- clergy and religious organizations,
- volunteer groups that work with the elderly and chronically ill,
- nursing home professional associations.

By using these resources, you will tap into a community of people who understand nursing homes and have a good deal of knowledge about the homes in your area. You should now be able to make a list of the homes in your area which have good reputations.

Other Information You Will Need

There are also some types of basic information that should help you narrow your list of nursing homes. Consider some of these factors—a quick phone call to the nursing home should answer these concerns:

Religious and Cultural Preferences. If you have religious or cultural preferences, contact the nursing homes on your list and see if they offer the type of environment which you would prefer.

Medicare and Medicaid Participation. If you will be using Medicare or Medicaid, make certain that the nursing homes on your list accept Medicare or Medicaid payment. Often, only a portion of the home is certified for Medicare or Medicaid, so make sure that the home has Medicare or Medicaid "beds" available. For more information how Medicare and Medicaid pay for nursing home care, scroll to the end of this section.

HMO Contracts. If you belong to a managed care plan that contracts with a particular nursing home or homes in your area, make sure the homes you are considering have contracts with your HMO.

Availability. Make certain that the nursing homes on your list will have space available at the time you might need to be admitted.

Special Care Needs. If you require care for special medical conditions or dementia, make sure that the nursing homes on your list are capable of meeting these special circumstances.

Location. If you have a large number of nursing home choices, it is usually a good idea to consider nursing homes that your family and friends can visit easily.

Why is location important? In most cases, it is a mistake to select a nursing home that is difficult to visit on a regular basis. Frequent visits are the best way to make sure that you or your relative does well in the nursing home. Visitors are important advocates for chronically ill residents. Frequent visits often make the transition to the nursing home easier for new residents and their families.

You will now be able to figure out which homes in your area may or may not be worth visiting. You will also now be better informed when you begin visiting your area's nursing homes.

Paying for Nursing Home Care

Nursing home care is expensive (a skilled nursing home will cost about $200 a day in many parts of the country). For most people, finding ways to finance nursing home care is a major concern. There are several ways that nursing home care is financed:

Personal Resources. About half of all nursing home residents pay nursing home costs out of personal resources. When most people enter nursing homes, they usually pay out of their own savings. As personal resources are spent, many people who stay in nursing homes for long periods eventually become eligible for Medicaid.

Long-Term Care Insurance. Long-Term Care Insurance is private insurance designed to cover long-term care costs. Plans vary widely, and you would be wise to do some research before purchasing any long-term care policy. Generally, only relatively healthy people may purchase long-term care insurance. For further information on this type of insurance, contact the National Association of Insurance Commissioners and ask for their free booklet, *The Shopper's Guide to Long-Term Care Insurance.* Call (816) 374-7259 for your copy.

331

Medicaid. Medicaid is a State and Federal program that will pay most nursing home costs for people with limited income and assets. Eligibility varies by state, and you should check into your state's eligibility requirements before assuming that you are either eligible or ineligible. Medicaid will only pay for nursing home care provided in Medicaid-certified facilities.

Medicare. Under certain limited conditions, Medicare will pay some nursing home costs for Medicare beneficiaries who require skilled nursing or rehabilitation services. To be covered, you must (after a qualifying hospital stay) receive the services from a Medicare-certified skilled nursing home. HCFA's book, *Your Medicare Handbook*, discusses the conditions under which Medicare will help pay for nursing home costs in a Medicare-certified nursing home. To obtain a free copy of *Your Medicare Handbook*, call (800) 638-6833.

Medicare Supplemental Insurance. This is private insurance (often called Medigap) that pays Medicare's deductibles and co-insurances, and may cover services not covered by Medicare. Most Medigap plans will help pay for skilled nursing care, but only when that care is covered by Medicare.

In addition, some people have nursing home costs covered, or partially covered, by managed care plans or employer benefit packages.

If you have any questions about how you will pay for nursing home care, what coverage you may already have, or whether there are any government programs that will help with your expenses, there are people who can help. Your State's Insurance Counseling and Assistance (ICA) program has counselors ready to help you figure out how you can finance your long-term care.

Visiting Nursing Homes

The nursing home visit is probably the most important step in selecting the right nursing home. A visit provides you with an opportunity to talk to nursing home staff and, more importantly, with the people who live and receive care at the nursing home.

When you visit the nursing home, you will probably be given a formal tour. While this may be a very useful introduction to the home, it is important that you are not overly influenced by a guided tour. When the tour is over, return to some of the places where staff are caring for residents. Be ready to ask the staff members who are caring for residents questions about their jobs and how they feel about caring for people with so many different needs. A checklist at the end of this chapter will give you some more ideas on what questions to ask.

Near the beginning of your visit, spend some time examining the nursing home's most recent survey report. By law, this report must be posted in the nursing home in an area that is accessible to visitors and residents. Surveyors compile a survey report that lists areas in which the nursing home is cited for deficient practices. Keep these deficiencies in mind as you visit the nursing home, and see whether the home has corrected the deficient practices listed on the survey report.

Over the last decade, different laws and regulations have been enacted to raise the standards of nursing home care, particularly with respect to quality of life. *The law now requires that residents receive the necessary care and services that will enable them to reach and maintain their highest practicable level of physical, mental and social well-being.* In addition, civil rights law ensures equal access in all nursing homes regardless of race, color or national origin.

Ask residents questions about the nursing home. Learn what they like and what their complaints are. Ask visitors or volunteers similar questions. The checklist at the end of this chapter will give you some additional ideas about what types of questions you should ask.

What Is a Survey?

All nursing homes that are certified to participate in the Medicare or Medicaid programs are visited by a team of trained State surveyors approximately once a year. These surveyors (like inspectors) examine the home over several days and inspect the performance of the nursing home in numerous areas—including quality of life and quality of care. At the conclusion of the survey, the team reports its findings. Nursing homes with deficiencies are subject to fines and other penalties if they are not corrected.

Quality of Life

When visiting nursing homes, pay special attention to quality of life issues. People who are admitted into nursing homes do not leave their personalities at the door. Nor do they lose their basic human needs for respect, encouragement, and friendliness. All individuals need to retain as much control over the events in their daily lives as possible.

Nursing home residents should have the freedom and privacy to attend their personal needs—from managing their own finances (if mentally able) to decorating their rooms with favorite items. They should also be able to participate in their care planning and retain the right to examine their medical records. Residents may only be restrained when medically necessary (see the end of this chapter for more information on restraint usage). Most importantly, staff must always respect the dignity of each individual resident.

To check to see if the nursing home respects the dignity of each individual, look into these questions:

- Are staff members courteous to residents and is the home's management responsive to concerns raised by residents?

- Does the nursing home provide a variety of activities and allow residents to choose the activities they want to attend?

- Does the nursing home provide menu choices or prepare special meals at the request of residents? (Sample the food if possible.)

- Are family members encouraged to visit, and are they allowed to visit in privacy when requested?

The checklist at the end of this chapter lists other topics you should consider when assessing whether the nursing home is sensitive to quality of life. Also, check Step 6 below for additional information on the rights of residents and family members.

Quality of Care

Unless you have a medical or social work background, it might be difficult to assess how well the nursing home provides high quality health care to its residents. However, there are still a number of actions you can take to evaluate whether the home is providing high quality health care.

- Check the survey report and see if the home was cited for deficient practices in any quality of care areas.

- Ask about the home's staffing, and ask residents if the staff are available when needed. Make sure that you are comfortable with the number of residents assigned to each nurse and nurse aide. Be aware that there might be less staff at night or on the weekends.

- If you have any special care needs (e.g., dementia, ventilator dependency), it is generally a good idea to make sure that the home has experience in working with people who have had the same condition.

- Even if you have a trusted doctor, ask about the nursing home's physician and how often he or she visits the home. Since the home's doctor may be called in case of emergencies, you should be confident that the home's doctor can take care of resident needs.

By law, nursing homes must complete a comprehensive assessment for every new resident within two weeks of admission. The home also must complete a care plan that is designed to help each resident reach or maintain his or her highest level of well-being. Ask the home about its care planning process and make sure you agree with the home's philosophy. Remember that residents who have meaningful activities and are as independent as possible are generally better able to maintain their health.

The Nursing Home Checklist

At the end of this chapter you will find a nursing home checklist. As you visit several homes, it might become difficult to keep all of your observations straight, so fill out the checklist shortly after every visit. Make copies of this checklist, so that you can fill out a separate checklist for every nursing home that you visit. Blank spaces have been left at the bottom of the page for you to add your own concerns to this list. If you have any gut feelings or additional observations, write them down also.

After visiting several homes and filling out the checklist, you should be ready to decide on a short list of homes that might be a good choice for you or your relative. When you narrow your list down to a small number, it is time to conduct follow-up analysis.

Step 5: Follow-up Analysis

Now that you have narrowed your search down to a short list of nursing homes, it is time to revisit some of the earlier steps. Contact the people in your network (from step 1) and make sure they are comfortable with your short list. See if they have any additional information to offer about the homes on your short list.

Follow-up Visits

You should visit the nursing homes on your short list at least one more time (or as many additional times as you think necessary). Make sure that you see the home at least once in the evening and/or on a weekend because staffing is frequently different at these times. Also, your follow-up visit should include attending a meeting of the nursing home's resident council and/or family council. These meetings will give you a unique look at the concerns of the residents and/or their families. If the nursing home does not have resident or family councils, that might tell you something about the philosophy of the home's management.

Follow-up visits should be conducted at different times of the day than your first visit. Be sure at least one of your visits was during the late morning or midday, so you can observe residents when they are out of bed, eating, and attending activities. Continue to ask questions, and take special note of the differences between the nursing homes left on your short list.

After your follow-up visits, you should be able to narrow your short list down to a few nursing homes. At this point it still may be difficult to pick one. A final call to the ombudsman and the other people who provided you with information in the past might help. If you have any additional questions, do not hesitate to contact or visit the nursing home again.

You should now be ready to select the nursing home that is best able to meet your needs. The final decision may still be difficult, and it is possible that more than one nursing home will be a good choice for you. However, you should now have enough information to be confident that you are making the wisest possible choice.

Step 6: After Admission

Even if you made a well-reasoned choice and selected a nursing home only after following the steps discussed in this chapter, it is possible that you may not be entirely satisfied with your choice. New nursing home residents may go through a difficult adjustment period, even if the nursing home is doing all that it can.

Be aware that the law gives you and your relatives specific rights in the nursing home. You should be ready to hold the nursing home accountable if it is not honoring the rights of residents and family members. A summary of these rights is detailed below.

Resident Rights In a Nursing Home

Some people think that nursing home residents surrender the right to make medical decisions, manage funds, and control their activities when they enter a nursing home. This is not true. As a nursing home resident, you have the same rights as anyone else, and certain special protections under the law. The nursing home must post and provide new residents with a statement that details each resident's rights. New residents also have these specific rights.

Respect. You have the right to be treated with dignity and respect. You have the right to make your own schedule, bed-time, and select the activities you would like to attend (as long as it fits your plan of care.) A nursing home is prohibited from using physical and chemical restraints except when necessary to treat medical symptoms (see the Reader Notice at the end of this chapter for more information on restraints.)

Services and Fees. The nursing home must inform you, in writing, about its services and fees before you enter the home. Most facilities charge a basic rate that covers room, meals, housekeeping, linen, general nursing care, recreation, and some personal care services. There may be extra charges for personal services, such as haircuts, flowers, and telephone.

Managing Money. You have the right to manage your own money or to designate someone you trust to do so. If you allow the nursing home to manage your personal funds, you must sign a written statement that authorizes the nursing home to manage your finances, and the nursing home must allow you access to your funds. Federal law requires that the home protect your funds from any loss by having a bond or similar arrangement.

Privacy, Property, and Living Arrangements. You have the right to privacy. In addition, you have the right to keep and use your personal property, as long as it does not interfere with the rights, health, or safety of others. Your mail can never be opened by the home unless you allow it. The nursing home must have a system in place to keep you safe from neglect and abuse, and to protect your property from theft. If you and your spouse live in the same home, you are entitled to share a room (if you both agree to do so).

337

Guardianship and Advanced Directives. As a nursing home resident, you are responsible for making your own decisions (unless you are mentally unable). If you wish, you may designate someone else to make health care decisions for you. You may also draw up advance directives. A Durable Power of Attorney will become your legal guardian if you ever become incapable of making your own decisions. You may also make your end of life wishes known in a living will.

Getting help with legal documents. Depending upon your State's laws, you may need a lawyer to draw up a Durable Power of Attorney order or a living will. Check with your local Office on Aging to find out if your state has any legal assistance services that help with preparing these documents. You will find the phone number for your local Office on Aging in the Blue Pages of your phone directory.

Visitors. You have the right to spend private time with the visitors of your choice at any reasonable hour. You have the right to make and receive telephone calls in privacy. The nursing home must permit your family to visit you at any time. Any person who provides you with health or legal services may see you at any reasonable times. Of course, you do not have to see anyone you do not wish to see.

Medical Care. You have the right to be informed about your medical condition, medications, and to participate in your plan of care. You have the right to refuse medications or treatments, and to see your own doctor.

Social Services. The nursing home must provide each resident with social services, including counseling, mediation of disputes with other residents, assistance in contacting legal and financial professionals, and discharge planning.

Moving Out. Living in a nursing home is voluntary. You are free to move to another place. However, nursing home admission policies usually require that you give proper notice that you are leaving. If you do not give proper notice, you may owe the nursing home money based on the home's proper notice rules. Residents whose nursing home services are covered by Medicare and Medicaid do not have to give the nursing home proper notice before moving out.

Discharge. The nursing home may not discharge or transfer you unless:

- it is necessary for the welfare, health, or safety of others,
- your health has declined to the point that the nursing home cannot meet your care needs,
- your health has improved to the extent that nursing home care is no longer necessary,
- the nursing home has not received payment for services delivered,
- the nursing home ceases operation.

If you have any concerns about the nursing home in which you live, call your local long-term care ombudsman.

Your Rights as a Relative

Relatives and friends have rights too. Family members and legal guardians have the right to privacy when visiting the nursing home (but only when requested by the resident.) They also have the right to meet with the families of other residents. If the nursing home has a family council, you have the right to join or address this group.

By law, nursing homes must develop a plan of care for every resident. Family members are allowed to assist in preparing the development of this care plan, with the resident's permission. In addition, relatives who have legal guardianship of nursing home residents have the right to examine all medical records concerning their loved one. If you are a resident's legal guardian, Federal law gives you the right to make important decisions on behalf of your relative.

It is important to remember that relatives play a major role in making sure that residents are receiving good care. You can make sure your loved one is receiving good care by visiting often, expressing your concerns whenever they arise, and being active in the nursing home's family council (or helping to start a family council if the nursing home does not have one.)

Remember that if your concerns are not being addressed by the nursing home or if you have a complaint, there are people who can help. Contact your state long-term care ombudsman.

Nursing Home Checklist

The checklist beginning on the next page is designed to be used in concert with the Health Care Financing Administrations booklet, *The Guide to Choosing a Nursing Home*. This booklet can be obtained by calling (800) 638-6833.

Nursing Home Checklist

This checklist is designed to help you evaluate and compare the nursing homes that you visit. It would be a good idea to make several copies of this checklist, so that you will have a new checklist for each home you visit. After you have completed checklists on all the nursing homes you plan on visiting, compare your checklists. Comparisons will be helpful in selecting the nursing homes that might be the best choice for you.

Part 1: Basic Information

Name of
Nursing Home: _____

Address: _____

        _____

Phone: _____

Cultural/Religious Affiliation (if any):   _____

Medicaid Certified?	Yes	No
Medicare Certified?	Yes	No
Admitting New Residents?	Yes	No
Convenient Location?	Yes	No
Is home capable of meeting your special care needs?	Yes	No

For parts two through five, rate the nursing home on a scale from one to ten, with ten being a perfect score.

Part 2: Quality of Life

1. Are residents treated respectfully
    by staff at all times?   1 2 3 4 5 6 7 8 9 10

2. Are residents dressed
    appropriately and well-groomed?   1 2 3 4 5 6 7 8 9 10

3. Does staff make an effort to meet
    the needs of each resident?   1 2 3 4 5 6 7 8 9 10

4. Is there a variety of activities to
    meet the needs of individual
    residents?   1 2 3 4 5 6 7 8 9 10

5. Is the food attractive and tasty?
    (sample a meal if possible)   1 2 3 4 5 6 7 8 9 10

6. Are resident rooms decorated
    with personal articles?   1 2 3 4 5 6 7 8 9 10

7. Is the home's environment
    homelike?   1 2 3 4 5 6 7 8 9 10

8. Do common areas and
    resident rooms contain
    comfortable furniture?   1 2 3 4 5 6 7 8 9 10

9. Does the facility have a family
    and residents' council?   1 2 3 4 5 6 7 8 9 10

10. Does the facility have contact
    with outside groups of volunteers?   1 2 3 4 5 6 7 8 9 10

Part 3: Quality of Care

11. Does staff encourage residents
    to act independently?   1 2 3 4 5 6 7 8 9 10

12. Does facility staff respond quickly
    to calls for assistance?   1 2 3 4 5 6 7 8 9 10

13. Are residents and family involved
    in resident care planning?   1 2 3 4 5 6 7 8 9 10

341

14. Does the home offer appropriate
    therapies (physical, speech, etc.)?   1 2 3 4 5 6 7 8 9 10

15. Does the nursing home have
    an arrangement with a nearby
    hospital?   1 2 3 4 5 6 7 8 9 10

Part 4: Safety

16. Are there enough staff to appro-
    priately provide care to residents?   1 2 3 4 5 6 7 8 9 10

17. Are there handrails in the
    hallways and grab bars in
    bathrooms?   1 2 3 4 5 6 7 8 9 10

18. Is the inside of the home in
    good repair and exits clearly
    marked?   1 2 3 4 5 6 7 8 9 10

19. Are spills and other accidents
    cleaned up quickly?   1 2 3 4 5 6 7 8 9 10

20. Are the hallways free of
    clutter and well-lighted?   1 2 3 4 5 6 7 8 9 10

Part 5: Other Concerns

21. Does the home have outdoor areas
    (patios, etc.) for resident use?   1 2 3 4 5 6 7 8 9 10

22. Does the home provide an
    updated fist of references?   1 2 3 4 5 6 7 8 9 10

23. Are the latest survey reports
    and lists or resident rights posted?   1 2 3 4 5 6 7 8 9 10

24. (Your Concern)

25. (Your Concern)

Additional Comments: _____

_____

Reader Notice

The Health Care Financing Administration (HCFA), the Federal Agency that oversees Medicare and Medicaid, wants you to be aware of the two issues involving nursing homes. First, nursing homes cannot require pre-payment from residents who are relying on Medicare or Medicaid to pay for their nursing home services. Second, nursing homes may not use physical or chemical restraints on residents, except when medically necessary.

Pre-Payment. If you are a Medicare or Medicaid beneficiary applying for admission to a nursing facility for care that will be covered by Medicare or Medicaid, it is unlawful for the facility to require you to pay a cash deposit. Federal law prohibits nursing facilities from requiring a pre-payment as a condition of admission for care covered under either Medicare or Medicaid. The facility may, however, request that a Medicare beneficiary pay coinsurance amounts and other charges for which a beneficiary is liable. You pay those charges as they become due, not before. A facility may also require a cash deposit before admission if your care will not be covered by either Medicare or Medicaid.

Restraints. You should also be aware that Federal Law prohibits nursing homes from using physical or chemical restraints on residents for discipline or for the convenience of nursing home staff. Restraints increase the chances that residents will develop incontinence, impaired circulation, and swelling. Restrained residents also tend to suffer decreased functional ability, lower self-esteem, and feelings of depression, anger, and stress. Restrained residents are not safer than they would be if left unrestrained. Restrained individuals are more likely to suffer serious injuries when they fall. It is important that nursing home residents, whenever possible, be left unrestrained.

Restraints may be used only when necessary to treat medical symptoms. Physical restraints include articles, such as belts or vests, that secure a resident's limbs or bind a resident to a bed, chair, or other stationary item. In addition, common nursing home items, such as lap trays and bed rails, when employed solely to keep a resident from moving about, are considered restraints. Chemical restraints include drugs that are administered to keep a resident subdued.

If you know of a nursing facility that is improperly demanding pre-payments or restraining residents, you should contact your State's Long Term Care Ombudsman. You will find their phone number and address in the "Additional Help and Information" section of this book.

Chapter 35

Alzheimer's Disease and Related Dementias: Legal Issues in Care and Treatment

Preface

This report focuses upon legal issues arising in the context of Alzheimer's disease, matters that affect the person with the disorder, his or her family, health care professionals, and society at large. It contains a series of public policy recommendations for actions that are designed to resolve the problems that now arise in the context of judgments of legal competency and medical diagnoses of probable Alzheimer's disease (AD) or other related dementing disorders (ADRD). [The abbreviation ADRD is used when referring to the dementias as an undifferentiated group of disorders with similar manifestations, e.g., the population considered to show the cognitive impairments of dementia as a result of either Alzheimer's disease or related disorders. The abbreviation AD is used when referring to features, such as neuropathological changes, thought to be specific to the Alzheimer's disease process rather than true of dementias in general.]

Introduction

Alzheimer's disease (AD) currently affects an estimated 4 million Americans. Manifested initially by mild forgetfulness, this devastating

Excerpted from *A Report to Congress of the Advisory Panel on Alzheimer's Disease: Alzheimer's Disease and Related Dementias: Legal Issues in Care and Treatment*, December 1994. For a copy of the complete report including footnotes, references, and appendices contact the Alzheimer's Disease Education and Referral Center (800) 438-4380.

disease eventually erodes all cognitive and functional abilities, leading to total dependence on caregivers and, ultimately, to death. The prevalence of AD increases dramatically with age. Persons age 65 to 74 have a 1 in 25 chance of having AD; for those 85 and older, the likelihood rises to a staggering level, approaching 1 in every 2 persons. Those age 85 and over represent the most rapidly growing sector of the American population, portending a dramatic increase in the overall number of cases of AD in the coming decade.

Persons with Alzheimer's disease and related dementias (ADRD) often are unaware of the toll taken by the multiple effects of the disease process at work within them. Initially, they evidence increasing "forgetfulness"; over time, they find themselves unable to work or to manage home life and personal care. Eventually, the inexorable course of the disease leads to loss of cognition and total dependence. On average, an individual's progressive incapacitation, with the attendant dependency and need for family or other forms of care, may last 6 to 8 years. At times, it can extend decades. In the progression of the disorder, persons with AD lose their ability to make decisions about even the most basic aspects of daily living: when and what to eat; how to dress; how to groom; how to toilet. They become dependent upon 24-hour supervision and need more intensive therapeutic interventions, most often aimed not at the disease itself, but at its secondary behavioral and psychiatric symptoms of agitation, wandering, and inappropriate behavior.

Intervention most often first comes from family and other informal caregivers. The families of those with Alzheimer's disease experience increasingly substantial burdens as the result of the caregiving role. In an effort to delay institutional care, spouses and other family members often attend to the AD patient in the home, at the cost of lost wages, lost jobs, and lost time to tend to one's own needs. The incidence of compromised physical and mental health among family caregivers is significant as well. While respite care, adult day programs, and other community-based health care services may help reduce the growing pressure experienced by family caregivers, these services are of limited availability in many areas and are not sought by many family caregivers.

One of the most common results of this increased caregiver burden is placement in long-term care facilities, adding to the family burden in economic terms. Indeed, AD is one of the late life health problems most greatly feared by American families, due both to the enormous suffering it causes and to the significant costs it incurs. Persons with ADRD often require extended periods of nursing home care; when coupled with their lost income and the lost income of family caregivers, the result may be economic disaster. For many persons with AD, the last years of life are spent in a long-term care facility, the costs of which are borne primarily by today's welfare system.

In its previous reports, the Panel considered a host of medical, ethical, and health economic issues arising at their interface with Alzheimer's disease. We have examined issues of eligibility, health care financing, and professional training. Panel reports have shed light on the special concerns of ethnic and minority populations facing AD; and we have wrestled with issues of values that control caregiving decisions made by and for persons with ADRD. In this report, we turn to legal issues, another area of growing concern in the care and treatment of AD. Central to the discussion are questions of autonomy and incapacity, medical decisionmaking, and long-term care.

The Law and Alzheimer's Disease

Today, the U.S. legal system contains very little codified "law" specific to Alzheimer's disease and related dementias, notwithstanding the fact that these disorders are thought to affect over 4 million AD patients and perhaps again as many family caregivers and to cost nearly $100 billion dollars annually. Relatively few statutes, whether at the Federal, state, or local jurisdictional level, contain any reference to Alzheimer's disease itself. A nationwide computer-based research inquiry conducted by the Panel found that in 1993, only 85 Federal and 200 state statutes in any area of jurisprudence included a specific reference to Alzheimer's disease. A preponderance of these statutes provide only for the establishment or operation of government task forces or panels on Alzheimer's disease rather than for the regulation of a substantive area of law. The research query also searched court decisions of record. Of over one half million decisions recorded by the Westlaw legal computer system, only 260 decisions include any reference to Alzheimer's disease per se. Of these 260 identified cases, 50 contain only passing reference to AD. It should be noted that this figure may be somewhat conservative. A second computer-aided search, using the term senile dementia, a term formerly used to describe what we know today as ADRD, identified an additional 130 cases, again a very small number. The search demonstrates the paucity of legal precedent in the area of ADRD, suggesting also that future decisions or statutes likely will not be based on precedent.

While little statutory, case, or regulatory law deals directly with Alzheimer's disease, a number of general areas of law have a significant effect upon persons with Alzheimer's disease and their families. The balance of this report will focus on those issues, among them legal issues bearing on autonomy and incapacity, and on medical decision-making.

Autonomy and Incapacity

A fundamental principle of the U.S. legal system is that people are autonomous—entitled to make their own decisions, whether in minor matters such as choosing what to eat, read, or wear, or in major issues such as deciding whether to marry, move from one's home, or refuse medical treatment for a terminal illness. To the greatest possible extent, our legal system supports the concept of self-determination. The legal system begins from the presumption that all persons have both the right and the ability to make their own choices and decisions, so long as those determinations are within the law. This legal presumption remains in effect until a court determines otherwise, based on fact finding and due process.

While legal statutes place a premium on autonomy and self-determination, they also recognize that a range of impairments may render a person incapable of independent decisionmaking, causing them to present a potential hazard to themselves or to others. Physical or mental impairments—among them, Alzheimer's disease or related dementias, stroke, mental illness, developmental disability—may limit a person's capacity to make choices or to undertake activities in one or more areas of life. To respond to questions of impaired decisionmaking ability, our legal system has adopted two separate approaches to the problems that arise in the wake of "incapacity" or "incompetence" (hereafter referred to collectively as "incapacity") to make decisions as the result of that impairment.

First, the legal system has established methods through which persons voluntarily may delegate certain of their decisionmaking rights to others. This arises most often when a risk of incapacity is recognized, such as when a medical diagnosis of a mentally disabling disorder is made early in its course (discussed below in Voluntary Transfers of Decisionmaking). For people who have never been alert (unimpaired) or who, when alert, made no provisions for transfer of decisionmaking, the law provides a second means of transfer. Under this alternative approach, an impaired individual's rights are removed involuntarily and given to another (discussed below in Involuntary Transfers of Decisionmaking).

Critical to the voluntary or involuntary transfer of decisionmaking is the legal determination regarding capacity or incapacity. With either approach, the legal system must establish, through a formal set of procedures, whether a person has the ability to make his or her own reasoned decisions. No single standard has been codified for this legal determination. Rather, the courts broadly look to ascertain whether the person in question understands the basic nature of the decision or decisions being made, reaches his or her decision or decisions in a reasoned manner, and understands the consequences of the determination.

Alzheimer's disease presents particularly complex problems for the legal system in efforts to make determinations of capacity or incapacity. The disease is difficult to diagnose in its early stages. To date, a review of court opinions of record suggests that little, if any, uniformity exists in either how the diagnosis of AD is established or how its severity is measured.

In most of the cases reviewed, the sitting judges simply appear to have relied upon physician or psychologist statements regarding the degree of mental impairment. The testifying expert most often was not asked about past experience or education in working with AD patients. More often than not, the expert appears not to have been asked how the diagnosis was reached. In the few cases in which specific information regarding the diagnostic process was elicited from the expert witness, the diagnosis most often was based upon test scores (usually, the Mini-Mental State Examination—MMSE) and on positron emission tomography (PET) and magnetic resonance imaging (MRI) scans.

The Panel observes that this approach to the assessment of legal capacity in persons with AD poses a number of problems, including: (a) reliance on a medical evaluation in the absence of specifically identified tests; (b) adequacy of the diagnostic screens, if used; (c) the familiarity of the medical witness with current practices in diagnosis and evaluation of potential AD; (d) reliability of determinations made through an evaluation performed at a distinct point in time; and (e) absence of measures of judgment.

From a clinical perspective, the determination that an individual may be suffering from the early stages of AD cannot be made easily or lightly, given its profound consequences for individuals and families alike. For this reason alone, courts should not be satisfied with a suggested diagnosis of AD in the absence of clear medical evidence to support that diagnosis. As will be discussed in greater detail below, even when the diagnosis of AD has been established, a presumption of incapacity would be premature.

While the MMSE and other mental status tests are useful to distinguish normal from impaired cognitive function, they are not necessarily the best tests against which to evaluate the specific cognitive losses and loss of judgment that arise in AD. Research has found that results on this and other similar global measures of mental status may be affected by specific non-cognitive characteristics of the person being evaluated, such as physical health, socioeconomic status, and education. For example, a person with AD who had attained a high level of education may test relatively high on a cognitive screen; yet the score may be low relative to the person's score when healthy. Significant cognitive loss may be present but may not be identified through screening measures since scores from these tests are judged against a scale that has been set to a relatively low common denominator. Similarly, persons with low education may have relatively low cognitive screen scores, but may not be suffering from AD. Moreover, in AD, particularly in its earlier stages, capacity may vary from day to day or even from morning to night; a single test instrument administered on a one-time basis may not reflect the overall state of impairment or lost judgment.

A host of significant diagnostic advances over the decade have led to the availability of more accurate evaluative techniques to aid in the establishment of a diagnosis of AD, whether for use in clinical care or in court-related evaluations of impairment. The Alzheimer's Association, in collaboration with the National Institutes of Health's National Institute of Neurological Disorders and Stroke (NINDS), has developed diagnostic criteria that have been found to have an 80-90 percent accuracy rate, a standard with a higher degree of certainty than found when relying on standard mental status examinations. Recent basic research findings suggest that new and more precise tools may not be long in development.

However, even the most accurate measure of lost cognitive capacity or the diagnosis of AD itself provides insufficient information upon which to make a legal determination of lost capacity. The concepts of cognition and judgment—the latter being the focus of the legal proceeding—are not synonymous. In addition to cognitive and neuropsychological assessment, other aspects of judgment should be evaluated through the assessment of occupational capacity or other measures of the practical aspects of functioning. Moreover, in forming a legal opinion of capacity, courts should evaluate historical evidence from the individual in question and informed others (such as family) as well as direct information regarding the individual's ability to make choices, understand the questions at hand, and comprehend the outcomes of those choices. Through such means, courts will be able to distinguish more clearly between the loss of memory ("forgetfulness" or early cognitive impairment) and judgment.

Other difficulties in the legal determination of capacity among persons with ADRD extend to the knowledge base of the medical experts and family of the person in question. The expertise and background of the medical witness, oftentimes a family doctor who has treated the patient for years, may not reflect current knowledge of the diagnosis and treatment of AD. This may lead to untoward findings. For example, one of the primary and early effects of the disease—forgetfulness—does not affect a person's ability to make informed decisions in the early stages of AD; yet evidence of forgetfulness may be central in the legal decisionmaking process. Similarly, family caregivers may have conflicting interests in the outcome, particularly if caregiving has become particularly burdensome to them.

Each of these questions arises in the conduct of a legal evaluation of capacity in a person with AD, without regard to the degree to which the disease has progressed. With the exception of the latest stages of the disease, during which time the individual in question most likely has lost the ability to recognize family or to communicate with any clarity, the questions are no easier to answer. The middle phase of the disease—a period that varies widely from AD patient to AD patient, given the 6-20-year span of the disease—is characterized by significant personality change and loss of judgment and memory, notwithstanding the fact that both speech and mobility remain intact. At this stage, courts and family alike may find it difficult to determine whether an AD patient's decisions are an expression of a desire for continued autonomy, or are a reflection of the disease process itself.

For example, concerned caregivers (family, health care professional, or adult protective services worker) may believe a person with AD to be unable to live alone safely because of the risk of malnutrition, disease, fire, wandering, or other similar hazards resulting from the increased inability to provide self-care or to avoid simple dangers. The person with AD may refuse a move to a supervised living setting, such as a personal care facility or a nursing home. In such cases, a court will be asked to determine whether this person is making a reasoned decision and, therefore, exercising personal autonomy in refusing the move. If the court determines that legal capacity and judgment

351

are present, the person in question will be allowed the risk of self-harm to safeguard his or her personal autonomy. If, on the other hand, the court determines that the person no longer is able to make appropriate decisions, the court will order the person to be placed in the supervised living setting, protecting the person under the state's "parens patriae" or "beneficence" powers.

As discussed in the Third Report of the Advisory Panel on Alzheimer's Disease, the Panel believes that, to the extent possible, the autonomy of a person with AD should be preserved for as long as possible. However, the Panel also recognizes that, at varying times in the course of AD in any one individual, the ability to make decisions, to self-direct daily activities, and to conduct one's life becomes so severely impaired that it becomes dangerous or hazardous to self or to others. While it is the responsibility of the courts to determine the point at which people with AD can no longer continue to act autonomously and decisions affecting their lives must be made by others, the Panel has observed that the information upon which these decisions are made is not necessarily complete or based upon state-of-the-art knowledge of the nature of AD. Moreover, little uniformity exists in how the legal system manages questions of capacity in persons with AD.

For these reasons, the Panel hopes to bring greater assurance of autonomy for the AD patient for the greatest length of time and greater uniformity and clarity to the process of legal determinations of capacity through a number of recommendations:

- Current best medical opinion holds that clinical diagnoses of Alzheimer's disease should be established through careful clinical evaluation at several different points in time. That evaluation should include, but not be limited to: (a) cognitive screening instruments (such as the MMSE); (b) NINDS/ADRDA Alzheimer's screening criteria, including other neuropsychological assessment tools; and (c) measures of practical aspects of functioning, such as occupational evaluations. In addition, the assessment would be incomplete in the absence of historical evidence provided by the person in question or informed individuals, such as family and personal physician. The same determining procedures and methods should be employed across legal jurisdictions to bring greater uniformity to legal decisionmaking about AD patients' capacity.

- Insofar as medical and legal determinations of cognitive ability and judgment are concerned, it is important to separate the two

352

concepts for the purpose of evaluating capacity. Judgment and cognitive ability are not synonymous terms; there is a difference between lost memory and lost judgment. Thus, AD's early feature of memory loss alone does not necessarily compromise a person's ability to make informed decisions or to express preferences; impairment of judgment arises in the course of the disease, not necessarily at its diagnosis. Courts should weigh this distinction carefully in competence determinations. Families and medical professionals, too, should be better informed about these distinctions.

• The complexity of capacity determinations for persons with AD suggests that greater uniformity in evaluations and the concomitant need for evaluations at multiple points in time are needed. A person with AD may be competent for certain purposes at a given time, yet found incompetent for other purposes at the same time. For this reason, the Panel recommends that courts consider implementing regularly scheduled reassessments of the legal capacity of persons with ADRD until such time as verbal and communication skills are irrevocably lost, thereby preserving autonomy in as many areas as possible for as long as possible. The Panel concurs that when these skills are determined to be lost irrevocably, repeated determinations of decisionmaking ability no longer are necessary. Given the large number of persons likely to be adjudicated in such a system, states may wish to establish special court diversion programs that utilize a uniform set of criteria and procedures to determine issues of capacity in persons with ADRD.

Voluntary Transfers of Decisionmaking

All states permit the establishment of voluntary legal arrangements—such as durable powers of attorney and trusts—through which a person can delegate to another the right to make certain decisions on his or her behalf. Historically, such arrangements have dealt primarily with financial matters; more recently, courts have broadened the interpretation of these arrangements to include delegation of broad personal and health care decisionmaking as well.

The most useful of these devices is the durable power of attorney. All states authorize their use for the purposes of delegating authority to manage financial and property matters. Though more than 40 states further authorize their use for purposes of delegating medical and personal decisions, other states make specific and separate statutory provisions for health care decisionmaking. Under a properly drafted general power of attorney, an agent may pay the bills of the impaired person, manage his or her property, provide for the person's dependents, and maintain his or her affairs to protect the impaired person's post-death estate plan. In states that permit powers of attorney to be used for medical and personal surrogate decisionmaking, the agent of a properly drawn power of attorney also may be able to consent to or to refuse medical treatment, hire medical personnel, and decide where the impaired person will live. (This last issue may require court approval, particularly for nursing home placement. Statutes vary from state to state.)

Trusts, while more complex and used most often for traditional estate planning purposes, also can provide for the complete management of the financial affairs of an incapacitated person and his or her dependents. Joint asset holdings, not a true delegation of authority but a means of sharing "ownership" of funds, may provide a means of simple estate planning and protection against incapacity. Through this mechanism, the healthy owner of a jointly held asset, such as a bank account, may be willing and able to use the assets to pay for the care of the impaired "partner." Unfortunately, this may not always be the case. Thus, this mechanism should be used with caution.

The great advantage of establishing these devices is that they allow a person who may later become incapacitated to determine who will act on his or her behalf. The documents upon which these arrangements are based can provide direction as to the decisions the giver wishes to have made. These devices, when properly drawn or established, generally avoid the need for future court intervention. However, these instruments require advance planning, an activity in which many people do not engage for a variety of reasons. Moreover, the person entering into such advance planning must have the legal ability to make his or her own decision at the time the document is executed. The Panel notes again that a person in the early stages of Alzheimer's disease retains the legal right to make his or her own decisions absent a court finding of incapacity and may well have the current ability to establish voluntary delegations of decisionmaking.

The Panel has found that the use of voluntary transfers of decisionmaking is meager, at best, whether used for the purposes of property and finances or for the purposes of medical and personal decisions. It is unclear whether these devices are not used because people are unaware of them, are unwilling (or emotionally unable) to confront their potential mortality, or perceive them to be too expensive to undertake. Whatever the reason, the Panel believes these voluntary transfers represent an important element in the maintenance of autonomous decisionmaking by persons with ADRD. Decisions made before issues of capacity arise are carried through by others on behalf of the incapacitated person in the manner specified in advance of the loss of judgmental and cognitive capacity. The use of such advance voluntary transfers can help avoid the need for involuntary guardianships once an individual has become incapacitated by AD. For this reason, the Panel makes a series of recommendations regarding this issue.

- As the Panel found in its third report with respect to persons with AD and as held as a key tenet of jurisprudence for the general population, individual autonomy and the right to make decisions should be granted primacy over the desires of others; these personal rights also should be safeguarded for as long as legally and medically possible. For these reasons, the Panel recommends that the legal and medical communities work together to reach consensus on a specific set of tools through which the legal system may better be able to ascertain whether a person of uncertain cognitive status retains the legal capacity to enter into agreements of any sort, including the legal delegation of decisionmaking. Standardization of these procedures nationwide is indicated, since the incidence and prevalence of AD do not vary widely from state to state. The needs of AD patients in Portland, Maine, are the same as those in Portland, Oregon.

- Greater education is needed about the utility and appropriateness of voluntary transfers of authority. Simple descriptions of what these mechanisms are and how they can be undertaken should be provided. Such information should be placed in the context of the nature of ADRD, its course, and its potential consequences on individual autonomy and decisionmaking. As discussed in greater detail later in this chapter, material on this subject could be included in the larger public education document that the Panel has recommended be developed for dissemination not only by ADRD-related programs, but also by the Administration on Aging through its legal services programs, Area Agencies on Aging, and multipurpose senior centers.

- Because persons diagnosed in the early stages of AD often retain the ability to undertake voluntary transfers of decisionmaking, health care professionals working with such persons should provide information about the mechanisms through which such voluntary delegations may be made. This is particularly important in states in which durable powers of attorney may be used to guide medical decisions at later stages of the disease process. From the perspective of the person with AD, the most important aspect of a voluntary transfer may be the early designation of a trusted, knowledgeable, specific surrogate decisionmaker in the event of incapacity. Professional societies, continuing education programs, and medical schools should help educate physicians to issues regarding voluntary transfers, since physicians often represent the most significant contact point for older Americans outside the family structure. In this way, physicians may help assure patient autonomy for as long as possible, ensuring that patient desires are met even when decisionmaking capacity has been lost. The early establishment of a voluntary transfer can safeguard against the need for such determinations at the point of hospital admission, a time not ideal for patient-centered decisionmaking.

Involuntary Transfers of Decisionmaking

In the absence of a legally binding voluntary arrangement as described above, court intervention is required when a person becomes incapacitated and a decision regarding his or her care or finances must be made. Most often a court's determination that an impaired person has become legally incapacitated is made on a prospective basis; from the moment of the court decision, the impaired person may no longer make decisions that are legally binding. These court actions often are referred to as "protective proceedings," and are divided into two separate categories. When a court determines that a person no longer is able to make personal decisions regarding matters such as where to live, whether to seek medical care (discussed in greater detail below), whether to marry, divorce, or seek other legal action, the court will appoint a surrogate decisionmaker in a guardianship proceeding. In contrast, conservatorships are legal proceedings to establish incapacity and to identify a surrogate decisionmaker for a person who no longer can manage financial matters such as bill paying, making investments, or selling realty.

Typically, these legal proceedings are brought before the probate or chancery court of the county in which the impaired person lives or owns property. Some variation exists among the states regarding the rights and procedures under which these hearings are convened. However, in general, the court first determines whether the impaired person can still manage his or her personal and financial affairs. If the court finds the person to be incapacitated, it then appoints either a guardian or conservator—or both—to make decisions on the impaired person's behalf.

In the past, courts generally gave guardians and conservators the authority to make all personal and financial decisions on the impaired person's behalf. More recently, however, a growing number of states have adopted laws that permit courts within the state's jurisdiction to restrict the powers to be granted to guardians and conservators, allowing the impaired person to continue to make specific classes of decisions not yet affected by incapacity. At least in theory, such laws support the Panel's articulated view that, to the extent practicable and for as long as possible, a person should be entitled to the maintenance of autonomy and self-direction. These laws seem particularly appropriate to persons with Alzheimer's disease, especially in view of the disease's relatively slow progression and the varying degrees of capacity that may be accepted by courts in making capacity determinations about different kinds of decisions. However, in the absence of research, the effectiveness of partial guardianships and conservatorships in the maintenance of personal autonomy is untested.

It is clear to the Panel that the use of voluntary transfers of decisionmaking should be encouraged. Unless the loss of cognition and judgment inherent in a diagnosis of AD is planned for through the exercise of such voluntary legal arrangements, then the courts, not the person with AD, are likely to decide who will become the surrogate decisionmaker and the range of that person's authority.

Medical Decisionmaking

Making decisions about one's own medical matters may be among the most personal of rights. Because the concept of autonomy is at its very roots, the U.S. legal system long has held that patients must be allowed to choose the medical care and treatment that they will receive. Unfortunately, the nature of Alzheimer's disease is such that patients are faced with a diminishing ability to make decisions at the very time that medical interventions are becoming increasingly complex and more difficult for the lay person readily to understand. When working with AD patients over time, health care providers must determine anew at each visit whether the AD patient retains the ability to decide care and, if not, who should be called upon to make decisions on that patient's behalf. The family and friends of the person with Alzheimer's disease are confronted yet again by the nature of the disease and its inevitable progression when they are asked, perhaps for the first time, to make care decisions.

The Patient or Presumed Patient

The general rule of law states that a person is presumed legally able to make his or her own decisions until a court determines otherwise. While the presumption may be and has been challenged in court, the law strongly suggests that the benefit of doubt should be given to the patient, thereby preserving the right to decide his or her own care or, in medico/legal terms, to give "informed consent," for so long as an opinion can be expressed. Surprisingly, few court cases have discussed precisely what standards should be used to determine a patient's mental capacity to consent to health care. However, the limited case law reviewed by the Panel suggests that the test is whether the patient is of sufficient mind to reasonably understand his or her condition, the nature and effect of the proposed treatment, and the attendant risks in pursuing—and not pursuing—such treatment. Because of our system's preference for autonomy and the very personal nature of the consequences of receiving or refusing medical care, an individual's own decisions about medical care should be given the greatest weight for as long as the patient is able to express a preference.

Advance Directives

At a point in time that varies with the speed of the course of disease, a person with AD will become unable to make his or her own medical decisions. Each of the 50 states now has statutes that permit the establishment of voluntary arrangements to delegate at least some medical decisionmaking rights to others. These arrangements, referred to as "advance directives," are written documents that a patient signs while competent; they direct how health care treatment decisions will be made in the event of future incapacity. Two types of advance directives have been established under law:

- A *Power of Attorney for Medical Care* is a document granting an agent (or "advocate") the right to make some or all medical decisions on the patient's behalf should the patient become ill. All of the states but Alabama have statutes that permit a person to delegate medical decisions to another through a special health care power of attorney or as part of a general power of attorney (discussed earlier in this chapter).

- *A Living Will* is a document providing specific instructions to physicians about an individual's wishes regarding medical care in the event the person becomes too ill to articulate such preferences. Forty-eight states have Living Will statutes.

- In the new proposed uniform statute, the separate concepts of the living will and the power of attorney for medical care are joined in a single document called an advance directive. That concept has been adopted in statutes in Arizona, Connecticut, Florida, Maryland, New Jersey, Oklahoma, Oregon, and Virginia.

These two types of directive often are combined in a single document that contains both a designation of an agent who will carry out the patient's wishes and a set of instructions to physicians who are about to provide care and treatment.

State statutes are not consistent in the delineation of the range of powers that may be given by a person in an advance directive. In general, however, such directives may authorize decisions regarding care (selecting who may provide services to the patient), custody (selecting the site at which the care is given), and medical treatment (selecting the diagnostic, surgical, therapeutic, or other procedures provided by health care workers at the differing sites). An interesting issue that may arise in the area of treatment advance directives is the question of experimental treatments for persons who might wish to become research participants. Greater attention should be paid to this last issue, particularly with respect to AD patients, whose loss of legal capacity may occur relatively early in the disease course.

Advance directives can be used and often are used to consent to life-sustaining treatment. They also can be used to refuse life-sustaining treatment at an identified point in the course of an illness; most advance directives are created for this very reason. While all states authorize the creation of advance directives, the extent to which they are actually in use is not known. What research has shown is that surrogate decisionmakers often do not choose the course of action identified as by the patient as preferred. Thus, given the irreversible nature and destruction of cognitive ability inherent in AD, the Panel believes it critical that people express their wishes regarding care: (1) if they have received a tentative or confirming diagnosis of the disorder in its early stages; or (2) if there is any concern about potential future loss of cognitive ability.

Refusing Medical Treatment

U.S. law now has clarified that individuals have the right to refuse medical treatment in appropriate circumstances. In the *Cruzan v Director, Missouri Department of Health* decision of 1991, the U.S. Supreme Court recognized that the right to refuse medical treatment is protected under the Constitution, although it is not an absolute right without qualification. The Court recognized that states do have a legitimate interest in preserving life, preventing suicide, maintaining the integrity of the health care profession, and protecting the rights of minors or other third parties entitled to support and care. These state interests must be balanced against patient autonomy, and often are included in the statutes that permit the creation of advance directives.

In light of these protective but sometimes conflicting interests, states have general freedom to make their own rules regarding treatment refusal. One area in which substantial differences exist among the states is whether the artificial provision of hydration and nutrition falls within the definition of medical treatment, and whether, as such, it then can be refused in an advance directive. In the *Cruzan* case, the Supreme Court drew no distinction between hydration and nutrition and any other forms of medical treatment, leaving the determination a medical one. Nevertheless, a dwindling number of state statutes continue either to limit or to prohibit the right to refuse such treatment.

Health care providers have expressed concerns that honoring advance directives may result in liability. So far, this concern appears to be unfounded. Advance directive statutes often include provisions that release a provider from civil or criminal liability if a directive has been followed in good faith. Extant court cases do not suggest substantial risk to the health care provider, either. Based on information compiled by the State Justice Institute, only one appellate court case was found to involve criminal charges being brought against a provider for heeding an advance directive; moreover, the charges brought in the case later were dismissed. Similarly, the State Justice Institute review found only a single civil suit brought against a provider for honoring an advance directive; five separate cases have been brought against providers for refusing to honor an advance directive and continuing treatment.

The nature of AD can present problems in the use of advance directives. These devices, whether by statutory language or by drafting, may restrict the right to refuse medical treatment to cases of terminal illness. Family members and others who must act on the patient's behalf find it difficult to know how AD falls within this definition, considering the uncertainty regarding its progression. In the Panel's opinion, AD, today, must be considered a terminal illness; end-stage AD is no less terminal than end-stage cancer or heart disease. The Panel understands that the uniform act on advance directives recently adopted by the National Commissioners of Uniform State Law removes the requirement that end-stage disease be certified. However, until the model statute is adopted by each of the 50 states, the Panel believes that determination of what constitutes "end-stage" AD should be the province of the treating physician. The Panel further suggests that individual physicians, courts, and families should be granted broad permission to establish when an advance directive of a person with ADRD should be honored. Dialogue on this issue is key to successful resolution in the best interests of the patient and society as a whole.

Treating in the Absence of Advance Directives

When a patient cannot make his or her own decisions and no advance directive has been set in place, health care providers often are uncertain whether they must seek judicial involvement before providing treatment. In some situations, the patient's condition or behavior may make such a step unnecessary. For example, the law long has recognized that informed consent need not be obtained in an emergency. Similarly, consent may be implied when a patient seeks or manifests a willingness to submit to treatment; however, case law does not elucidate clearly the parameters within which these exceptions are legally acceptable.

In some states, a "family consent" statute further diminishes the need for judicial involvement. In the absence of an advance directive, such a statute typically gives authority to make medical decisions for an incapacitated patient to family members; priority is given to the closest relative.

Reliance on state statutes and court proceedings to determine the appropriateness of medical treatment in the absence of advance directives occurs less frequently than one would suspect by relying on media accounts (e.g., Cruzan, Quinlan, etc.). To date, most frequently, medical decisionmaking for incapacitated people is made informally by families in the absence of specific legal authority or basis for making decisions except their concern and knowledge of the patient's wishes. While this approach may not be supported by clear legal authority, reliance upon family decisionmaking is widespread, not only acknowledged but approved by some courts. This practice also is supported by the landmark Federal report, *The President's Commission for the Study of Ethical Problems in Medicine and Biomedical and Behavioral Research: Deciding To Forego Life-Sustaining Treatment,* 1983, and is incorporated in many hospital practice guidelines.

When relying upon informal decisionmakers, health care providers may need to determine who among the family members is the most appropriate to act on the patient's behalf. In most circumstances, the spouse is the preferred first choice. State case decisions often uphold the right of one spouse to act for the other under certain circumstances. The spouse generally also has the highest priority among family members for court appointment as guardian, should legal authorization be sought or required. However, if the spouse is ill or a history of neglect or domestic relations complaints is present, health care providers and courts alike may well question whether the spouse is the best candidate for the role as surrogate decisionmaker.

In the absence of a spouse, adult children generally are the next choice. Unfortunately, the law provides little help in determining which child to rely upon, should there be disagreement between or among them. Again, health care providers should be alert to possible indications of abuse, neglect, or other family difficulties. As the Panel observed in its third report, it is critical to assure against competing interests when it becomes necessary to rely on family or informal caregiver decisionmaking. For this reason, the Panel emphasizes the need for health care professionals to engage in regular conversations about these difficult medical issues with their patients with suspected or diagnosed AD. By placing greater emphasis upon the importance of advance directives, physicians and other health care professionals might help assure that a patient's desires are articulated before issues of capacity arise and long before the need for medical intervention occurs.

Federal Involvement in Medical Decisionmaking

In 1990, the U.S. Congress adopted the Patient Self-Determination Act, which requires all Medicare or Medicaid certified health care organizations, including hospitals, nursing homes, home health agencies, hospices, and prepaid organizations, to:

i. give all patients written information regarding their rights under state law to make decisions about medical care, including, in particular, the rights to refuse medical treatment and to prepare or have honored written instructions outlining their wishes;

ii. have written policies and procedures about the use of "advance directives";

iii. include the "advance directive" in the medical record of any patient who has made one; and,

iv. educate the facility's staff and the community on issues regarding advance directives.

This law could help increase the awareness and the use of advance directives and not interfere with states' rights to codify state health care law. The statute's laudable goals, however, will be met only if people indeed receive and understand the information regarding their medical decisionmaking rights, and if the means necessary to establish their wishes are readily accessible.

In its Third Report, the Panel identified a number of principles that should guide overall decisionmaking in the care of AD patients:

- Place high priority on the values of patients and families.
- Emphasize quality of life, broadly defined, over mere survival.
- Encourage resolution of value conflicts among patients, families, and care providers through early education and other mechanisms outside the court system.

The Panel believes that these same principles should guide the medical decisionmaking that occurs in the care and treatment of Alzheimer's patients. To that end and as stated earlier in this chapter, the Panel recommends that given the nature and destruction of cognitive ability inherent in AD, people should be encouraged to express their wishes regarding care through the use of advance directives. Such directives are warranted whether the individual is at risk of AD, has received a tentative or confirming diagnosis of the disorder, or if there is any concern about potential loss of cognitive ability in the future.

However, while patient values—expressed through such advance directives—should be foremost in medical decisionmaking, the Panel concedes that much is not known about how individual decisions about treatment preferences may change over time. For example, an advance directive issued in anticipation of AD may be far different from one that might be issued after confirmatory diagnosis of the disorder. For this reason, the Panel believes that greater research is warranted regarding the stability of treatment preferences over time. Such research could help ascertain whether advance directives should be reevaluated and altered at the will of the person with AD at various points in the disease process. Further, by suggesting the use of advance directives, the Panel is also arguing for further basic and clinical research that may lead to the detection of AD in its very earliest stages, before questions that could cloud the validity of an advance directive arise, such as issues of capacity or cognitive status.

Yet, even with an advance directive in place, its utility has been limited by the laws governing such documents. Most often, a right to refuse treatment (contained in an advance directive) is limited to cases of terminal illness. Unfortunately, neither case history nor general practice of medicine or law is clear regarding precisely how AD falls within that definition. In the Panel's view, until such time as the uniform act on advance directives is enacted in each state, both those rendering treatment to AD patients and those defining statutes governing the right to refuse treatment today must consider AD to be a terminal illness. End-stage AD should be treated in the same way as end-stage heart disease or cancer; advance directives should be honored based on the treating physician's determination that the illness has reached its final stage. As observed in its previous reports, the Panel recognizes the difficulties inherent in linking such policy principles to clinical care or personal decisions by individual patients and families. Nonetheless, the issue remains one of values, and those of the individual with AD should remain paramount in the medical and legal decisionmaking processes.

Conclusion

This report represents the culmination of several years of Advisory Panel deliberations regarding legal issues affecting the care and treatment of people with Alzheimer's disease. The issues are complex, ranging from questions of autonomy and capacity to medical treatment and the right to refuse that treatment. The lengthy trajectory of AD further complicates how decisions regarding the legal rights of a person with AD are to be protected and how that person's safety is also to be maintained. The Panel's Third Report emphasized the role of values in the care and treatment of persons with AD. Values form an overarching theme in this report as well, including the values implied in law and statute, the values inherent in the voluntary transfer of decisionmaking, the values held by formal and informal caregivers, and the values contained in advance directives.

The legal implications of Alzheimer's disease have not been clarified in case law to date. However, as the numbers of persons with AD rises, the need for more reasoned and medically sound mechanisms to determine issues of capacity and stage of illness is heightened. To that end, the Panel has made a host of recommendations regarding legal capacity and medical decisionmaking in AD care and treatment.

- Medical and legal determinations of cognitive ability and judgment are not synonymous. Courts should weigh this distinction in competence determinations; families and medical professionals should be better informed of the differences.

- Greater uniformity in medical evaluations and the conduct of evaluations at different points in time can help ensure that the autonomy of a person with AD may be maintained for as long as possible.

- The legal and medical communities should work together to reach consensus on specific nationally applicable tools through which the legal system may be able to ascertain whether a person of uncertain cognitive status retains the legal capacity to make his or her own decisions.

- The use and appropriateness of voluntary transfers of authority should be the subject of education for older persons and their families, through not only ADRD-related organizations, but programs working with older Americans in general, whether at the Federal, state, or local levels. Health professionals, too, should be educated about such mechanisms and should provide information about them to their patients or clients. Professional societies, continuing education programs, and medical schools can be helpful in this effort.

- The use of advance directives should be encouraged for those at risk of or those diagnosed with AD. Through improved methods of early detection of AD the timely issuance of such directives can be facilitated. Until such time as the model uniform act on advance directives is adopted by each of the states, the use of advance directives, however, must be accompanied by acceptance of the Panel's view that there is such a concept as "end-stage" AD and that the trajectory of AD today is no different from that of a patient diagnosed with incurable heart disease or cancer.

The Panel believes that enactment of the recommendations contained in this report will be beneficial not only to large numbers of ADRD patients and their families, but also to the wider community. It calls upon those in the medical and legal professions to begin to grapple with the legal issues surrounding Alzheimer's disease from the perspective of the patient and family, urging greater education of older Americans and caregivers to legal mechanisms available to preserve individual autonomy in the event of lost cognitive capacity due to ADRD.

Part Five

Additional Help and Information

Chapter 36

Alzheimer's Disease and Related Disorders: Terms You Should Know

acetylcholine: a neurotransmitter that plays an important role in learning and memory; found in reduced levels in the brains of Alzheimer's victims.

activities of daily living (ADLs): basic activities that are important to self care, such as bathing, dressing, using the toilet, eating, and getting in and out of a chair.

akinesia: impaired body movement.

Alzheimer's Disease Associated Protein (ADAP): a protein that seems to appear only in the tissue of people with Alzheimer's. It has been found in both the brain and spinal fluid.

amyloid: See beta amyloid.

amyloid precursor protein (APP): a normal, essential substance made by brain cells that contain beta amyloid. In Alzheimer's, APP is cut and releases beta amyloid. Beta amyloid then forms clumps called senile plaque.

antioxidants: substances that deactivate oxygen free radicals.

Compiled from NIH Pub. Nos. 94-3676 and 95-3782 and National Institute of Neurological Disorders and Stroke (NINDS) fact sheet on Huntington's Disease, April 1998.

apoE4: one form of the apoE gene (see apolipoprotein E), which produces the protein apolipoprotein E4; this form of the gene occurs more often in people with Alzheimer's disease than in the general population. The other two forms of the gene, apoE2 and apoE3, may protect against the disease.

apolipoprotein E (ApoE): a protein that ferries cholesterol through the bloodstream. The ApoE gene has three variants (or alleles), E2, E3, and E4. Each person inherits an allele from each parent. Ninety percent of the population inherit one copy of ApoE3, and 60 percent inherit two copies.

autosomal dominant disorder: a non-sex-linked disorder that can be inherited even if only one parent passes on the defective gene.

axon: the tube-like part of a neuron that transmits outgoing signals to other cells.

basal ganglia: a region located at the base of the brain composed of four clusters of neurons, or nerve cells. This area is responsible for body movement and coordination.

behavioral symptoms: symptoms of Alzheimer's disease that are troublesome for family and professional caregivers, such as wandering, pacing, agitation, screaming, and aggressive reactions.

beta amyloid: a protein found in dense deposits forming the core of neuritic plaques.

blood-brain barrier: a group of mechanisms that keep some substances in the bloodstream from entering cells in the brain.

calcium channel blocker: a drug that stops calcium from entering cells.

capillaries: the smallest blood vessels, which route blood to individual cells.

caregiver: anyone who provides care to a physically or cognitively impaired person, including both family and other caregivers at home and professional caregivers in health care settings.

caudate nuclei: part of the striatum in the basal ganglia. See basal ganglia, striatum.

cell: the smallest unit of a living organism that is capable of functioning independently.

cerebral cortex: the part of the brain most involved in learning, language, and reasoning.

cholinergic: pertaining to acetylcholine; the cholinergic system includes the neurons that contain acetylcholine and the neurons and proteins that are stimulated or activated by acetylcholine.

chorea: uncontrolled body movements. Chorea is derived from the Greek word for dance.

chromosome: a threadlike structure in the nucleus of a cell containing genes. Humans have 23 pairs of chromosomes, one set from the mother, one from the father. Chromosomes are composed of deoxyribonucleic acid (DNA) and proteins and, under a microscope, appear as rod-like structures. See deoxyribonucleic acid (DNA), gene.

clinical trial: a carefully controlled study designed to test whether an intervention, such as a drug, is safe and effective in human beings.

cognitive functions: all aspects of thinking, perceiving, and remembering.

computerized tomography scan (CT or CAT scan): a diagnostic test that uses a computer and x-rays to obtain a highly detailed picture of the brain.

cortex: part of the brain responsible for thought, perception, and memory. See basal ganglia.

cortisol: the major natural glucocorticoid (GC) in humans. It is the primary stress hormone.

dementia: significant loss of intellectual abilities such as memory capacity, severe enough to interfere with social or occupational functioning.

371

dendrites: the branch-like extension of neurons that receive messages from other neurons.

deoxyribonucleic acid (DNA): a large double stranded molecule within chromosomes; the substance of heredity containing the genetic information necessary for cells to divide and produce proteins. DNA carries the code for every inherited characteristic of an organism; sequences of DNA make up genes. See gene.

dominant: a trait that is apparent even when the gene for that disorder is inherited from only one parent. See autosomal dominant disorder, recessive, gene.

Familial Alzheimer's disease (FAD): an early-onset form of Alzheimer's disease that appears to be inherited. In FAD, several members of the same generation in a family are often affected.

free radicals: see oxygen free radicals.

gene: the biologic unit of heredity, each gene is located at a definite position on a particular chromosome and is made up of a string of chemicals, called bases, arranged in a certain sequence along the DNA molecule. See deoxyribonucleic acid (DNA).

gene mutation: an abnormality in the sequence of bases of a gene.

glucose metabolism: the process by which cells turn food into energy.

hippocampus: an area buried deep in the forebrain that helps regulate emotion and memory.

huntingtin: the protein encoded by the gene that carries the Huntington Disease defect. The repeated CAG sequence in the gene causes an abnormal form of huntingtin to be formed. The function of the normal form of huntingtin is not yet known.

kindred: a group of related persons, such as a family or clan.

magnetic resonance imaging (MRI): a diagnostic and research technique that uses radiowaves, magnetic fields, and computer analysis to create a picture of body tissues and structures, including brain anatomy. MRI can now also be used to measure brain activity.

magnetic resonance spectroscopy imaging (MRSI): a research technique that allows scientists to measure concentrations of substances in the brain.

marker: a piece of DNA that lies on the chromosome so close to a gene that the two are inherited together. Like a signpost, markers are used during genetic testing and research to locate the nearby presence of a gene. See chromosome, deoxyribonucleic acid (DNA).

metabolism: the normal process of turning food into energy.

mitochondria: microscopic structures inside cells where glucose metabolism takes place; energy-producing bodies within cells that are the cells' "power plants."

multi-infarct dementia: dementia brought on by a series of strokes.

mutation: in genetics, any defect in a gene. See gene.

myoclonus: a condition in which muscles or portions of muscles contract abnormally.

nerve growth factor (NFG): a substance that occurs naturally in the body and enhances the growth and survival of cholinergic nerves.

neuritic plaques: deposits of amyloid mixed with fragments of dead and dying neurons.

neurofibrillary tangles: collections of twisted nerve cell fibers or paired helical filaments found in the cell bodies of neurons in Alzheimer's disease.

neuron: a nerve cell, the basic impulse-conducting unit of the nervous system. Nerve cells communicate with other cells through an electrochemical process called neurotransmission.

neuroscientist: a scientist who studies the brain.

neurotoxic: poisonous to nerves or nerve tissue.

neurotransmitter: a chemical messenger between neurons that transmits nerve impulses from one cell to another; a substance that is released by the axon of one neuron and excites or inhibits activity in a neighboring neuron.

neurotrophic factors: a family of substances that promote growth and regeneration of neurons.

nucleus basalis of Meynert: a small group of cholinergic nerve cells in the forebrain and connected to areas of the cerebral cortex.

oxygen free radicals: oxygen molecule with an unpaired electron that is highly reactive, combining readily with other molecules and sometimes causing damage to cells. See also antioxidants.

paired helical filaments: twisted fibers making up neurofibrillary tangles.

pallidum: part of the basal ganglia of the brain. The pallidum is composed of the globus pallidus and the ventral pallidum. See basal ganglia.

PET scan: see positron emission tomography.

phospholipids: molecules of fat in cell membranes.

plaques: see neuritic plaques.

positron emission tomography (PET): an imaging technique that allows researchers to observe and measure brain activity by monitoring blood flow and concentrations of substances such as oxygen and glucose in brain tissues. PET produces three-dimensional, colored images of chemicals or substances functioning within the body. These images are called PET scans.

prevalence: the number of cases of a disease that are present in a particular population at a given time.

protease: an enzyme that splits a protein into smaller sections.

protein: a molecule made up of amino acids arranged in a specific order which is determined by a gene. Proteins include neurotransmitters, enzymes, and hundreds of other substances.

pseudodementia: a severe form of depression resulting from a progressive brain disorder in which cognitive changes mimic those of dementia.

putamen: an area of the brain that decreases in size as a result of the damage produced by Huntington's Disease.

receptor: recognition sites on cells that cause a response in the body when stimulated by certain chemicals called neurotransmitters. They act as on-and-off switches for the next nerve cell. See neuron, neurotransmitters.

recessive: a trait that is apparent only when the gene or genes for it are inherited from both parents. See dominant, gene.

respite care: temporary relief from the burden of caregiving provided in the home, a nursing home, or elsewhere in a community.

senile chorea: a relatively mild and rare disorder found in elderly adults and characterized by choreic movements. It is believed by some scientists to be caused by a different gene mutation than that causing Huntington's Disease.

senile dementia: an outdated term, previously used for dementia in old age.

single photon emission computerized tomography (SPECT): an imaging technique that allows researchers to monitor blood flow to different parts of the brain.

special care unit: a long-term care facility with environmental features and/or programs designed for people with dementia.

SPECT: see single photon emission computerized tomography.

spectroscopy: see magnetic resonance spectroscopy imaging.

striatum: part of the basal ganglia of the brain. The striatum is composed of the caudate nucleus, putamen, and ventral striatum. See basal ganglia, caudate nuclei.

sundowning: the tendency for the behavioral symptoms of Alzheimer's disease to grow worse in the afternoon and evening.

synapse: the minute gap between nerve cells across which neurotransmitters pass.

tangles: see neurofibrillary tangles.

tau: a protein that is a principal component of paired helical filaments in neurofibrillary tangles.

trait: any genetically determined characteristic. See dominant, gene, recessive.

transgenic mice: mice that receive injections of foreign genes during the embryonic stage of development. Their cells then follow the "instructions" of the foreign genes, resulting in the development of a certain trait or characteristic. Transgenic mice can serve as an animal model of a certain disease, telling researchers how genes work in specific cells.

ventricles: cavities within the brain that are filled with cerebrospinal fluid. In Huntington's Disease, tissue loss causes enlargement of the ventricles.

Chapter 37

A Guide to Federal Programs for Alzheimer's Disease Patients

Foreword

This guide is a roadmap to federally sponsored activities relating to Alzheimer's disease and related disorders. It presents a diverse picture of efforts including biomedical, behavioral, social, and services research; delivery, financing, and evaluation of services; education and training of health and social service personnel; collection, production, dissemination, and evaluation of information; and collection and analysis of data.

Many of the activities and programs described focus specifically on Alzheimer's disease. Others have a broader focus on health or aging research or services that may include Alzheimer's disease. Some, but not all, involve activities in specific States and communities.

The information is organized to emphasize the unique roles of the various agencies comprising the Federal Government's Alzheimer's disease initiative, with descriptions of specific programs and activities listed under their primary sponsor. Listings of field centers, project sites, and other local and regional resources supported by Federal agencies are also provided.

Excerpted from *Alzheimer's Disease: A Guide to Federal Programs*, Alzheimer's Disease Education and Referral Center (ADEAR), National Institute on Aging (NIA), NIH Pub. No. 93-3635, December 1993; updated and verified in September 1998.

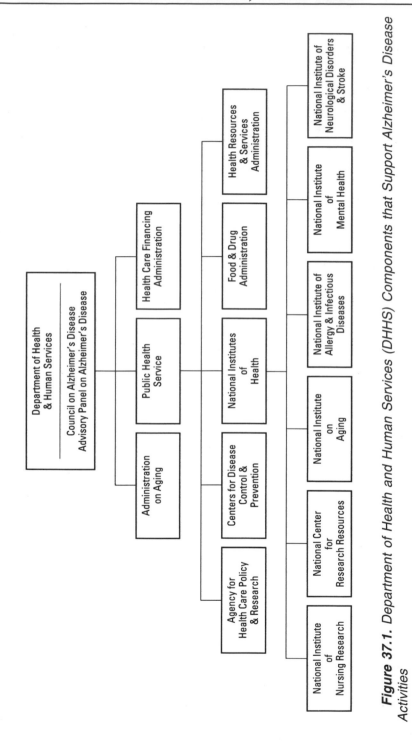

***Figure 37.1.** Department of Health and Human Services (DHHS) Components that Support Alzheimer's Disease Activities*

Agency Programs and Activities

Administration on Aging
Public Affairs Office
Department of Health and Human Services
330 Independence Avenue SW
Washington, DC 20201
(202) 401-4143

Purpose

The Administration on Aging (AoA) develops programs and coordinates delivery of community services specified by the Older Americans Act through a national network of 57 State agencies on aging and more than 657 Area Agencies on Aging (AAAs). AoA also supports research and demonstration projects and other initiatives designed to develop and strengthen family- and community-based care.

Programs and Activities

Title III Services. Title III of the Older Americans Act of 1965 provides Federal grants to the States for developing a comprehensive and coordinated system of services to help older people live independently in their communities and homes. States designate AAAs within their jurisdictions to deliver these services. The Older Americans Act gives priority to older people with the greatest economic or social needs. It specifically establishes AAAs as a source of support for families and people with Alzheimer's disease and related disorders, as well as to frail older people.

Many services provided by AAAs under Title III are essential to maintaining the ability of people with Alzheimer's disease to live in the community. The exact mixture of services varies by AAA and is subject to funding constraints. However, all AAAs offer the following:

- Nutrition services—congregate and home-delivered meals
- Access services—transportation, outreach, and information and referral
- In-home services—homemaker and home health aides, visiting and telephone reassurance, chore maintenance, in-home respite care, and home modification
- Community services—adult day care, senior centers, legal assistance, adult protective services, and caregiver support groups

Support for Providers of In-Home Services

The 1992 amendments to the Older Americans Act authorize grants to States to provide supportive activities to those who deliver in-home services to frail older people, including people with Alzheimer's disease. Supportive activities may include training and counseling, technical assistance in forming and operating support groups, information about services to families and providers, and lists of respite care providers.

Eldercare Locator

Along with the National Association of State Units on Aging and the National Association of Area Agencies on Aging, AoA cosponsors the Eldercare Locator, a nationwide telephone service that provides information about services offered by State and area agencies in particular communities. The toll-free number for Eldercare Locator is 800-677-1116.

Alzheimer's Disease Projects

Alzheimer's disease projects sponsored by AoA have produced useful information and important innovations in several areas. They have contributed especially to the development of comprehensive community-based systems of care, programs to support family caregivers, and services to meet the special needs of minority caregivers.

These projects have expanded the knowledge and understanding of Alzheimer's disease among service providers, demonstrated ways to deliver care and disseminate information, and increased State and AAA capabilities in Alzheimer's disease training and service coordination.

Minority Access Projects

Since 1990, AoA has supported three projects to demonstrate ways to improve access to services by minority persons with Alzheimer's disease and their caregivers. These projects are developing innovative and effective ways to meet the special information needs of minority persons.

National Eldercare Campaign

In 1991, AoA launched the National Eldercare Campaign in an effort to increase and improve home care and community-based services for vulnerable older people at risk of losing their self-sufficiency.

Currently, two special efforts in the campaign focus on Alzheimer's disease: establishment of a network of Eldercare Institutes, including a National Eldercare Institute on Long-Term Care and Alzheimer's Disease, and a Community Eldercare Awareness Campaign, a collaborative effort between AoA and the Alzheimer's Association.

National Eldercare Institute on Long-Term Care and Alzheimer's Disease. The National Eldercare Institute on Long-Term Care and Alzheimer's Disease was established in 1992 at the University of South Florida's Suncoast Gerontology Center in Tampa. Its mission is to improve coordination and cooperation among all components of the long-term care system to ensure that frail elders, caregivers, and people with Alzheimer's disease are better served. Areas of concentration for the institute include caregiving and caregiver issues and development of in-home and community-based long-term care services. To help each State and AAA meet the needs of older people at risk, AoA sponsors 13 National Eldercare Institutes that provide technical assistance, research, policy analysis, training, information exchange, best practice models, and public information.

This eldercare institute builds on the efforts of another AoA initiative: the National Resource Center on Alzheimer's Disease (NRCAD), also based at the Suncoast Center from 1988 through 1991. Also a source of information and technical support for State agencies, NRCAD assisted States in planning, developing, and implementing coordinated community-based long-term care and support programs for older people.

Current practices in caregiving support for families of people with Alzheimer's disease were synthesized in a center-produced monograph entitled *Alzheimer's Disease: Caregiver Practices, Programs and Community-Based Strategies*. The monograph, which has been widely disseminated throughout the United States, is available from the National Eldercare Institute.

National Eldercare Institute on
Long-Term Care and Alzheimer's Disease
University of South Florida
Suncoast Gerontology Center
MDC Box 50
12901 Bruce B. Downs Boulevard
Tampa, FL 33612
(813) 974-4355
(81) 974-4251 fax

Community Eldercare Awareness Campaigns. In 1992, AoA provided funding to the Alzheimer's Association to develop and test innovative strategies for building eldercare coalitions through community awareness activities. The Alzheimer's Association selected five sites for building coalitions and organizing Community Eldercare Awareness Campaigns to effect community change for at-risk older people and their caregivers. Sites selected represent a diverse set of communities with significant populations of older people at risk; for example, physically or cognitively impaired, minority, low income, and/or isolated.

Through training, technical assistance, and grants to five of its local chapters, the Alzheimer's Association hopes to: (1) show how unmet needs of at-risk older people and their caregivers impact the economic and social well-being of an entire community, and (2) involve and empower at-risk older people and their caregivers who are now excluded from community decision-making by their physical and cognitive impairments.

The campaigns are expected to produce results at two levels—in communities where the campaigns are organized and as a model to replicate in other communities and by other organizations. A number of products will be developed through the campaigns that will be distributed to Alzheimer's Association chapters and other aging and nonaging organizations, including a training manual for campaign coordinators, a community awareness organizing kit, materials on how to organize high-visibility events, and materials for support group leaders, aging service providers, religious leaders, and others who work directly with frail elderly and their caregivers.

Community Eldercare Awareness Campaigns
Project Management and Coordination
Alzheimer's Association Public Policy Office
Suite 710, 1319 F Street NW
Washington, DC 20005
(202) 393-7737
(202) 393-2109 fax
e-mail: pp@alz.org
website: www.alz.org

Dementia Care and Respite Services Program

From 1988 to 1992, AoA, the Robert Wood Johnson Foundation (RWJF), and the Alzheimer's Association joined forces to help people with Alzheimer's disease and their families throughout the Nation. The focus of these joint efforts was a multimillion-dollar demonstration known as the Dementia Care and Respite Services Program. The program was designed to demonstrate that nonprofit daycare centers can provide financially viable day programs and other respite and health-related services needed by people with dementia and their caregivers. Of the 19 RWJF-funded projects, 9 were cofunded with AoA and 9 were cofunded with the Alzheimer's Association.

Dementia Care and Respite Services Program
Direction and Technical Assistance
Department of Psychiatry and Behavioral Medicine
Wake Forest School of Medicine
Medical Center Boulevard
Winston-Salem, NC 27157-1087
(336) 716-4551
website: www.wfusm.edu

Partners in Caregiving

Following the demonstration's success, RWJF announced a new grant program Partners in Caregiving: The Dementia Services Program. This program provides technical assistance and funding to help 50 adult daycare centers develop and strengthen innovative center-based, in-home, and other respite programs for people with dementia and other chronic conditions. Participating sites were announced in 1993.

Information Dissemination

AoA publishes *Aging*, a quarterly magazine with news and features from the aging services field. For more information, contact:

Aging
Administration on Aging
330 Independence Avenue SW
Washington, DC 20201
(202) 619-0441

Training materials and reports developed through AoA programs are available from:

Division of Dissemination and Utilization
Administration on Aging
330 Independence Avenue SW
Washington, DC 20201
(202) 619-0441

Publications about AoA are available from:

Office of External Affairs
Administration on Aging
330 Independence Avenue SW
Washington, DC 20201
(202) 619-7501

Agency for Health Care Policy and Research

Information and Publications Division
Executive Office Center
2101 East Jefferson Street, Suite 501
Rockville, MD 20852
(301) 594-1368
(301) 594-2283 fax
website: www.ahcpr.gov

Purpose

The purpose of the Agency for Health Care Policy and Research (AHCPR) is to enhance the quality, appropriateness, and effectiveness of health care services and to improve access to that care. Created in 1989, AHCPR is the Federal Government's focal point for medical effectiveness and health services research.

Programs and Activities

Center for General Health Services Intramural Research. The Center for General Health Services Intramural Research undertakes health policy research and analysis that address issues of concern to the Federal Government and provides technical assistance to Federal agencies and other public and private organizations involved in financing or delivering health care.

National Medical Expenditure Survey. The National Medical Expenditure Survey (NMES) was first conducted in 1977 and repeated in 1987. The most recent expenditure survey was conducted in the field from 1987 to 1989. NMES collects data on how Americans use medical services, how much they pay for care, and how these expenditures are financed.

NMES obtained data from 15,000 households and 35,000 persons, documenting through repeated interviews the health and medical care experiences of the group during a complete calendar year. Household data were augmented by information from providers, employers, and insurers. A separate but similar household survey of American Indians and Alaska Natives was conducted at the same time.

NMES also included a separate survey of nursing homes and homes for the mentally retarded that collected information on 11,000 residents and new admissions during the same target year. Thus, NMES is an important source of information on the use, cost, and financing of both home-based and institutional long-term care services for people with Alzheimer's disease and related dementias.

Currently, data are being collected from NMES on the insurance status and coverage of people with dementia. The survey is also being used by AHCPR to identify the characteristics of household and institutional care and the implications of household care for the family, including the impact on earnings and the cost of provider services.

AHCPR is also considering issues for the next NMES, to be conducted in 1995. One area of particular concern is how to measure cognitive impairment in a large national survey. A series of studies will be undertaken to determine how to distinguish between degenerative and nondegenerative dementias, acute and chronic conditions, functional and organic conditions, and level of impairment.

- *Availability of Specialty Units.* In 1990, based on NMES, estimates were published by AHCPR of the availability in 1987 of special nursing home programs for people with Alzheimer's disease, along with projections of availability in 1991, based on the expansion plans of reporting facilities. The report, "Current and Projected Availability of Special Nursing Home Programs for Alzheimer's Disease Patients," is available from AHCPR.

- *Eligibility for Long-Term Care Services.* While home care services could be expanded to help meet the growing demand for long-term care services, there is concern about the costs of such services if they are targeted too broadly. AHCPR has compared the effects on the size of eligibility pools of using cognitive impairment, disruptive behaviors, and limitations in activities of daily living as eligibility criteria. Findings are discussed in the report "Cognitive Impairment and Disruptive Behaviors Among Community-Based Elderly Persons: Implications for Targeting Long-Term Care," available from AHCPR.

- *Employed Caregivers.* AHCPR has also studied the competing demands of employment and informal caregiving responsibilities. It

385

found that those who care for older people with behavioral problems are more likely to be employed than caregivers of disabled older people without behavioral problems.

Center for General Health Services Extramural Research. The Center for General Health Services Extramural Research supports a broad range of health services and health care technology research, demonstration, and evaluation, including projects to examine the quality and availability of services for people with a dementing disease. The center is particularly interested in the effectiveness of special care units and diagnostic techniques and the relative costs of alternative services for people with dementia.

Office of the Forum for Quality and Effectiveness in Health Care. The Office of the Forum for Quality and Effectiveness in Health Care is responsible for facilitating the development, review, and updating of clinically relevant guidelines to assist health care practitioners in the prevention, diagnosis, treatment, and management of clinical conditions. The office also develops performance measures, standards of quality, and evaluation criteria through which health care practitioners and others may review the provision of health care and ensure its quality. The goal of these activities is to enhance the quality, appropriateness, and effectiveness of health care.

- *Panel on Screening for Alzheimer's Disease and Related Disorders.* AHCPR commissions panels to develop clinical guidelines on selected diseases and disorders, including the Panel on Screening for Alzheimer's Disease and Related Disorders, which was convened in 1992. The panel has 16 members, including representatives from social work, nursing, psychology, internal medicine, neurology, geriatrics, and consumer groups.

  AHCPR panels draft guidelines after reviewing scientific literature and available scientific evidence and evaluating the possible benefits, harms, health outcomes, and costs associated with various interventions. As part of the process of developing clinical guidelines, AHCPR panels solicit comments and information from interested individuals and organizations.

  Panel chairpersons, who are critical to the guideline development process and its products, are selected on the basis of relevant experience, recognition in the field, record of leadership in relevant activities, demonstrated capacity to lead group decision making, demonstrated capacity to respond to consumer concerns, and prior experience in developing guidelines for the clinical conditions in question.

To comment, or for more information on the Panel on Screening for Alzheimer's Disease and Related Disorders, contact:

> Center for Practice and Technology Assessment
> Agency for Health Care Policy and Research
> 2101 East Jefferson Street, Suite 401
> Rockville, MD 20852
> (301) 594-4015; (301) 594-4027 fax
> website: www.ahcpr.gov

Information Dissemination

As clinical guidelines are completed, AHCPR disseminates them to practitioners and other users. Organizations of health care practitioners, health care consumers, peer reviewers, accrediting bodies, academic medical centers, medical educators, researchers, payers, and other appropriate groups are encouraged to disseminate guidelines to members and constituents.

Guidelines are also presented in print and through other media, and they are made available through libraries and indexing services. AHCPR plans to publish guidelines developed by the Alzheimer's disease screening panel for consumers, as well as for physicians and nurses.

For information on AHCPR clinical guidelines, reports from NMES, and other publications currently available, contact the Information and Publications Division. The address is given at the beginning of this entry.

Centers for Disease Control and Prevention
Office of Public Inquiries
1600 Clifton Road NE
Atlanta, GA 30333
(404) 639-3534

Purpose

The Centers for Disease Control and Prevention (CDC) is part of the Public Health Service (PHS) under the Department of Health and Human Services (DHHS). It collects and publishes data on national disease trends, epidemics, and environmental health problems and administers block grants to States for preventive services and national health education programs. Within CDC, the Center for Chronic Disease Prevention and Health Promotion and the National Center for Health Statistics (NCHS) have an active interest in Alzheimer's disease.

Programs and Activities

Center for Chronic Disease Prevention and Health Promotion. The Center for Chronic Disease Prevention and Health Promotion translates chronic disease preventive practices, behaviors, and policies into widespread public health strategies through epidemiologic, behavioral, and laboratory investigations, and State and community demonstrations and interventions. The Aging and Statistics Branch (ASB) has responsibility for Alzheimer's disease.

Division of Chronic Disease Control and Community Intervention
Health Care and Aging Studies Branch
Mail Stop K45
4770 Buford Highway NE
Atlanta, GA 30341-3724
(770) 488-5532; (770) 488-5964 fax

- *Healthy People 2000.* As part of the DHHS Healthy People 2000 initiative, ASB is working toward the goal of having primary health providers screen older people during 60 percent of visits to identify cognitive problems, including Alzheimer's disease. ASB is also working to establish a baseline estimate of how frequently providers screen for cognitive problems.

- *Report on Alzheimer's Disease Survival and Mortality.* In 1990, ASB used death certificates from each State to report on the prevalence of Alzheimer's disease as an underlying cause of death from 1979 through 1987. "Mortality from Alzheimer's disease— United States, 1979-87" appeared in the *Journal of the American Medical Association* on January 16, 1991 (vol. 265, no. 3, page 313). Using data from hospital records, State registries, and death certificates, ASB is working toward providing more reliable estimates of the prevalence and incidence of Alzheimer's disease.

- *Support of Programs in State Health Departments.* Since 1988, ASB has taken an active role in initiating State Alzheimer's disease projects. ASB serves as a consultant to State health departments developing Alzheimer's disease registries and information networks, at the same time promoting standardization of diagnostic methodologies. ASB also provides mechanisms for sharing information and experience among States.

- *National Center for Health Statistics.* The National Center for Health Statistics (NCHS) collects, analyzes, and distributes data on health in the United States. NCHS produces and distributes a variety of statistical reports on mortality, resource use, data evaluation and methods research, analytical and epidemiological studies, and other topics related to health. NCHS' Clearinghouse on Health Indexes helps administrators and researchers develop health measures and also provides annotated bibliographies and referrals.

  National Center for Health Statistics
  6525 Belcrest Road
  Hyattsville, MD 20782
  (301) 436-8500
  website: www.cdc.gov/nchswww

- *National Nursing Home Survey.* National Center for Health Statistics (NCHS) has issued a series of reports from the 1985 National Nursing Home Survey (NNHS). NNHS is a nationwide sample (excluding Alaska and Hawaii) of nursing and related care homes, their residents, patients discharged, and staff, conducted periodically by NCHS. One report, "Mental Illness in Nursing Homes, 1985," presents data on residents with organic brain syndromes, including Alzheimer's disease, in nursing homes.

Information Dissemination

For information on NCHS statistical reports and publications, contact CDC at the address listed at the beginning of this entry.

Department of Justice
Office of Public Affairs
Room 1228, 10th Street and Constitution Avenue NW
Washington, DC 20530
(202) 514-2007; (202) 514-5331
www.usdoj.gov

Purpose

The Department of Justice (DoJ) enforces Federal laws, represents the Government in Federal cases, and interprets laws under which other departments act.

Programs and Activities

Office of Juvenile Justice and Delinquency Prevention.

- *Training and Dissemination of Technical Assistance Division Project Safe Return.* In 1992, Congress authorized the Missing Alzheimer's Alert Program (now Project Safe Return) within the Office of Juvenile Justice and Delinquency Prevention (OJJDP). Project Safe Return is a national program to facilitate the identification and safe return of missing memory-impaired persons who, because of dementia, are at risk of wandering from the safety of their homes and families. The Alzheimer's Association was designated to operate the program through its nationwide network of 220 local chapters and 6 area resource centers (ARCs).

The program is designed to:

- Create a central, computerized registry of information on memory-impaired persons and a national toll-free telephone line to access the registry

- Establish an identification system with identification jewelry and clothing labels purchased and distributed through a central service

- Create educational and informational materials for use and distribution by participating chapters, which will focus on training law enforcement officers and emergency personnel and support for families and other caregivers of missing registrants

Project Safe Return is the first step in a multiyear strategy to offer broader protection and increased safety for the growing number of people with Alzheimer's disease. For more information on Project Safe Return, contact:

Alzheimer's Association
919 North Michigan Avenue, Suite 1000
Chicago, IL 60611-1676
(800) 272-3900
(312) 335-8700 phone
(312) 335-1110 fax
website: www.alz.org

Information Dissemination

National Institute of Justice, National Criminal Justice Reference Service. The National Institute of Justice's National Criminal Justice Reference Service (NCJRS) provides database searches on elder abuse and other topics related to Alzheimer's disease. Contact NCJRS by writing or calling:

NCJRS Department
P.O. Box 6000
Rockville, MD 20850
800-851-3420
(301) 519-5212 fax
website: www.jcjrs.org

To use NCJRS automated fax on demand service, call 1-800-851-3420 and select option 1.

Department of Veterans Affairs
Public Information Office
810 Vermont Avenue NW
Washington, DC 20420
(202) 273-5400
website: www.va.gov.com

Purpose

The Department of Veterans Affairs (VA) provides benefits to military service veterans and their dependents. These benefits include educational assistance, vocational rehabilitation, home loans, and comprehensive dental and medical care in outpatient clinics, Veterans Administration medical centers (VAMCs), and nursing homes around the country.

Programs and Activities

Office of Geriatrics and Extended Care. In view of the growing number of older veterans (currently more than a quarter of the veteran population is over 65 years old), the VA actively promotes interdisciplinary geriatric and gerontological programs through which many medical and health students learn to care for people with Alzheimer's disease, and supports a number of special services for people with dementia.

- *Geriatric Research, Education, and Clinical Centers Program.* Geriatric Research, Education, and Clinical Centers (GRECCs) train practitioners, teachers, and researchers in the field of geriatrics. The program began in 1975; there are 16 GRECCs now in operation. Each GRECC conducts biomedical, clinical, and health services research in a defined area of aging; educates health professionals; and develops clinical models to improve care of older veterans. Four GRECCs currently focus on various aspects of Alzheimer's disease and related dementias.

  GRECCs Active in Alzheimer's Disease:

  California
  Palo Alto GRECC
  VAMC, 3801 Miranda Ave.
  Palo Alto, CA 94304
  (650) 493-5000
  (650) 855-9437 fax

  Minnesota
  Minneapolis GRECC
  VAMC, One Veterans Drive
  Minneapolis, MN 55417
  (612) 725-2051
  (612) 725-2084 fax

  Massachusetts
  Bedford GRECC
  VAMC, 200 Springs Road
  Bedford, MA 01730
  (781) 275-7500
  (781) 787-3537 fax

  Washington
  Seattle GRECC
  VAMC, 1660 S.Columbian Way,
    182B
  Seattle, WA 98108
  (206) 764-2308
  (206) 764-2569 fax

- *Health Care Services for Veterans with Dementia.* Programs for veterans with dementia are located throughout the VA network of health care facilities, which include medical centers, outpatient clinics, nursing homes, domiciliaries, hospital-based home care programs, adult day health programs, and community residential care programs. Most VAMCs operate respite care programs, which primarily provide relief for family caregivers of veterans, and many have active geriatric evaluation and management programs. The VA also contracts with community facilities for hospital care, nursing home care, and adult day health care and provides assistance to States for care of veterans in State veteran domiciliaries and nursing homes.

- *Multiphase VAMC Dementia Survey.* In 1988 and 1989, the VA surveyed all medical centers to determine the number and types of special dementia programs they offered. The survey showed that 31 out of 172 facilities had inpatient dementia units at that time, while 22 had outpatient dementia programs, 25 had dementia assessment clinics, and 8 facilities had established dementia registries. These services were concentrated in 56 VA facilities, approximately 33 percent of VAMCs.

  In 1990, the VA collected data on resources allocated for the care of people with dementia from a sample of centers with special programs. The information from this second phase of the VAMC Dementia Survey will be used in program planning for dementia, as well as in determining specific educational needs of health care providers in Alzheimer's disease and related dementias.

  Also in 1990 and 1991, in the third phase of its survey, the VA obtained information from existing special care units (SCUs) in VAMCs regarding process of care, staffing patterns, and cost of care in such units. A total of 13 VAMCs were visited from among the 31 facilities identified as having an SCU in the first phase of the survey. A uniform survey instrument was used to collect data on multiple variables at each site. Results of this survey are being used in the current development of flexible guidelines for VA inpatient dementia units.

Office of Research and Development.

- *Intramural Research.* Areas of interest related to Alzheimer's disease in the VA's intramural research program include:

  - Epidemiology of dementia—clinical and genetic heterogeneity, registries, ethnic comparisons

  - Etiology and pathogenesis—biomarkers, mechanisms of neural degeneration, neurochemical models, immune responses

- Diagnosis—chemical markers, differential diagnosis, neuroimaging, medical correlates, cerebrospinal fluid (CSF) markers

- Clinical course—cognitive deficits, patterns of memory loss, behavioral changes, sleep disturbances, assessment instruments

- Treatment—wandering behavior, music therapy, physostigmine, tacrine, milacemide, calcium channel blockers

- The family—impact on older women caregivers, impact on children, risk factors in caregiving, grief, coping strategies

- Systems of care—comparison of SCUs, institutional versus home care, adapted work, cost of care

Office of Academic Affairs.

- *Physician Residency Program in Geriatrics.* This program began in 1978 as a fellowship program and is the largest agency-sponsored geriatrics training program in the Nation. It has played a critical role in developing this new medical specialty in the United States and gaining recognition for it from the Accreditation Council for Graduate Medical Education. By the end of 1990, over 40 VAMCs had accredited geriatric programs strongly integrated with each affiliate's internal medicine base. Graduates serve as medical school faculty, medical directors of nursing homes, directors of aging centers, and staff geriatricians.

- *Geriatric Psychiatry Fellowship Program.* This program provides psychiatrists with expertise in two areas: (1) diagnosis and treatment of older people with dementia and other psychiatric problems, and (2) teaching and conducting research.

- *Research Training for Psychiatrists.* This 3-year program teaches VA psychiatrists techniques and approaches that enable them to contribute to the biological understanding of psychiatric illnesses. Although not specifically a geriatric program, some of the fellows work on age-related research, such as neuroendocrine regulation in Alzheimer's disease.

- *Clinical Pharmacology Fellowship Program.* In this program, postresidency physicians work to advance knowledge about drug interactions, adverse reactions, and risks to patients. This is a 2-year program, with an option for a third year.

* *Geropsychology Postdoctoral Fellowship Program*. This program is designed to increase the number of VA psychologists trained in the psychological care and treatment of geriatric patients. As of fiscal year 1994, 10 VAMCs will offer these 1-year fellowships.

* *Gerontologic Nurse Fellowship Program*. This program prepares geriatric nurse clinicians, educators, administrators, and researchers for leadership positions in geriatrics and long-term care. The program provides a 2-year fellowship for graduate nursing students enrolled in qualified doctoral-level nursing programs and whose doctoral dissertations focus on clinical research in geriatrics or gerontology.

* *VA/Robert Wood Johnson Clinical Scholars Program*. Fellows in this program complete projects concerning some aspect of health services research. At least one of the six clinical scholars selected each year has specialized in geriatrics.

* *Interdisciplinary Team Training Program*. The Interdisciplinary Team Training Program (ITTP) is an educational program that provides didactic and clinical instruction to VA faculty, practitioners, and affiliated students from three or more health professions. Its purpose is to develop a cadre of health practitioners with the knowledge and competencies required to provide interdisciplinary team care to meet the wide spectrum of health care and service needs of veterans. This team training focuses on select VA priority areas of need, such as geriatrics. ITTP also provides training to other VAMCs and serves as a role model for affiliated students. ITTP sites:

Alabama

Birmingham VAMC
700 South 19th Street
Birmingham, AL 35233
(205) 933-8101
(205) 933-4484 fax

Arizona

Tucson VAMC
3601 South Sixth Avenue
Tucson, AZ 85723
(520) 792-1450
(520) 629-1811 fax

Arkansas

John L. McClellan Memorial
    Veterans Hospital
4300 West 7th Street
Little Rock, AR 72205-5484
(501) 661-1202
(501) 688-1629 fax

California

Palo Alto VAMC
3801 Miranda Avenue
Palo Alto, CA 94304
(650) 493-5000
(650) 855-9437 fax

Sepulveda VAMC
16111 Plummer Street
Sepulveda, CA 91343
(818) 891-7711
(818) 895-9519 fax

Florida

James A. Haley Veterans' Hospital
13000 Bruce B. Downs Boulevard
Tampa, FL 33612
(813) 972-2000
(813) 972-7680 fax

New York

Buffalo VAMC
3495 Bailey Avenue
Buffalo, NY 14215
(716) 834-9200
(716) 862-3433

Oregon

Portland VAMC
P.O. Box 1034
Portland, OR 97207
(503) 220-8262
(503) 721-1053

Pennsylvania

Coatesville VAMC
1400 Black Horse Hill Rd.
Coatesville, PA 19320
(610) 384-7711
(610) 383-0207

Tennessee

Memphis VAMC
1030 Jefferson Avenue
Memphis, TN 38104
(901) 523-8990
(901) 577-7241

Utah

Salt Lake City VAMC
500 Foothill Drive
Salt Lake City, UT 84148
(801) 582-1565

- *Continuing Education.* The VA provides continuing education at all VAMCs and operates a network of continuing education field units, including:

    - Seven regional medical education centers (RMECs) located throughout the country

- A continuing education center (CEC) located in St. Louis, Missouri, which coordinates national training programs in priority areas identified by the VA Undersecretary for Health

- Two dental education centers (DECs), one engineering training center (ETC), and seven Cooperative Health Manpower Education Programs (CHEPs), which support remote area VAMCs that do not have formal medical school affiliations.

Libraries, medical media, television production studios, education specialists, and curriculum designers are also integral to accomplishing the VA's education mission.

A number of continuing education programs focus on caring for people with Alzheimer's disease and related dementias. In addition, five of the VA's national training programs have focused on geriatrics or aging: health care problems of the elderly, ambulatory care and the elderly, geriatric evaluation and management teams, nursing home care of the mentally ill, and medication management in the elderly.

- Regional Medical Education Centers (RMECs)

Alabama

Birmingham VAMC
700 South 19th Street
Birmingham, AL 35233
(205) 933-8101
(205) 933-4484

California

Long Beach VAMC
5901 East 7th Street
Long Beach, CA 90822
(562) 494-2611

Minnesota

Minneapolis VAMC
One Veterans Drive
Minneapolis, MN 55417
(612) 725-2000

New York

Northport VAMC
79 Middleville Road
Northport, NY 11768
(516) 261-4400
(516) 754-7905 fax

North Carolina

Durham VAMC
508 Fulton Street
Durham, NC 27705
(919) 286-0411
(919) 286-6825 fax

Ohio

Cleveland VAMC
10701 East Boulevard
Cleveland, OH 44106
(216) 791-3800
(216) 421-3001 fax

Utah

Salt Lake City VAMC
500 Foothill Drive
Salt Lake City, UT 84148
(801) 582-1565

- Continuing Education Center (CEC)

Missouri

St. Louis VAMC
915 North Grand Avenue
St. Louis, MO 63125
(314) 652-4100

Information Dissemination

The VA has produced and distributes the following information resources:

- *Dementia: Guidelines for Diagnosis and Treatment* (October 1989), a manual

- *Guide for Families Caring for Persons with Dementia-Related Diseases*, a series of 21 caregiver education pamphlets (August 1989) developed by the Minneapolis GRECC

Limited quantities of these publications were produced. For information on availability, write:

Department of Veterans Affairs
Office of Geriatrics and Extended Care, 114-B
810 Vermont Avenue NW
Washington, DC 20420

Three videotapes were developed by the Bedford Division of the Boston GRECC:

- "Alzheimer's Disease and the Family Conference"

- "Alzheimer's Disease: Managing the Later Stages in the Health Care Setting"

- "Alzheimer's Disease: Managing the Later Stages in the Home"

Further information about these videotapes is available from:

National Technical Information Service (NTIS)
U.S. Department of Commerce
Springfield, VA 22161
(800) 788-6282
(703) 321-8547 fax
website: www.ntis.gov

Food and Drug Administration
Office of Consumer Affairs
Room 16-85
5600 Fishers Lane
Rockville, MD 20857
(301) 827-5006
(301) 443-9767 fax

Purpose

The Food and Drug Administration (FDA) conducts research and develops standards on the composition, quality, and safety of drugs, cosmetics, medical devices, radiation-emitting products, foods, food additives, and infant formulas; develops labeling and product standards conducts inspections of manufacturers; issues orders to companies to recall and/or cease selling or producing hazardous products; and enforces rulings and recommends action to the Justice Department. FDA has 157 district and local offices across the country.

FDA acts as public health protector by ensuring that all drugs on the market are safe and effective. Relating to Alzheimer's disease, FDA is responsible for evaluating and regulating clinical trials on experimental drugs and biological products, and also for ensuring the quality and safe of drugs used to treat behavioral symptoms of the disease.

Programs and Activities

Division of Neuropharmacological Drug Products Center for Drug Evaluation and Research.

- *Review of New Drugs*. By law, in order to be marketed, all new drugs must be approved by FDA as being "safe and effective." In deciding whether to approve a drug, FDA weighs "risk versus benefit"—determining whether the drug produces the intended benefits without causing side effects that outweigh those benefits.

FDA's review process begins when a sponsor has completed initial testing of a new drug in animals and is ready to begin clinical trials with humans. The sponsor submits an investigational new drug (IND) application to FDA, providing results of laboratory and animal research and information on previous use of the drug in humans. The sponsor also provides details on how clinical trials will be conducted.

Within 30 days, FDA must let the sponsor know whether, in its judgment, the testing the sponsor proposes is sufficiently safe. If so, the IND is placed "in effect" and the clinical study may proceed. If not, FDA may place the study on hold until the sponsor makes needed changes.

Clinical trials are normally done in three phases involving progressively larger numbers of people. The clinical trial process, which can take from several months to several years, includes evaluation of both short- and long-term safety, effectiveness, and optimal dosage.

After completing clinical trials, a sponsor submits a new drug application (NDA) to FDA. The NDA is assigned to one of seven review divisions depending on the type of drug. FDA decides to approve a new drug if there is substantial evidence that it is effective and safe under the conditions of use in the proposed labeling. The review process may take from several months to several years. The drug evaluation process often includes an advisory committee of experts, especially if a major scientific or public controversy is involved or if special regulatory requirements are being considered.

- *Expanded Access to Promising Experimental Drugs*. FDA published a regulation in 1987 to provide expanded access to promising experimental drugs so that desperately ill patients can benefit from those drugs earlier than was possible before. In 1992, an experimental treatment for Alzheimer's disease, THA, was made available under expanded access policy for the first time.

- *Monitoring Drugs on the Market*. After a drug is approved for marketing, the agency collects and analyzes tens of thousands of reports each year on drugs to monitor for unexpected adverse reactions.

Information Dissemination

FDA is a leading source of health information for consumers and health professionals. FDA publishes a bimonthly magazine, *FDA Consumer,* and also distributes reprints of several articles about Alzheimer's disease. Another FDA publication is the *FDA Drug Bulletin,* which provides more than a million doctors and other health professionals with the latest information on drugs, biologics, and radiological and medical devices. For more information, contact the Office of Consumer Affairs listed at the beginning of this entry.

Health Care Financing Administration
Office of Public Affairs
6325 Security Boulevard
P.O. Box 1721
Baltimore, MD 21207
Medicare Hotline: 800-638-6833
website: www.hcfa.gov

Purpose

The Health Care Financing Administration (HCFA), which oversees the Medicare and Medicaid programs, was established to combine health financing and quality assurance programs in a single agency.

Programs and Activities

Medicare and Medigap Regulation. Medicare is the primary health insurance program for people age 65 and older and those with certain disabilities. Medicare coverage provides for acute hospital care, physician services, brief stays in skilled nursing facilities, and short-term skilled home care related to a medical problem. Medicare coverage is determined by the nature of the services required by the patient, not the specific diagnosis. Coverage is restricted to medical care and does not include the long-term care services that people with Alzheimer's disease need at home or in nursing facilities. While there is no medical treatment for Alzheimer's disease, Medicare does cover treatment of other medical problems that people with Alzheimer's disease might have.

Together with the States, HCFA sets guidelines for and regulates the market for Medigap insurance policies, which provide private supplementary coverage for Medicare enrollees.

For more information on Medicare or Medigap insurance, call HCFA's toll-free Medigap Hotline listed above, or write to the Office of Public Affairs at the above address.

Medicaid. Medicaid covers health services for low-income individuals and families. While Medicaid is coordinated by HCFA, the program is administered by the States, and coverage and eligibility requirements vary from State to State. People with Alzheimer's disease may receive nursing home benefits and, in some States, limited community long-term care services once they meet a State's financial eligibility requirements for Medicaid. These services are provided, however, at the option of the State and are not mandated by Federal law.

Medicaid Home and Community-Based Waivers (2176 Waivers). Since 1982, HCFA has been granting specific waivers to States permitting Medicaid coverage and reimbursement for home and community-based services provided to people who would otherwise need care in a nursing home or other institutional setting.

People with Alzheimer's disease or related dementias and their families who are eligible for Medicaid, and who are in localities and States covered under the waiver program, are provided special services such as adult day care, respite care, personal care, and case management services to delay or prevent institutionalization.

Home and Community Care for the Frail and Functionally Disabled Elderly. Provisions of the Omnibus Reconciliation Act of 1990 allow States to provide home and community care to functionally disabled older people, defined as financially eligible people age 65 and older who require substantial assistance in performing two of three specified activities of daily living (toileting, transferring, and eating). The act establishes somewhat more liberal criteria for people with a primary or secondary diagnosis of Alzheimer's disease, who qualify if they require substantial assistance (including verbal reminding or physical cueing) or supervision in performing two of five specified activities of daily living (bathing, dressing, toileting, transferring, and eating). Unlike other Medicaid benefits, however, Federal funds for this State option are capped at a specific level.

402

State Medicaid Offices

Alabama

Alabama Medicaid Agency
P.O. Box 5624
Montgomery, AL 36103-5624
(334) 242-5000

Alaska

Div. of Medical Assistance
Dept. of Health and Social
 Services
P.O. Box 110660
Juneau, AK 99811-0660
(907) 465-3355
(907) 465-2204 fax

Arizona

Arizona Health Care Cost
 Containment System
701 East Jefferson
P.O. Box 25520
Phoenix, AZ 85002-5520
(602) 417-4680
(602) 252-3636 fax

Arkansas

Office of Medical Services
Arkansas Dept. of Human
 Services
P.O. Box 1437, Slot 1100
Little Rock, AR 72203-1437
(501) 682-8292
(501) 682-1197 fax

California

Dept. of Health Services
714 P Street, Room 1253
Sacramento, CA 95814
(916) 654-0391
(916) 657-1156 fax

Colorado

Health Care Financing and
 Policy
1575 Sherman Street, 10th
 Floor
Denver, CO 80203-1714
(303) 866-6092
(303) 866-4411 fax

Connecticut

Department of Social Ser-
 vices
25 Sigourney Street
Hartford, CT 06106
(860) 424-4908
(860) 464-5114 fax

Delaware

Department of Health and
 Social Services
Delaware State Hospital
P.O. Box 906
New Castle, DE 19720
(302) 577-4901
(302) 577-4899 fax

District of Columbia

Medical Services Adminis-
 tration
D.C. Department of Health
2100 Martin Luther King,
 Jr., Ave. SE, Suite 302
Washington, DC 20020
(202) 727-0735
(202) 610-3209 fax

Florida

Agency for Health Care Administration
2728 Fort Knox Boulevard
Building 3
Tallahassee, FL 32308
(850) 488-3560
(850) 414-1721 fax

Georgia

Georgia Department of
Medical Assistance
#2 Peach Tree Street
Atlanta, GA 30303
(404) 656-4479
(404) 651-6880 fax

Hawaii

Dept. of Social Services
820 Mililani St., Suite 606
Honolulu, HI 96813-2938
(808) 586-5391
(808) 586-5389 fax

Idaho

Bureau of Medicaid Policy
and Operations
Dept. of Health and Welfare
P.O. Box 83720
Boise, ID 83720-0036
(208) 334-5795
(208) 332-7342 fax

Illinois

Medical Operations
Illinois Dept. of Public Aid
201 S. Grand Avenue East
Springfield, IL 62763-0001
(217) 782-2570
(217) 52407114 fax

Indiana

Medicaid Policy and Planning
Indiana Family and Social
Services Administration
Room W382
Indianapolis, IN 46207-7083
(317) 233-4455
(317) 233-7382 fax

Iowa

Dept. of Human Services
Hoover State Office Bldg.,
5th Floor
Des Moines, IA 50319-0114
(515) 281-8794
(515) 281-7791 fax

Kansas

Commission of Adults and
Medical Services
Docking State Office Bldg.,
Room 628-S
915 Harrison Street
Topeka, KS 66612
(785) 296-3981
(785) 296-4813 fax

Kentucky

Dept. of Medicaid Services
275 East Main Street,
6th Floor West
Frankfort, KY 40621
(502) 564-4321
(502) 564-0509 fax

Louisiana

Bureau of Health Services
Financing
P.O. Box 91030
Baton Rouge, LA 70821-9030
(504) 342-3891
(504) 342-3893 fax

Maine

Bureau of Medical Services
Dept. of Human Services
State House Station #11
249 Western Avenue
Augusta, ME 04333
(207) 287-2093
(207) 287-2675 fax

Maryland

Department of Health and
  Mental Hygiene
201 West Preston Street
Baltimore, MD 21201
(410) 676-4664
(410) 333-7687 fax

Massachusetts

Department of Transitional
  Assistance
600 Washington Street
Boston, MA 02111
(617) 348-8500
(617) 348-8575 fax

Michigan

Department of Community
  Health
P.O. Box 30479
Lansing, MI 48909
(517) 335-5001
(517) 335-5007 fax

Minnesota

Health Care Administration
Dept. of Human Services
444 Lafayette Road, 6th Floor
St. Paul, MN 55155-3848
(612) 296-3386
(612) 297-3230 fax

Mississippi

Division of Medicaid
Office of the Governor
Suite 801, Robert E. Lee Bldg.
239 North Lamar Street
Jackson, MS 39201-1399
(601) 359-6050
(601) 359-6048 fax

Missouri

Division of Medical Services
Dept. of Social Services
P.O. Box 6500
Jefferson City, MO 65102
(573) 751-6922
(573) 751-6564 fax

Montana

Health Policy Services
Department of Public Health
  and Human Services
1400 Broadway
Helena, MT 59601
(406) 444-4141
(406) 444-1861 fax

Nebraska

Medicaid Division
Dept. of Social Services
P.O. Box 95026
Lincoln, NE 68509-5026
(402) 471-9718
(402) 471-9092 fax

Nevada

Nevada Medicaid
Welfare Division, Dept. of
  Human Resources
2527 North Carson Street
Carson City, NV 89710
(702) 687-4378
(702) 687-8727 fax

New Hampshire

Department of Health and
    Human Services
Office of Health Manage-
    ment
Medicaid Administration
    Bureau
6 Haze Drive
Concord, NH 03301-6521
(603) 271-4353
(603) 271-4376 fax

New Jersey

Division of Medical
    Assistance and Health
    Services
P.O. Box 712
7 Quakerbridge Plaza
Trenton, NJ 08625
(609) 588-2600
(609) 588-3583 fax

New Mexico

Medical Assistance Division
Department of Human
    Services
P.O. Box 2348
Santa Fe, NM 87504-2348
(505) 827-3106
(505) 827-3185 fax

New York

New York State Department
    of Health
Empire State Plaza, Corning
    Tower
40 North Pearl Street
Albany, NY 12237-0001
(518) 474-2011
(518) 474-5450 fax

North Carolina

Division. of Medical
    Assistance
Dept. of Human Resources
P.O. Box 29529
Raleigh, NC 27626-0529
(919) 733-2060
(919) 733-6608 fax

North Dakota

Dept. of Human Services
600 E. Boulevard Avenue
Bismarck, ND 58505-0261
(701) 328-3194
(701) 328-1544 fax

Ohio

Office of Medicaid
Dept. of Human Services
31st Floor
30 East Broad Street
Columbus, OH 43266-0423
(614) 644-0140
(614) 752-3986 fax

Oklahoma

Oklahoma Health Care
    Authority
4545 N. Lincoln Boulevard,
    Suite 124
Oklahoma City, OK 73105
(405) 530-3373
(405) 530-3478 fax

Oregon

Dept. of Human Resources
500 Summer Street
Salem, OR 97310-1014
(503) 945-5772
(503) 373-7689 fax

Pennsylvania

Dept. of Public Welfare
Office of Medical Assistance
   Programs
Room 515
Health & Welfare Building
P.O. Box 2675
Harrisburg, PA 17105-2675
(717) 787-1870
(717) 787-4639 fax

Puerto Rico

Office of Economic
   Assistance to the
   Medically Indigent
Department of Health
Call Box 70184
San Juan, PR 00936
(809) 765-1230
(787) 250-0990 fax

Rhode Island

Department of Human
   Services
600 New London Avenue
Cranston, RI 02920
(401) 464-3575
(401) 464-3677 fax

South Carolina

Department of Health and
   Human Services
P.O. Box 8206
Columbia, SC 29202-8206
(803) 253-6100
(803) 253-4137 fax

South Dakota

Program Administrator
Dept. of Social Services
Office of Medical Services
700 Governors Drive
Pierre, SD 57501-2291
(605) 773-3495
(605) 773-5246 fax

Tennessee

Bureau of Medicaid
729 Church Street
Nashville, TN 37247-6501
(615) 741-0213
(615) 741-0882 fax

Texas

Dept. of Human Services
Mail Code W513
P.O. Box 149030
Austin, TX 78714-9030
(512) 424-6517
(512) 424-6585 fax

Utah

Div. of Health Care Financing
Utah Department of Health
P.O. Box 143101
Salt Lake City, UT 84114-3101
(801) 538-6406
(801) 538-6099 fax

Vermont

Office of VT Health Access
Dept. of Social Welfare
Medicaid Division
103 South Main Street
Waterbury, VT 05676-0276
(802) 241-2880
(802) 241-2897 fax

Virginia

Virginia Dept. of Medical
  Assistance Services
Suite 1300
600 East Broad Street
Richmond, VA 23219
(804) 786-8099
(804) 371-4981 fax

Virgin Islands

Bureau of Health Insurance
  and Medical Assistance
Suite 302
Frostco Center 2
10-3A Altona
St. Thomas, VI 00802
(809) 774-4624
(809) 774-4918 fax

Washington

Medical Assistance Adminis-
  tration
Department of Social and
  Health Services
P.O. Box 45080
Olympia, WA 98504-5080
(360) 902-7807
(360) 902-7588 fax

West Virginia

Department of Health and
  Human Resources
Bureau for Medical Services
Building 6, State Capitol
  Complex
Charleston, WV 25305
(304) 926-1700
(304) 926-1833 fax
website: wvonline.com

Wisconsin

Bureau of Health Care
  Financing
Division of Health and
  Social Services
1 West Wilson, Room 250
Madison, WI 53701-0309
(608) 266-2522
(608) 266-1096 fax

Wyoming

Division of Health Care
  Financing
6101 Yellowstone Road
Cheyenne, WY 82002
(307) 777-7531
(307) 777-6964 fax

Office of Demonstrations and Evaluations. The Office of Demonstrations and Evaluations supports analyses, experiments, demonstrations, and pilot projects primarily to provide information that assists in administration of the Medicare and Medicaid programs.

- *Medicare Alzheimer's Disease Demonstration.* In an effort to learn about the kinds of services used by people with dementia and their families, Congress included a provision in the Omnibus Budget Reconciliation Act of 1986 to establish the Medicare Alzheimer's Disease Demonstration. The purpose of this project, which began in May 1989 [and was completed in 1993], is to determine the effectiveness, cost, and impact on health status and functioning of providing comprehensive services to Medicare beneficiaries with Alzheimer's disease or related disorders.

Two models of care are being studied under this project. Both models provide case management—assessment, care planning, service arrangement, and client monitoring—and a variety of in-home and community-based services that are not covered under Medicare, such as adult day care, homemaker/personal care services, companion services, family counseling, and caregiver education and training. The two models vary according to the intensity of the case management clients receive and the amount of reimbursement available for demonstration services: Model A (1:100 case manager/client ratio, $300 monthly expenditure cap); and Model B (1:30 case manager/client ratio, $500 monthly expenditure cap).

Social/Health Maintenance Organization Demonstration. HCFA is targeting late 1993 to begin selecting grantees for a second demonstration project to apply the Social/Health Maintenance Organization (S/HMO) model in multiple communities. The S/HMO is a novel concept for financing and expanding long-term care coverage benefits that HCFA first tested at four sites from 1985 to 1990. Through the S/HMO, Medicare pays a fixed monthly capitation (per enrollee) amount, so that beneficiaries are eligible to receive a package of long-term care benefits, as well as medical and acute care.

On the basis of the experience of the first S/HMO demonstration, the follow-up project will place special emphasis on integrating chronic and acute care benefits. Findings that are relevant to people with Alzheimer's disease and their families are likely to emerge.

Community Care for Alzheimer's Disease and Related Disorders. With funding from HCFA, the Urban Institute is analyzing and comparing data for people with and without cognitive impairments who were involved in the National Long-Term Care Channeling Demonstration Project, conducted between 1980 and 1985. The two specific objectives of the current project are: (1) to determine the range of services used, sources used, and costs of care to community residents with cognitive impairments due to Alzheimer's disease and related disorders; and (2) to determine the risks of these residents entering nursing homes as a function of their physical and mental health status.

409

Adult Day Center Census. Section 208 of the subsequently repealed Medicare Catastrophic Care Act mandated a study to provide Congress with information on the services, scope and availability, costs and financing, quality assurance mechanisms, and users of services for adult daycare centers. The final report, "The National Adult Day Center Census—89, A Descriptive Report," was completed in 1990. The study was conducted by a research team from the Institute for Health and Aging at the University of San Francisco and the National Institute of Adult Daycare, and jointly funded by HCFA and the American Association of Retired Persons (AARP). Of over 2,000 operating centers that were identified, 1,425 centers completed the survey. According to the results, one-third of participants in daycare programs suffer from Alzheimer's disease or related disorders.

Program of All-Inclusive Care for the Elderly. Section 9412 of Public Law 99-509 directs HCFA to conduct a demonstration called the Program of All-Inclusive Care for the Elderly (PACE), which replicates the model of care developed by On Lok Senior Health Services in San Francisco. This model program, which delivers services to very frail community-dwelling older people through managed care, began in 1990 and is currently operating at nine sites. Plans are underway to test the PACE model in five more communities.

The PACE model includes as core services adult day health care and multidisciplinary case management through which access and allocation of all health and long-term care services are arranged. Physician, therapeutic, ancillary, and social support services are provided at the adult daycare center whenever possible. Hospital, nursing home, home health, and other specialized services are provided by the community. Transportation is also provided to all enrolled members who require it.

Though not dealing exclusively with people with Alzheimer's disease, most PACE enrollees are cognitively impaired, and some findings relevant to people with dementia are expected to emerge.

- PACE Sites:

California

On Lok Senior Health Services
1441 Powell Street
San Francisco, CA 94133
(415) 989-2578
(415) 292-8675 fax

Colorado

Total Longterm Care, Inc.
1801 East 19th Avenue, #608
Denver, CO 80218
(303) 839-7540
(303) 869-1843 fax

Massachusetts

East Boston Neighborhood
    Health Center
Elder Service Plan
10 Gove Street
East Boston, MA 02128
(617) 569-5800
(617) 539-5454 fax

New York

Comprehensive Care
    Management
2401 White Plains Road
Bronx, NY 10467
(718) 515-8600
(718) 881-1028 fax

Oregon

Providence Elderplace
1235 NE 47th Avenue,
    Suite 220
Portland, OR 97213
(503) 215-7550
(503) 215-7543 fax

Texas

Bienvivir Senior Health
    Services
6000 Welch Street, Suite A-2
El Paso, TX 79905
(915) 779-2555
(915) 779-1753 fax

Information Dissemination

HCFA publishes statistical information and reports on its research and demonstration projects. It also publishes a quarterly journal, the *Health Care Financing Review*. For more information, contact HCFA's Office of Public Affairs listed at the beginning of this entry.

Health Resources and Services Administration

Public Information Office
5600 Fishers Lane
Rockville, MD 20857
(301) 443-2086
(301) 433-1989 fax
website: www.hrsa.dhhs.gov

Purpose

The Health Resources and Services Administration (HRSA) administers Federal health services programs related to access, quality, equity, and cost of health care. HRSA supports State and community efforts to deliver care to underserved areas and to groups with special health needs.

Two bureaus within HRSA have programs related to Alzheimer's disease—the Bureau of Health Professions and the Bureau of Primary Health Care.

411

Programs and Activities

Bureau of Health Professions. The Bureau of Health Professions supports education and training of students in the health professions through scholarships, loans, traineeships, financial assistance to schools, and development of regional resources.

- *Geriatric Education Center Program.* Begun in 1983, the Geriatric Education Center (GEC) program strengthens multidisciplinary training of health professionals in the diagnosis, treatment, and prevention of disease, including Alzheimer's disease and other health concerns of older people. Functioning within a defined geographic area, each GEC provides services to and establishes collaborative relationships among the health education community within that area. This educational community includes organizations or institutions (both affiliated and unaffiliated with a GEC or its parent organization) that sponsor formal and informal educational programs and activities for faculty, students, and practitioners in health care.

These GECs train health professions faculty to prepare students to address the special health problems of older adults. Other GEC program activities include multidisciplinary curriculum development, consultation, information dissemination, technical assistance, and continuing education for health care practitioners.

The ultimate goal of the GEC program is to improve the quality of health care for the expanding older population by enhancing the knowledge and skills of health professionals in geriatrics.

GEC programs include workshops, seminars, conferences, and fellowships. Programs are offered in nursing, medicine, dentistry, social work, psychology, rehabilitation, pharmacology, and long-term care administration. Most GECs have activities relating to Alzheimer's disease.

GECs:

Florida

Miami Area GEC
University of Miami
1400 NW 10ᵗʰ Ave. (M-865)
Miami, FL 33136
(305) 547-6270
(305) 243-4804 fax

Minnesota

Minnesota Area GEC
University of Minnesota
Box 197 Mayo
420 Delaware Street SE
Minneapolis, MN 55455
(612) 624-3904
(612) 624-8448

Mississippi

Mississippi GEC
University of Mississippi
    Medical Center
2500 North State Street
Jackson, MS 39216-4505
(601) 984-6190
(601) 984-6659 fax

Ohio

Western Reserve GEC
12200 Fairhill Road
Cleveland, OH 44120
(216) 368 5433
(216) 368-3118 fax

Oklahoma

Oklahoma GEC
University of Oklahoma
P.O. Box 26901, VAMC 11G
Oklahoma City, OK 73190
(405) 271-8558
(405) 271-3887 fax

Oregon

Oregon GEC
Portland VAMC—Mail Code
    P 3 OGEC
P.O. Box 1034
Portland, OR 97207-1034
(503) 721-7821
(503) 220-3471

Pennsylvania

Delaware Valley
    Mid-Atlantic GEC
University of Pennsylvania
Institute on Aging
3615 Chestnut Street
Philadelphia, PA 19104
(215) 898-3174

Pennsylvania (continued)

GEC of Pennsylvania
University of Pittsburgh
121 University Place
Pittsburgh, PA 15260
(412) 624-5533

Virginia

Virginia GEC
P.O. Box 980228
520 North 12th Street,
    Room B19
Richmond, VA 23298
(804) 828-9060
(804) 828-7905 fax
website: www.vcu.edu

Washington

Northwest GEC
University of Washington,
    HL-23
Seattle, WA 98195
(206) 685-7478

Wisconsin

Wisconsin GEC
Marquette University
Academic Support Facility,
    Room 160
P.O. Box 1881
Milwaukee, WI 53201-1881
(414) 288-3712
(414) 288-1973
website:
    www.marquette.edu/
    wgec

Bureau of Primary Health Care. The Bureau of Primary Health Care promotes the availability of primary, community, and preventive health services, and services for underserved populations.

- *Grants for State Alzheimer's Disease Programs.* In 1990, the Home Health Care and Alzheimer's Disease Amendments to the Public Health Service Act established the Alzheimer's Demonstration Grant Program in the Bureau of Primary Health Care's Division of Programs for Special Populations. The objectives of the program were:

  - To demonstrate how existing public and private nonprofit resources within a State may be more effectively identified, used, and coordinated to deliver appropriate respite care and supportive services to people with Alzheimer's disease and related dementias and their families and caregivers.

  - To identify gaps in the services existing within the community and, where possible, to develop creative approaches to bridge these gaps.

  - To identify and develop strategies to overcome barriers that exist in accessing these services.

The program awarded grants in 1992 to nine State government agencies, the District of Columbia, and Puerto Rico to help them plan, establish, and conduct:

- Diagnostic and treatment services
- Care management
- Respite care
- Day care
- Home health care
- Companion services
- Personal care
- Legal counseling
- Education
- Information dissemination and referral

Alzheimer's Demonstration Grant Program Grantees

California

State of California Department of Health Services
Alzheimer's Disease Program
MS 725, P.O. Box 942732
Sacramento, CA 94234-7320
(916) 327-4662; (916) 327-7763 fax
website: www.dhs.cahwnet.gov/org/ps/cd.c/cdcb/alzheimers/alzindex.htm

District of Columbia

Government of the District of Columbia
DC Office on Aging
441 4th Street NW, Suite 9005
Washington, DC 20005
(202) 724-5622
(202) 724-4979
website: www.ci.washington.dc.us

Florida

Florida Department of Elder Affairs
Division of Programs
440 Esplande Way, Suite 152
Tallahassee, FL 32399-7000
(850) 414-2000
(850) 424-2004 fax
website: www.state.fl.us/doea/doea.html

Maine

State of Maine Department of Human Services
Bureau of Elder and Adult Services
State House Station 11
Augusta, ME 04333-0011
(207) 624-5335
(207) 624-5361
website: www.state.me.us/dhs/beas

Montana

Senior and Long-Term Care
P.O. Box 4210
Helena, MT 59604-4210
(406) 444-4077
(406) 444-4473 fax

Puerto Rico

Puerto Rico Governor's Office of Elderly Affairs
P.O. Box 50063
Old San Juan Station, PR 00902
(787) 721-4560

Information Dissemination

For more information on HRSA programs and publications, contact the Public Information Office listed at the beginning of this entry.

National Center for Research Resources
Building 12A
12 South Drive, MSC 5662
Bethesda, MD 20892-5662
(301) 435-0791
(301) 480-3661 fax
website: http://www.ncrr.nih.gov

Purpose

The National Center for Research Resources (NCRR), a component of the National Institutes of Health (NIH), supports intramural and extramural biomedical research that includes clinical trials, development and studies of animal and other disease models, basic biomedical research, and instrumentation research. NCRR also supports the operation of instrumentation and computer facilities as well as research centers in academic institutions with large minority enrollments.

Programs and Activities

General Clinical Research Center Program. The General Clinical Research Center (GCRC) program supports a national network of centers, which are usually configured as physically separate units within the hospitals at academic medical centers. The primary mission of GCRC is to provide equipment and other resources to investigators who receive their primary support from other components of NIH, other Federal and State agencies, and the private sector.

Most GCRCs generally provide both inpatient and outpatient research facilities within a university-associated hospital setting. The network of GCRCs supports multifaceted research on diseases affecting both children and adults. GCRC research efforts related to Alzheimer's disease range from studies on pathogenesis to clinical drug trials. A list of GCRCs that conduct research on Alzheimer's disease follows.

- GCRCs Active in Alzheimer's Disease

Alabama

University of Alabama at Birmingham GCRC
3-West Jefferson Tower
625 South 19th Street
Birmingham, AL 35233-6909
(205) 934-4852

California

University of California, Los Angeles GCRC
27-066 CHS
10833 LeConte Avenue
Los Angeles, CA 90095-1697
(310) 825-5225

University of California, San Diego GCRC
UCSD Medical Center
200 W. Arbor Drive, #8341
San Diego, CA 92103
(619) 543-6180

Maryland

Johns Hopkins University GCRC
Johns Hopkins University School of Medicine
4940 Eastern Avenue
Baltimore, MD 21224
(410) 550-1850

Massachusetts

Massachusetts Institute of Technology GCRC
50 Ames Street, E17-445
Cambridge, MA 02139
(617) 253-3091

New York

Mt. Sinai School of Medicine GCRC
1184 Fifth Avenue
Box 1027
New York, NY 10029
(212) 241-6045

North Carolina
Duke University GCRC
Duke University Medical Center
Box 3854, 3540 Rankin CRC
Durham, NC 27710
(919) 684-3806
website: www.duke.edu/rankincru

Texas
University of Texas Southwestern Medical Center (Dallas)
    GCRC
5323 Harry Hines Boulevard
Dallas, TX 75235-8891
(214) 590-7783
website: www.crcdec.swmed.edu

Vermont
University of Vermont GCRC
Baird 7
Medical Center Hospital of Vermont
Burlington, VT 05401
(802) 656-2793

Information Dissemination

A directory that describes the program in more detail and lists all GCRCs is available from the Public Information Office at the address listed at the beginning of this entry.

National Institute on Aging
Public Information Office
Building 31, Room 5C27
31 Center Drive
Bethesda, MD 20892
(800) 222-2225
(301) 496-1752
(301) 496-1072 fax

also:
(800) 438-4380 (ADEAR—Alzheimer's Disease Education and Referral Center)

Purpose

The National Institute on Aging (NIA), part of the National Institutes of Health (NIH), is the Federal Government's principal agency for conducting and supporting biomedical, social, and behavioral research on the aging processes and the diseases and special problems of older people.

NIA is also the lead agency in Federal efforts on Alzheimer's disease, housing the Office of Alzheimer's Disease Research (OADR). OADR promotes and encourages the advancement of Alzheimer's disease research programs supported by NIA and NIH, other Federal and State agencies, and private organizations. Within NIA, OADR advises the director and other staff on Alzheimer's-related issues and coordinates and monitors NIA's Alzheimer's disease research activities.

OADR manages an NIH Coordinating Committee on Alzheimer's Disease, and also supports cooperative and collaborative efforts, prepares plans and reports, and organizes national and international conferences and workshops.

Programs and Activities

Neuroscience and Neuropsychology of Aging Program; Dementias of Aging Program. The Neuroscience and Neuropsychology of Aging (NNA) program fosters extramural research and training to further the understanding of aging processes in the structure and functioning of the nervous system. Within NNA, the study of Alzheimer's disease and other disorders associated with the aging nervous system is the special focus of the Dementias of Aging program.

The Dementias of Aging program has four components: basic research, population studies, clinical studies, and research centers. The focus is on basic, clinical, and epidemiological studies of the etiology, diagnosis, and treatment of Alzheimer's disease and other dementias, as well as treatable brain disorders of older people.

Basic Research. The Basic Research program supports research on the etiology of Alzheimer's disease and other age-related neurodegenerative disorders. This research includes studies to identify genes associated with inherited forms of these diseases and biochemical and molecular genetic analysis of the components of amyloid plaques, neurofibrillary tangles, and other abnormal structures found in the brains of people with Alzheimer's disease. Since it has not been proven that plaques and tangles are direct causes of Alzheimer's disease neuropathology, the Basic Research program is also studying other processes and factors that may be involved in nerve cell damage, including cellular communication, the production and processing of proteins, immune system functions, brain metabolism, toxins, and infections.

Population Studies. The Population Studies program supports research in the epidemiology of Alzheimer's disease and on models for large-area registries for Alzheimer's disease and other dementing diseases of later life. Areas of special interest include:

- Domestic, cross-cultural, and international epidemiological studies of age-specific incidence, prevalence rates, and risk factors

- Development and testing of registries for dementing diseases

- Research on the natural histories, clinical courses, comorbid conditions, and causes of death of specific dementing diseases

- Familial studies

- Development of sensitive and specific cognitive and diagnostic screening instruments for heterogeneous and culturally varied populations

Clinical Studies. The Clinical Studies program supports research on diagnosing, treating, and managing people with Alzheimer's disease. The goal of research on diagnosis is to develop reliable and valid diagnostic procedures and instruments. To meet this goal, researchers are seeking preclinical and antemortem biological, chemical, and behavioral markers. They are also testing neuropsychological batteries and brain-imaging techniques and studying the relationship between clinical symptoms and brain pathology.

The Clinical Studies program is also conducting preclinical animal studies and clinical drug trials to find ways to interrupt the course of the disease and, ultimately, prevent it. Research also focuses on managing the behavioral manifestations of Alzheimer's disease—including wandering, insomnia, pacing, agitation, feeding and dressing difficulties, and urinary and fecal incontinence—through drug therapy and behavioral and environmental interventions.

Research Centers. Since 1985, the Alzheimer's Disease Centers (ADC) program has supported a multifaceted approach to research on Alzheimer's disease. This program provides clinical services, conducts basic and clinical research, disseminates professional and public information, and sponsors educational activities. The ADC program also provides core resources to serve as a foundation for developing expanded multidisciplinary research activities on Alzheimer's disease.

Currently, 28 centers are operating at major medical institutions across the Nation. While each of the 28 centers has its unique areas of emphasis, one of the ADC program's advantages is the opportunity it provides for collaborative studies that draw upon the expertise of scientists from many different disciplines. The common goal of the ADC program is to enhance research on Alzheimer's disease by providing a network for sharing new ideas as well as research results.

To expand diagnostic and treatment services in rural and minority communities, and to collect research data from a more diverse population, in 1990 NIA began establishing satellite clinics affiliated with the ADC program. Contact information could be verified for 25 such centers in 1998.

- ADC and Satellite Diagnostic and Treatment Centers

    Alabama

    University of Alabama at Birmingham
    Department of Neurology
    454 Sparks Center
    1720 Seventh Avenue S
    Birmingham, AL 35294
    (205) 934-3847

    California

    University of California, Davis
    Department of Neurology
    Northern California Alzheimer's Disease Center
    Alta Bates-Herrick Hospital
    2001 Dwight Way
    Berkeley, CA 94704
    (510) 204-4444
    Satellites: Oakland, CA; Yolo County, CA

    University of California, Los Angeles
    Department of Neurology and Psychiatry
    710 Westwood Plaza
    Los Angeles, CA 90024-1759
    (310) 206-5238
    website: www.adc.ucla.edu

University of California, San Diego
Alzheimer's Disease Research Center
9500 Gilman Drive
LaJolla, CA 92093-0948
(619) 622-5800
Satellite: Imperial Valley, CA

University of Southern California
Ethel Percy Andrus Gerontology Center
University Park, MC-0191
3715 McClintock Avenue
Los Angeles, CA 90089-0191
(213) 740-7777
Satellite: California State University, Los Angeles, CA

Georgia

Decatur VA Medical Center
Rehabilitation Research and Development Center (151R)
1670 Clairmont Road
Decatur, GA 30033
(404) 728-5064
Satellite: DeKalb-Grady Neighborhood Health Center, Atlanta, GA

Illinois

Rush-Presbyterian/St.Luke's Medical Center
Rush Alzheimer's Disease Center
8 North
710 South Paulina Street
Chicago, IL 60612
(312) 942-4463

Southern Illinois University
Center for Alzheimer's Disease and Related Disorders
SIU School of Medicine
Third Floor
751 N. Rutledge
Springfield, IL 62702
(217) 782-8249
Satellite: Supports 14 hospitals and medical centers serving
95 counties

Indiana

Indiana University
Department of Pathology
MS-A142
Indiana University School of Medicine
635 Barnhill Drive, Room A142
Indianapolis, IN 46202-5120
(317) 278-2030

Kansas

University of Kansas Medical Center
Alzheimer's and Parkinson Disease Center
39th & Rainbow Boulevard
Kansas City, KS 66160-7314
(913) 588-6925
Satellite: Hays, KS

Kentucky

University of Kentucky
Sanders-Brown Research Center on Aging
101 Sanders-Brown Building
800 South Lime
Lexington, KY 40536-0230
(606) 323-6040
Satellites Prestonburg, KY; Hazard, KY; Glasgow, KY;
Johnson City, TN; clinics associated with University of Louisville Medical Center, Louisville, KY; Vanderbilt University
Medical Center, Nashville, TN; and Meharry Medical Center, Nashville, TN

Maryland

The Johns Hopkins Medical Institutions
The Johns Hopkins University
School of Medicine
558 Ross Research Building
720 Rutland Avenue
Baltimore, MD 21205-2182
(410) 955-1535
Satellite: Remote TV assessment project

Massachusetts

Harvard Medical School
Massachusetts General Hospital
Department of Neurology
ACC 830
Fruit Street
Boston, MA 02114
(617) 726-1728
Satellite: Southwestern Vermont Medical Center,
Bennington, VT

Michigan

University of Michigan
Department of Neurology
Michigan Alzheimer's Disease Research Center
3D03, 300 North Ingalls
Ann Arbor, MI 48109-0489
(734) 764-2190
Satellites: Lafayette Clinic, Detroit, MI; Munson Medical
Center, Munson, MI

Minnesota

Mayo Clinic Department of Health Sciences Research
Mayo Clinic
200 First Street SW
Rochester, MN 55905
(507) 284-1324
Satellites: Jacksonville, FL; Guam

Missouri

Washington University
Alzheimer's Disease Research Center
Washington University School of Medicine
4488 Forest Park Avenue, Suite 101
St. Louis, MO 63108
(314) 286-2881
Satellites: St. Louis Health Department, St. Louis Area
Agency on Aging, and St. Louis Regional Hospital; Iowa/
Missouri Consortium for Alzheimer's Disease Clinical Edu-
cation and Outreach

New York

Mt. Sinai School of Medicine
Bronx VA Medical Center
Department of Psychiatry
Mt. Sinai School of Medicine
1 Gustave Levy Place
New York, NY 10029
(212) 241-8329
Satellite: Elmhurst Hospital, Queens, NY

New York University
Aging and Dementia Research Center
Department of Psychiatry (HN312C)
NYU Medical Center
550 First Avenue
New York, NY 10016
(212) 263-5700
Satellite: Brooklyn Alzheimer's Disease Assistance Center,
SUNY Health Sciences Center

University of Rochester
Department of Neurobiology and Anatomy
University of Rochester
Medical Center
601 Elmwood Avenue, Box 603
Rochester, NY 14642
(716) 275-2581
Satellites: Rochester inner city in conjunction with Project
Reach; Bath, NY; Penn Yann, NY; Newark, NY

North Carolina

Duke University
The Joseph and Kathleen Bryan Alzheimer's Disease Re-
search Center at Duke University
Medical Center
2200 W. Main Street
Suite 230
Durham, NC 27705
(919) 286-3228

Ohio

Case Western Reserve University
Alzheimer's Disease Center
University Hospitals of Cleveland
2074 Abington Road
Cleveland, OH 44106
(216) 844-7360
Satellite: Lakewood Hospital, Cleveland, OH

Oregon

Oregon Health Sciences University
3181 South West Sam Jackson Park Road, L226
Portland, OR 97201
(503) 494-6976
Satellites: Multicultural Senior Center, Portland, OR;
Medford, OR

Pennsylvania

University of Pittsburgh
Alzheimer's Disease Research Center
200 Lothropp, 4th Floor
Pittsburgh, PA 15213
(412) 692-2700

Texas

Baylor College of Medicine
Alzheimer's Disease Research Center
Department of Neurology
One Baylor Plaza
Houston, TX 77030
(713) 798-6660

The University of Texas
Southwestern Medical Center at Dallas
Department of Neurology
5323 Harry Hines Boulevard
Dallas, TX 75235-9070
(214) 648-3198
website: www.swmed.edu
Satellites: W.W. Hastings Indian Hospital, Tahlequah, OK,
and Tulsa (OK) City-County Health Department; Dallas

County (TX) Mental Health and Mental Retardation Center
Elder Services; Tyler (TX) Regional Mental Health and
Mental Retardation Center

Washington
University of Washington
Mail Stop GG19
2707 Northeast Blakely
Seattle, WA 98195
(206) 543-6761
Satellite: Mobile unit serving several counties

Drug Discovery and Testing Program. To expand and expedite
the search for drugs to treat Alzheimer's disease, NIA supports
Drug Discovery Groups at six research centers, along with a 30-site
consortium for short-term clinical testing of potentially promising
compounds to slow Alzheimer's disease or relieve some of its symptoms.

The drug discovery project is designed to stimulate research into
the design, development, and testing of novel compounds aimed at
delaying, stopping, or, if possible, reversing the progressive decline
in the cognitive function of people with Alzheimer's disease. It is intended to go beyond efforts already underway at academic research
centers and in the pharmaceutical industry and concentrates on
projects of a more speculative, but potentially effective nature.

- **Drug Discovery Groups**

California
University of California,
    San Diego
9500 Gilman Drive
LaJolla, CA 92093
(619) 534-2305

University of Southern
    California
University Park,
    MC-0191
Los Angeles, CA 90089-0191
(213) 740-5662

Colorado
University of Colorado
Health Sciences Center
4200 East 9th Avenue
Denver, CO 80262
(303) 372-0000

Florida
University of Florida
Gainesville, FL 32610
(352) 392-3261

Illinois

Abbott Laboratories
9MN AP9A
100 Abbott Park Road
Abbott Park, IL 60064
(847) 937-6100

New York

Rockefeller University
1230 York Avenue
New York, NY 10021
(212) 327-8780

- ## Cooperative Clinical Testing Centers

Alabama

University of Alabama at
    Birmingham
Department of Neurology
454 Sparks Center
1720 Seventh Avenue South
Birmingham, AL 35294-0017
(205) 934-3847

California

San Diego VA Medical Cen-
ter
Department of Neurology
3350 LaJolla Village Drive
LaJolla, CA 92161
(619) 552-8585, ext. 3685

University of California,
    Irvine
College of Medicine
2205 Biological Science II
Irvine, CA 92717-4550
(949) 824-6119

University of Southern
    California
Department of Psychiatry
University Park Campus
Los Angeles, CA 90089
(213) 740-2311

Florida

University of Miami School
    of Medicine
MRI Building, 2nd Floor
4300 Alton Road
Miami Beach, FL 33140
(305) 674-2194

Suncoast Gerontology Center
MDC Box 50
12901 Bruce B. Downs Blvd.
Tampa, FL 33612
(813) 974-4355

Georgia

Emory Alzheimer's Disease
    Center
Wesley Woods Center
Department of Neurology
1365 Clifton Road
Atlanta, GA 30322
(404) 728-6682

Illinois

Rush-Presbyterian/
    St. Luke's Medical Center
8 North
710 South Paulina Street
Chicago, IL 60612
(312) 942-3350

Illinois (continued)

Southern Illinois University
Third Floor
751 Rutledge
Springfield, IL 62702
(217) 785-4468

Kansas

Kansas University Medical
    Center
39ᵗʰ & Rainbow Boulevard
Kansas City, KS 66160-7314
(913) 588-6970

Kentucky

University of Kentucky
Center on Aging
Sanders-Brown Building,
    Room 101
South Limestone Street
Lexington, KY 40536-0230
(606) 323-6040

Maryland

Johns Hopkins University
Department of Neurology
Francis Scott Key Medical
    Center
4940 Eastern Avenue, Rm 122
Baltimore, MD 21224
(410) 550-0592

Massachusetts

Harvard Medical School/
    Massachusetts General
    Hospital
Department of Neurology-
    ACC 830
Boston, MA 02114
(617) 726-1728

Massachusetts (continued)

University of Massachusetts
    Medical Center
Department of Neurology
55 Lake Avenue North
Worcester, MA 01665
(508) 856-3081

Michigan

University of Michigan
    Medical Center
Box 0316
Taubman Center, Room 1920
Ann Arbor, MI 48109-0316
(734) 936-9045

Minnesota

Mayo Clinic
Department of Neurology
200 First Avenue SW
Rochester, MN 55905
(507) 284-4006

University of Minnesota
    School of Medicine
FUMC
Box 295,
420 Delaware Avenue SE
Minneapolis, MN 55455
(612) 625-9900

Missouri

Washington University
The Jewish Hospital of St.
    Louis
216 South Kingshighway
    Boulevard
St. Louis, MO 63110
(314) 454-5605

New York

Bronx VAMC
130 W. Kingsbridge Road
Bronx, NY 10468
(718) 584-9000

Burke Rehabilitation
   Hospital
785 Mamaroneck Avenue
White Plains, NY 10605
(914) 948-0050

Columbia University
630 West 168th Street
New York, NY 10032
(212) 854-1754

New York University
   Medical Center
Department of Neurology
   (HN 314)
550 First Avenue
New York, NY 10016
(212) 263-5700

University of Rochester
   Medical Center
Monroe Community Hospital
435 East Henrietta Road
Rochester, NY 14620
(716) 274-6500

North Carolina

Duke University Medical
   Center
Box 2900
Durham, NC 27710
(919) 684-6274

Ohio

University Hospital
   Cleveland
Case Western Reserve
   University
2074 Abington Road
Cleveland, OH 44106
(216) 844-7360

Oregon

Oregon Health Sciences
   University
Department of Neurology
   L226
3181 Southwest Sam
   Jackson Park Road
Portland, OR 97201
(503) 494-6976

Pennsylvania

The Graduate Hospital
Department of Neurology
1 Graduate Plaza
Suite 900, Pepper Pavilion
Philadelphia, PA 19146
(215) 893-2440

University of Pittsburgh
   Hospitals
Suite 400
3600 Forbes Avenue
Pittsburgh, PA 15213
(412) 647-2160

Texas

Baylor College of Medicine
Suite 1801
6550 Fannin
Houston, TX 77030
(713) 798-7416

Texas (continued)

University of Texas
Southwestern Medical
   Center at Dallas
5323 Harry Hines Boulevard
Dallas, TX 75235-9070
(214) 648-3198
website: www.swmed.edu

Washington

University of Washington
Department of Psychiatry
   and Behavioral Sciences
RP-10
Seattle, WA 98195
(206) 768-5304

Awards for Leadership and Excellence in Alzheimer's Disease and Related Dementias. NIA makes Leadership and Excellence in Alzheimer's Disease (LEAD) and Related Dementia awards to senior researchers who have made distinguished achievements in biomedical research in areas relating to Alzheimer's disease and related disorders. Awards are used to support research and to train junior researchers. Recommendations for LEAD awards are made by the National Advisory Council on Aging. Awards are made for 1-year periods, and may be renewed for up to six additional consecutive 1-year periods.

Consortium to Establish a Registry for Alzheimer's Disease. Funded by NIA, the Consortium to Establish a Registry for Alzheimer's Disease (CERAD) is a project to develop a national registry of standardized data on Alzheimer's disease. CERAD involves the work of physicians and scientists at 31 university medical centers who are studying Alzheimer's disease. These investigators share their knowledge and resources in order to develop uniform methods of evaluating the clinical and neuropsychological status of people with Alzheimer's disease.

CERAD is organized into five task forces dedicated to the following purposes:

- Developing uniform assessments for the behavioral and neurological signs and symptoms of Alzheimer's disease

- Standardizing methods of measuring the neuropsychological manifestations of the illness

- Using magnetic resonance imaging to develop uniform rating scales for interpreting the presence and severity of the abnormalities seen in the brain

431

- Providing a standardized method for examining the brain at autopsy

- Establishing a data management center where statisticians, computer experts, and information specialists store, process, and analyze the information obtained from patients and volunteers enrolled as controls in the CERAD project

Other special areas of pursuit in CERAD include:

- Collecting information about Alzheimer's disease in African-Americans and Hispanic Americans

- Establishing criteria for postmortem diagnosis and obtaining autopsy examinations of both nondemented older people and people who had Alzheimer's disease

- Enhancing understanding of the relationship of neuroimaging findings to clinical and neuropathological alterations

- Translating the CERAD clinical and neuropsychological assessment package into other languages for testing Hispanic Americans and other ethnic groups

- **CERAD Principal Investigator**
  Albert Heyman, M.D.
  Duke University Medical Center
  Box 3203
  Durham, NC 27710
  (919) 286-4393
  (919) 286-9319 fax
  e-mail: nash0004@mc.duke.edu
  website: www.mc.duke.edu/depts/neurology/cerad.html
  Data collection for this project is complete.

Intramural Research Program. Scientists in the Intramural Research Program conduct research on the aging process, on age-associated diseases and disabilities, and on various interventions to prevent or reverse age-associated disabilities.

The Laboratory of Neurosciences (LNS) broad research program on Alzheimer's disease and other dementias of the elderly includes studies on diagnosis, clinical presentation, and treatment. Scientists at LNS are also investigating the brain and nervous system changes that take place during development and aging in both animals and humans, coordinating this research with clinical studies of dementia.

Ongoing LNS studies include a longitudinal study and drug trials to test potential treatments for memory loss and dementia. Volunteers participate in either or both types of studies based on interest and medical history. LNS seeks normal, healthy volunteers, as well as volunteers with memory loss, dementia, or depression.

> Laboratory of Neurosciences
> Brain Aging and Dementia
> Building 10, Room 6C414
> National Institutes of Health
> 9000 Rockville Pike
> Bethesda, MD 20892
> (301) 496-4754

Alzheimer's disease research is also a primary focus of the Molecular Neurobiology Unit located at NIA's Gerontology Research Center in Baltimore, Maryland. This unit pursues a basic program on brain aging, molecular changes in Alzheimer's disease, and various experimental interventions.

> Gerontology Research Center
> Johns Hopkins-Bay View Medical Center
> 5600 Nathan Shock Drive
> Baltimore, MD 21224
> (410) 558-8100

Behavioral and Social Research Program. The Behavioral and Social Research (BSR) program supports social and behavioral research and training on aging processes and the place of older people in society.

BSR supports numerous activities related to Alzheimer's disease, including research on reducing burdens of care for Alzheimer's disease and multidisciplinary studies on the design and effectiveness of specialized care units for people with dementia.

- *Special Care Units Initiative.* In Fiscal Year (FY) 1991, NIA began funding multicenter cooperative agreements on special care units (SCUs), the first set of coordinated research projects to identify the components of institutional care associated with "special care" and evaluate the impact on people with dementia, their families, and the health care system.

433

Investigators who are awarded cooperative agreements work with one another and with funding agency program administrators. Collaboration aims to standardize definitions of SCUs, data collection instruments, and analyses wherever possible. A companion initiative on strategies for reducing burdens of care experienced by families and other informal caregivers began in FY 1992. Additionally, NIA is sponsoring a newly established national working group of approximately 50 experts conducting Alzheimer's disease special care research. NIA is also exploring ways to work collaboratively with the Health Care Financing Administration (HCFA) on its Medicare Alzheimer's Disease Demonstration (see HCFA entry).

Information Dissemination

Alzheimer's Disease Education and Referral Center. NIA established the Alzheimer's Disease Education and Referral (ADEAR) Center in 1990 as authorized by Congress through Public Law 99-660, which called for the creation of "a clearinghouse on Alzheimer's disease...to compile, archive, and disseminate information... concerning Alzheimer's disease" for health professionals, people with Alzheimer's disease and their families, and the general public. The center is a national resource for information on diagnosis, treatment issues, patient care, caregiver needs, long-term care, education and training, research activities, and ongoing programs, as well as referrals to resources at both national and State levels.

With special emphasis on identifying and filling information gaps, the ADEAR Center produces and distributes educational materials such as brochures, factsheets, bibliographies, technical publications, and congressional reports. It also maintains the Alzheimer's disease subfile of the online Combined Health Information Database (CHID). CHID contains citations, abstracts, and availability information on patient brochures and factsheets, books and journal articles, audiovisuals, posters, program descriptions, and training materials. Health professionals may obtain searches of the Alzheimer's disease subfile of CHID from the center free of charge.

ADEAR Center staff respond to inquiries by telephone and in writing and are available to assist visitors in using the ADEAR Center library, which includes books, reprints, and reference works, as well as audiovisual equipment for viewing videotapes. The center actively develops collaborative relationships with Federal and State agencies and other intermediary groups, engaging in joint projects and exhibiting at major professional and voluntary meetings.

434

Publications distributed by the ADEAR Center include the *Progress Report on Alzheimer's Disease* and *Alzheimer's Disease: Fact Sheet*. The center also publishes *Connections*, a quarterly newsletter for professionals. For more information and list of ADEAR Center publications, contact:

ADEAR Center
P.O. Box 8250
Silver Spring, MD 20907-8250
(800) 438-4380

National Institute of Allergy and Infectious Diseases

Office of Communications
31Center Drive, MSC 2520
Building 31, Room 7A50
Bethesda, MD 20892-2520
(301) 496-5717

Purpose

The National Institute of Allergy and Infectious Diseases (NIAID), part of the National Institutes of Health (NIH), is the Federal Government's principal agency for research on the causes of allergic, immunologic, and infectious diseases and methods of diagnosing and treating these illnesses.

Programs and Activities

Division of Extramural Research. Alzheimer's disease-related research at NIAID concerns the role of viruses in diseases that affect the brain. This research focuses on scrapie, an infectious agent that produces dementia in animals. Although it is possible that Alzheimer's disease is caused by a communicable agent, this research is primarily based on the hope that the study of viral genetic elements in the brain will lead to a better understanding of the cause of Alzheimer's disease.

NIAID also supports other research concerned with understanding how viruses enter brain cells. Scientists hope to learn how viruses cause disease and the impact of their interaction with the immune system.

Division of Intramural Research. Much of NIAID's intramural research on Alzheimer's disease is conducted at the Institute's Rocky Mountain Laboratory:

435

NIAID Rocky Mountain Laboratory
903 South Fourth Street
Hamilton, MT 59840-2999
(406) 363-3211

Information Dissemination

For information on NIAID publications, contact the Office of Communications listed at the beginning of this entry.

National Institute of Mental Health
Public Inquiries Office
Room 7C-02, MSC 8030
5600 Fishers Lane Rockville, MD 20892-8030
(301) 443-4513

Purpose

The National Institute of Mental Health (NIMH) is part of the National Institutes of Health (NIH). NIMH conducts and supports research to learn more about the causes, prevention, and treatment of mental and emotional illness.

NIMH is committed to promoting and supporting research on multiple aspects of Alzheimer's disease, including work in the neurosciences, the behavioral sciences, and services research. The areas studied range from investigations of potential etiological factors to evaluations and cost-effectiveness studies of promising models for delivering services to people with Alzheimer's disease and their families.

Programs and Activities

Mental Disorders of the Aging Program. NIMH supports extramural Alzheimer's disease research through the Mental Disorders of the Aging Program, which specializes in research to learn how the aging process affects mental health and mental illness.

Studies supported by NIMH cover nearly all aspects of problems surrounding Alzheimer's disease. These include basic science research projects on the fundamental mechanisms of memory and learning as well as investigations into potential etiologic factors explored through neuroanatomy, biochemistry, genetics, electrophysiology and neuroradiography of the disease, and applied science projects focusing on diagnostic techniques and treatment approaches.

The following are specific areas of interest of NIMH:

- Etiology and pathogenesis—Down's syndrome and Alzheimer's disease, genetic studies, neurotransmitters, growth factors, immunocytochemical changes

- Diagnosis and clinical course—biological markers, EEG changes, cognitive screening instruments, evaluation of communication abilities

- Treatment—drug treatment of psychosis and behavioral problems, care in the nursing home, treatment of depression in Alzheimer's disease

- The family—psychosocial needs of family caregivers, health impact of caregiving, caregiving "careers"

- Systems of care—evaluating effectiveness of respite care workers, individual assessment and treatment planning, case management, and referral

- *Family Stress.* On an ongoing basis, NIMH sponsors an announcement soliciting grant applications entitled "Research on Family Stress and the Care of Alzheimer's Disease Victims." Grant recipients have explored such areas as the development of instruments to assess the level of caregiver stress, the effects of stress on caregivers' emotional and physical health, and the effectiveness of various family-based interventions and instruments. This research has contributed to major advances in each of these areas.

Clinical Research Centers. NIMH has established a group of six clinical research centers to explore various aspects of mental functioning in older people. Four of the centers concentrate on Alzheimer's disease research.

- **NIMH Clinical Research Centers**

  California

  Clinical Research Center for the Study of Senile Dementia
  Stanford University School of Medicine
  Stanford, CA 94305
  (650) 723-4000

New York

Geriatric Psychopharmacology Center
New York University Medical Center
550 First Avenue
New York, NY 10016
(212) 263-7300

Ohio

Clinical Research Center for the Study of Alzheimer's Disease
University Hospitals of Cleveland
2074 Abington Road
Cleveland, OH 44106
(216) 844-7360

Pennsylvania

Clinical Research Center on Depression in Residential Care
Facilities
Philadelphia Geriatric Center
5301 Old York Road
Philadelphia, PA 19141
(215) 456-2000

Diagnostic Centers for Familial Alzheimer's Disease. Under a cooperative agreement with the National Institute on Aging (NIA), NIMH funds diagnostic centers for familial Alzheimer's disease at three sites. The centers concentrate on identifying families and collecting diagnostic information and genetic materials for scientific research.

- **NIMH Diagnostic Centers.**

Alabama

University of Alabama
UAB Station
Birmingham, AL 35294
(205) 934-4011

Maryland

Johns Hopkins Hospital
600 North Wolfe, Osler 320
Baltimore, MD 21287-5371
(410) 955-6792

Massachusetts

Massachusetts General
   Hospital
Department of Psychiatry/
   Gerontology (149-9124)
Building 149,
13th Street
Charleston, MA 02129-2060
(617) 726-5571

438

Unit on Geriatric Psychopharmacology. As part of its Laboratory of Clinical Science Intramural Research Program, NIMH maintains a unit on geriatric psychopharmacology dedicated to the study of pharmacologic agents in treating Alzheimer's disease and other mental disorders of older people. These investigators are particularly interested in developing and testing innovative drugs that affect the biologic functioning of various disorders.

This research includes studies to identify early markers for Alzheimer's disease; short-range trials of potential therapeutic agents; and long-term trials with agents of definite theoretical or clinical interest. The unit is also interested in testing the efficacy of combination treatment strategies in Alzheimer's disease.

In addition, the intramural research program seeks to elucidate the frequent overlap of symptoms in people with depression and dementia. Researchers are tracking the variable mood states of people with dementia over time, are searching for clues as to when antidepressant treatment may be indicated, and are developing instruments to quantify and monitor the functional capacities of people with Alzheimer's disease.

Programs for Training Research, Clinical Research, Clinical Personnel, and Research Instrumentation. NIMH administers the Geriatric Mental Health Academic Award Program for psychiatrists and nurses. The purpose of the program is to assist in the development of research-oriented resource faculty members in geriatric mental health in academic settings. Alzheimer's disease is one of the areas addressed by these scientists.

NIMH also supports the development of young investigators with Research Scientist Development Awards, which are primarily focused on research and related educational activities in the area of Alzheimer's disease.

Several research training grants for institutional fellowship programs in geriatric mental health research are funded. NIMH currently supports seven institutional awards for fellowship programs in which the curriculum includes substantial attention to Alzheimer's disease. Seven research training grants in the areas of neuropsychology, neuroimmunology, and behavioral genetics have secondary relevance for Alzheimer's disease.

NIMH administers a three-part clinical training program in mental health and aging. Various mental health disciplines are funded, including individual faculty scholar awards, institutional clinical training grants for minority students, and general clinical training. Curricula address a range of areas, including Alzheimer's disease.

Through its Small Instrumentation Grants Program, NIMH awards grants to universities and hospitals. Recipients purchase equipment for basic research relevant to understanding the etiology of Alzheimer's disease.

Information Dissemination

Efforts include distribution of a factsheet on Alzheimer's disease written especially for families, dissemination of summaries of research findings on Alzheimer's disease, and the writing and editing of textbook chapters and books on Alzheimer's disease by NIMH staff in conjunction with researchers and clinicians in the field.

For information on NIMH publications, contact the Public Inquiries Office listed at the beginning of this entry.

National Institute of Neurological Disorders and Stroke
Information Office
Building 31, Room 8A16
31 Center Drive, MSC 2540
Bethesda, MD 20892-2540
(301) 496-5751

Purpose

The National Institute of Neurological Disorders and Stroke (NINDS), part of the National Institutes of Health (NIH), is the Federal Government's principal agency for research on the causes, prevention, detection, and treatment of neurological diseases and stroke.

Programs and Activities

Division of Demyelinating, Atrophic, and Dementing Disorders.

- *Research on Alzheimer's Disease.* As the principal supporter of neurological research in the United States, NINDS places a high priority on the study of Alzheimer's disease. In both intramural and extramural laboratories, NINDS-supported scientists are pursuing basic studies of brain and brain cell abnormalities associated with dementing disorders; in clinical settings, they are trying to improve the methods of diagnosis and treatment.

440

The following are specific areas of interest of NINDS:

- Epidemiology—genetics, maternal age, and other risk factors; cross-cultural comparisons

- Etiology and pathogenesis—twin studies, behavioral abnormalities in nonhuman aged primates, performance of memory tasks, neuronal size, cortical thickness, neuropathological and neurochemical abnormalities underlying behavioral deficits, neurotransmitter and neuroanatomical alterations in aged mice and monkeys, nerve growth factor

- Diagnosis—familial Alzheimer's disease (genetic linkage, identifying primary molecular events, defining clinical and biochemical disease progression, longitudinal investigations of affected and at-risk subjects), skin patterns, behavioral profiles, psychosocial aspects of presymptomatic testing, biochemical analysis of cerebrospinal fluid

- Clinical course—data from Bronx aging study, gender-based differences, correlations between neuropsychology and silent myocardial infarction, stability of cognition, inverse relationships between dementia and pathology in some groups, stability of general health, neuropathological, neurochemical, and molecular genetic correlations in normal and demented subjects

- Treatment—relation between transmitter system abnormalities and cognitive functional deficits, pathogenesis of selective neurodegeneration, heterogeneity of positron emission tomography (PET) abnormalities, spinal fluid transmitter levels, region-specific cognitive activation procedures with single photon emission computed tomography (SPECT)

- *Research Centers.* NINDS sponsors two centers with interests related to Alzheimer's disease and related disorders:

Florida

Research Center for Cerebral Vascular Disease
University of Miami School of Medicine
1501 NW 9th Avenue
Miami, FL 33136
(305) 547-6731

New York

Research Center for Cerebral Vascular Disease
Cornell University Medical College
1300 York Avenue
New York, NY 10021
(212) 746-5454

- *Training of Research and Clinical Personnel.* NINDS supports trainees and training programs through institutional grants and individual postdoctoral fellowships. NINDS also sponsors three programs designed to aid basic researchers and clinical investigators as they begin their scientific careers. One program supports young basic scientists, another supports young physicians, and the third supports physician researchers. Alzheimer's disease is included among the areas addressed by scientists in these programs.

- *Work Group on Diagnosis of Alzheimer's Disease.* Under the auspices of the Department of Health and Human Services Task Force (now Council) on Alzheimer's Disease, the Work Group on Diagnosis of Alzheimer's Disease was established by NINDS and the Alzheimer's Association. This workgroup provided scientists and physicians with a much-needed expert consensus on the criteria to distinguish probable, possible, and definite Alzheimer's disease. The "Report of the National Institute of Neurological and Communicative Disorders and Stroke-Alzheimer's Disease and Related Disorders Association Work Group under the Auspices of the Department of Health and Human Services Task Force on Alzheimer's Disease" was published in *Neurology* 34: 939-944, 1984. This report has become the standard used by neurologists to diagnose Alzheimer's disease. NINDS continues to sponsor conferences on etiology, pathogenesis, and treatment of Alzheimer's disease independently and in cooperation with other NIH components.

Information Dissemination

NINDS distributes publications that present up-to-date information on Alzheimer's disease. These publications and a collection of articles about Alzheimer's disease are available from the Information Office listed at the beginning of this entry.

National Institute of Nursing Research
Public Information Office
Building 31, Room 5B13
31 Center Drive, MSC 2178
Bethesda, MD 20892
(301) 496-0207

Purpose

The National Institute of Nursing Research (NINR), part of the National Institutes of Health (NIH), provides funding for nursing research and research training. Its programs include research in health promotion and disease prevention, acute and chronic illness, and delivery of nursing care.

Programs and Activities

Acute and Chronic Illness Branch.

- *Highlights of Research and Other Program Activities.* NINR's activities related to Alzheimer's disease focus on helping professional and informal caregivers cope with patients' loss of personality and abilities and their increasing care needs. Behavioral management is a primary topic, including drug therapy and behavioral strategies that can be used by families and professionals.

  The following are specific areas of interest of NINR:

  - Systems of care—effectiveness of special care units in long-term care facilities; effect of hospital discharge and planning procedures on hospitalized older patients, including those with Alzheimer's disease; patterns and processes of rural home care for older adults, including those with Alzheimer's disease
  - Family-based interventions—cultural factors affecting family caregiving, development of curriculum for instructing caregivers, and strategies of care

- *Fellowships, Career Development Awards, and Research Training.* An ongoing NINR program announcement, first issued in 1989, describes NINR interest in supporting pre- and postdoctoral fellowships and career development awards for qualified nurses interested in undertaking Alzheimer's disease and related disorders research training. Applicants for these fellowships are encouraged to seek training sponsors and sites that have established research programs with this focus.

  NINR also participates in a program announcement, along with the National Institute on Aging (NIA), the National Institute of

443

Mental Health (NIMH), and the Agency for Health Care and Policy Research (AHCPR) to seek research, career development, and research training applications on issues in caregiving for Alzheimer's disease and related disorders. The purpose of the program announcement is to provide a broad framework for specifying the range of caregiving, social, behavioral, economic, and health issues in Alzheimer's disease and related disorders.

Information Dissemination

NINR has worked with NIA's Alzheimer's Disease Centers (ADC) to develop educational materials focusing on the cognitive assessment and use of assessment data in managing home health care patients with Alzheimer's disease or related disorders. For more information, contact NIA's Alzheimer's Disease Education and Referral (ADEAR) Center at 800-438-4380.

Chapter 38

State Agencies on Aging

Designated by the Governor and State Legislature, State Agencies on Aging provide leadership and guidance to the agencies and organizations serving the elderly within their State. Serving as advocates for older people, the agencies oversee a complex, statewide service system designed to complement other human service systems. State Agencies on Aging foster the expansion of community-based services and provide policy direction and technical assistance to the Area Agencies on Aging within their States. To learn more about the State aging network, contact your State Agency on Aging.

Alabama

Alabama Commission on Aging
RSA Plaza, Suite 470
770 Washington Avenue
Montgomery, AL 36130
(334) 242-5743
(334) 242-5594 fax
e-mail: mbeck@coa.state.al.us
http://webserver.dsmd.state.al.us/coa

Alaska

Alaska Commission on Aging
Division of Senior Services
Department of Administration
P.O. Box 110209
Juneau, AK 99811-0209
(907) 465-3250
(907) 465-4716 fax
http://www.state.ak.us/local/akpages/ADMIN/dss/homess.htm

Excerpted from *Resource Directory for Older People*, National Institute on Aging, NIH Pub. No. 95-738, March 1996; contact information verified and updated in 1998.

Arizona

Aging and Adult Administration
Department of Economic Security
1789 W. Jefferson, Site Code 950A
Phoenix, AZ 85007
(602) 542-4446
(602) 542-6575 fax

Arkansas

Div. of Aging and Adult Services
Arkansas Dept. of Human Services
P.O. Box 1437, Slot 1412
1417 Donaghey Plaza
South Little Rock, AR 72203-1437
(501) 682-2441
(501) 682-8155 fax
http://ww.dhs.com

California

California Department of Aging
1600 K Street
Sacramento, CA 95814
(916) 322-5290
(916) 324-1903 fax
http://www.aging.state.ca.us

Colorado

Aging and Adult Services
Department of Human Services
110 16th Street, Suite 200
Denver, CO 80202
(303) 620-4147
(303) 620-4191 fax

Connecticut

Community Services Division of
Elderly Services
25 Sigourney Street
Hartford, CT 06106-5033
(860) 424-5277
(203) 424-4966 fax
e-mail: adultserv.dss@po.state.ct.us
http://ww.dss.state.ct.us

Delaware

Delaware Department of
Health and Social Services
Division of Services for Aging
and Adults with Physical
Disabilities
Second Floor Annex
1901 North DuPont Highway
New Castle, DE 19720
(302) 577-4791
or (800) 223-9074
(302) 577-4793 fax

District of Columbia

District of Columbia Office on
Aging
441 4th Street NW
Suite 900 South
Washington, DC 20001
(202) 724-5622
(202) 724-4979 fax
http://www.ci.washington.dc.us

Florida

Department of Elder Affairs
4040 Esplanade Way, Suite 152
Tallahassee, FL 32399-7000
(850) 414-2000
(850) 414-6216 fax
http://www.state.fl.us/doea/doea.
html

Georgia

Division of Aging Services
Dept. of Human Resources
Thirty Sixth Floor
2 Peachtree Street, NW
Atlanta, GA 30303
(404) 657-5258
(404) 657-5285 fax

Idaho

Idaho Commission on Aging
700 W. Jefferson, Room 108
P.O. Box 83720
Boise, ID 83720
(208) 334-3833
(208) 334-3033 fax

Illinois

Illinois Department on Aging
421 E. Capitol Avenue, Suite 100
Springfield, IL 62701-1789
(217) 785-2870
(312) 814-2630 Chicago Office
(217) 785-4477 fax

Indiana

Division of Disability, Aging and
  Rehabilitative Services
Br. of Aging and In-Home Services
402 West Washington Street
Indianapolis, IN 46207-7083
(317) 232-7122 or
toll free in-state (800) 545-7763
(317) 232-7867 fax

Iowa

Department of Elder Affairs
200 Tent Street, 3rd Floor
Des Moines, IA 50309-3609
(515) 281-5187 or
complaint hotline (800) 532-3213
(515) 281-4036 fax

Kansas

Department on Aging
New England Building
503 S. Kansas
Topeka, KS 66603-3404
(913) 296-4986
(785) 296-0256 fax

Kentucky

Kentucky Office of Aging
Cabinet for Families & Children
275 E. Main Street, 5th Floor W.
Frankfort, KY 40621
(502) 564-6930
(502) 564-4595 fax

Louisiana

Governor's Office of Elderly
  Affairs
P.O. Box 80374
Baton Rouge, LA 70898-0374
(504) 342-7100
(504) 342-7133 fax

Maine

Bureau of Elder and Adult
  Services
Department of Human Services
219 Capitol Street
State House, Station 11
Augusta, ME 04333-0011
(207) 624-8060
(207) 624-8124 fax

Maryland

Maryland Office on Aging
State Office Building, Rm 1007
301 West Preston Street
Baltimore, MD 21201-2374
(410) 767-1102
(410) 333-7943 fax

Massachusetts

Massachusetts Executive Office
  of Elder Affairs
One Ashburton Place, 5th Floor
Boston, MA 02108
(617) 727-7750
(617) 727-9368 fax

Michigan

Office of Services to the Aging
P.O. Box 30676
Lansing, MI 48909
(517) 373-8230
(517) 373-7876 Director
(517) 373-4092 fax

Minnesota

Minnesota Board on Aging
444 Lafayette Road
St. Paul, MN 55155-3843
(612) 296-2770 or (800) 882-6262
(612) 297-7855 fax
http://www.dhs.state.mn.us

Mississippi

Div. of Aging and Adult Services
750 North State Street
Jackson, MS 39202
(601) 359-4925
(601) 359-4370 fax
e-mail: elanderson@mdhs.state.
   ms.us
http://www.mdhs.state.ms.us

Missouri

Division on Aging
Department of Social Services
P.O. Box 1337
615 Howerton Court
Jefferson City, MO 65102-1337
(573) 751-3082
(573) 751-8687 fax

Montana

Office on Aging
Department of Family Services
P.O. Box 8005
Helena, MT 59604-8005
(406) 444-5900 or (800) 332-2272
(406) 444-5956 fax

Nebraska

Department on Aging
P.O. Box 95044
301 Centennial Mall
South Lincoln, NE 68509-5044
(402) 471-2307
(402) 471-4619 fax
http://www.hhs.state.ne.us

Nevada

Nevada Div. for Aging Services
340 North 11th Street, Suite 203
Las Vegas, NV 89101
(702) 486-3545
(702) 486-3572 fax

New Hampshire

Div. of Elderly and Adult Services
State Office Park South
115 Pleasant St. Annex Bldg. #1
Concord, NH 03301-3843
(603) 271-4680
(603) 271-4643 fax
http://www.nhworks.state.nh.us

New Jersey

New Jersey Division on Aging
Dept. of Community Affairs
12 Quakerbridge Plaza
Trenton, NJ 08625-0807
(800) 729-8820 or (609) 558-3139
(609) 633-6609 fax

New Mexico

State Agency on Aging
La Villa Rivera Building,
   Ground Floor
228 East Palace Avenue
Santa Fe, NM 87501
(505) 827-7640
(505) 827-7649 fax

New York

NY State Office for the Aging
2 Empire State Plaza
Albany, NY 12223-1251
(800) 342-9871 or (518) 474-8388
(518) 474-0608 fax
e-mail: feedback@aging.state.ny.us
http://www.aging.state.ny.us/
  nysofa

North Carolina

Division of Aging
Taylor Hall, Dorothea Dix
  Hospital Campus
693 Palmer Drive
Raleigh, NC 27603
(919) 733-3983
(919) 733-0443 fax

North Dakota

Department of Human Services
Aging Services Division
600 South 2nd St., Suite 1C
Bismarck, ND 58504-5729
(701) 328-8910
(701) 328-8989 fax

Ohio

Ohio Department of Aging
50 West Broad Street, 9th Floor
Columbus, OH 43215-5928
(614) 644-7967
(614) 466-5741 fax

Oklahoma

Services for the Aging
Department of Human Services
P.O. Box 25352
Oklahoma City, OK 73125
(405) 521-2281 or 521-2327
(405) 521-2086 fax

Oregon

Senior and Disabled Services
  Division
500 Summer Street NE, 2nd Floor
Salem, OR 97310-1015
(503) 945-5811
(503) 373-7823 fax
http://www.sdsd.hr.state.or.us

Pennsylvania

Pennsylvania Dept. of Aging
555 Walnut Street, 5th Floor
Harrisburg, PA 17101-1919
(717) 783-1550
(717) 783-6842 fax

Puerto Rico

Commonwealth of Puerto Rico
Governor's Office of Elderly
  Affairs
P.O. Box 50063, Old San Juan
  Station
San Juan, PR 00902
(787) 721-4560
(787) 721-6510 fax

Rhode Island

Department of Elderly Affairs
160 Pine Street
Providence, RI 02903-3708
(401) 222-2858

South Carolina

Department of Health and
  Human Services
Office on Aging
1801 Main Street
Columbia, SC 29203-8206
(803) 253-6177
(803) 253-4173 fax

South Dakota

Office of Adult Services and
  Aging
Richard F. Kneip Building
700 Governors Drive
Pierre, SD 57501-2291
(605) 773-3656
(605) 773-6834 fax

Tennessee

Commission on Aging
Andrew Jackson Building
500 Deaderick Street
9th Floor
Nashville, TN 37243-0860
(615) 741-2056
(615) 741-3309 fax

Texas

Department on Aging
P.O. Box 12786 Capitol Station
Austin, TX 78711
(512) 424-6840
(512) 424-6890 fax
e-mail: mail@pdoa.state.tx.us
http://www.pdoa.state.tx.us

Utah

Division of Aging and Adult
  Services
Box 45500
120 North 200 West
Salt Lake City, UT 84145-0500
(801) 538-3910
(801) 538-4395 fax
e-mail:
  helengoddard@email.state.
  ut.us

Vermont

Vermont Department of Aging
  and Disabilities
Dept. of Licensing and Protection
Waterbury Complex
103 South Main Street
Waterbury, VT 05671
(802) 241-2345
(802) 241-2358 fax
e-mail: dad@vt.us
http://www.state.vt.us

Virginia

Virginia Dept. for the Aging
1600 Forest Avenue
Suite 102, Preston Bldg.
Richmond, VA 23229
(804) 662-9333
(804) 662-9354 fax
http://www.aging.state.va.us

Virgin Islands

Virgin Islands Department of
  Human Services
Knud Hansen Complex
Building A
1303 Hospital Ground
Charlotte Amalie, VI 00802
(809) 774-1166
(809) 774-3466 fax

Washington

Aging and Adult Services
  Administration
Department of Social and
  Health Services
P.O. Box 45600, M/S 45600
Olympia, WA 98504-5600
(425) 493-2500
(306) 438-8633 fax

West Virginia

West Virginia Commission on
  Aging
Holly Grove, State Capitol
1900 Kanawha Boulevard East
Charleston, WV 25305-0160
(304) 558-3317
(304) 558-0004 fax
e-mail: hollygrove@juno.com

Wisconsin

Bureau of Aging and Long Term
  Care Resources (BALTCR)
Suite 300
217 South Hamilton
Madison, WI 53703
(608) 266-2536
(608) 267-3203 fax

Wyoming

Department of Health
Division on Aging
Hathaway Building, 1st Floor
2300 Capital Avenue
Cheyenne, WY 82002-0480
(307) 777-7986
(307) 777-5340 fax
e-mail:
  wmilto@missc.state.wy.us

Chapter 39

Directory of State Long-Term Care Ombudsman Programs

State Long-Term-Care Ombudsman Programs investigate and resolve complaints made by or on behalf of residents of nursing homes, board and care homes, and similar adult homes. The programs also promotes policies and practices to improve the quality of life, health, safety, and rights of these residents.

Alabama
State LTC Ombudsman
Commission on Aging
770 Washington Avenue
RSA Plaza
Suite 470
Montgomery, AL 36130
(334) 242-5743
(334) 242-5594 fax
e-mail: mbeck@coa.state.al.us
http://webserver.dsmd.state.al.
  us/coa

Excerpted from *Resource Directory for Older People*, National Institute on Aging, NIH Pub. No. 95-738, March 1996; contact information verified and updated in 1998.

Alaska
Office of the LTC Ombudsman
Alaska Commission on Aging
LTC Ombudsman Office
3601 C Street
Suite 260
Anchorage, AK 99503-5209
(907) 563-6393
(907) 561-3862 fax

Arizona
State LTC Ombudsman
Aging and Adult Administration
1789 West Jefferson
Site Code 950A
Phoenix, AZ 85007
(602) 542-4446
(602) 542-6575 fax

Arkansas

State LTC Ombudsman
Department of Human Services
State LTC Ombudsman Office
P.O. Box 1437
Slot 1412
1417 Donaghey Plaza
Little Rock, AR 72203-1437
(501) 682-2441
(501) 682-8155 fax
http://www.dhs.com

California

State LTC Ombudsman
California Department of Aging
1600 K Street
Sacramento, CA 95814
(916) 332-5290
(916) 324-1903 fax
http://www.aging.state.ca.us

Colorado

State LTC Ombudsman
The Legal Center
455 Sherman Street
Suite 130
Denver, CO 80203
(303) 722-0300
(303) 722-0720 fax

Connecticut

State LTC Ombudsman
Elder Services Division
25 Sigourney Street
10th Floor
Hartford, CT 06106-5033
(203) 424-5277
(203) 424-4966 fax
e-mail:
   adultserv.dss@po.state.ct.us
http://www.dss.state.ct.us

Delaware

State LTC Ombudsman
DH&SS Division
Services for the Aging and
   Disabled
1901 N. Dupont Hwy.
"T" Building
New Castle, DE 19710
(302) 453-3820
(302) 368-6565 fax

District of Columbia

State LTC Ombudsman
AARP-Legal Counsel for the
   Elderly
State LTC Ombudsman Office
601 E Street NW, 4th Floor,
   Building A
Washington, DC 20049
(202) 662-4933
(202) 434-6464 fax

Florida

State LTC Ombudsman
State LTC Ombudsman Council
600 S. Calhoun Street
Holland Bldg., Room 270
Tallahassee, FL 32301
(850) 488-2039
(850) 488-5657 fax

Georgia

LTC State Ombudsman
Division of Aging Services
2 Peachtree Street NW
36th Floor
Atlanta, GA 30303
(404) 657-5319
(404) 657-5285 fax

Hawaii

State LTC Ombudsman
Office of the Governor
Executive Office on Aging
250 South Hotel Street
Suite 109
Honolulu, HI 96813
(808) 586-0100
(808) 586-0185 fax
e-mail:
  eoa@mail.health.state.hi.us

Idaho

State LTC Ombudsman
Idaho Commission on Aging
P.O. Box 83720
3380 Americana Terrace, #120
Boise, ID 83720-0007
(208) 334-2220
(208) 334-3033 fax
e-mail: chart@icoa.state.id.us
http://www2.state.id.us/icoa

Illinois

State LTC Ombudsman
Illinois Department on Aging
421 East Capitol Avenue
Springfield, IL 62701
(217) 785-3140
(217) 785-4477 fax

Indiana

State LTC Ombudsman
Division of Aging and Rehabilitation Services
P.O. Box 708
402 West Washington Street,
  #W-454
Indianapolis, IN 46207-7083
(317) 232-7134
(317) 232-7867 fax

Iowa

State LTC Ombudsman
Iowa Dept. of Elder Affairs
Clemens Building
200 10th Street, 3rd Floor
Des Moines, IA 50309-3609
(515) 281-5187
(515) 281-4036 fax
e-mail:
  carl.mcpherson@dea.state.ia.us

Kansas

State LTC Ombudsman
Kansas Department on Aging
New England Building
503 S. Kansas
Topeka, KS 66603-3404
(785) 296-4986
(785) 296-0256 fax
e-mail:
  myrondunvan@aging.wpo.state.ks.us
http://www.aging.wpo.state.ks.us

Kentucky

State LTC Ombudsman
Division of Aging Services
State LTC Ombudsman Office
275 East Main Street, 5th Floor
West Frankfort, KY 40621
(502) 564-6930
(502) 564-4595 fax

Louisiana

State LTC Ombudsman
Governor's Office of Elderly
  Affairs
State LTC Ombudsman Office
412 North 4th Street, 3rd Floor
Baton Rouge, LA 70802
(504) 342-7100
(504) 342-7144 fax

Maine

State LTC Ombudsman Program
21 Bangor Street
P.O. Box 126
Augusta, ME 04332
(207) 621-1079
(207) 621-0509 fax

Maryland

Maryland Office on Aging
301 West Preston St., Rm. 1007
Baltimore, MD 21201
(410) 225-1100
(410) 333-7943 fax

Massachusetts

State LTC Ombudsman
Executive Office of Elder Affairs
One Ashburton Place, 5th Floor
Boston, MA 02108-1518
(617) 727-7750
(617) 727-9368 fax

Michigan

State LTC Ombudsman
Citizens for Better Care
State LTC Ombudsman Office
416 North Homer St., Suite 101
Lansing, MI 48912-4700
(517) 336-6753
(517) 336-7718 fax
e-mail: hturnham@aol.com

Minnesota

State LTC Ombudsman
Office of Ombudsman
85 East 7th Place, Suite 280
St. Paul, MN 55101
(612) 296-0382
(612) 297-5654 fax
http://www.dhs.state.mn.us/ag-
   ing/default.htm

Mississippi

State LTC Ombudsman
Div. of Aging and Adult Services
750 North State Street
Jackson, MS 39202
(601) 359-4926
(601) 359-4370 fax

Missouri

State LTC Ombudsman
Missouri Division of Aging
Department of Social Services
P.O. Box 1337
Jefferson City, MO 65102
(573) 751-3082
(573) 751-8687 fax

Montana

State LTC Ombudsman
Office on Aging
Department of Family Services
P.O. Box 4210
Helena, MT 59604-4210
(406) 444-4077
(406) 444-7743 fax

Nebraska

State LTC Ombudsman
Nebraska Department on Aging
301 Centennial Mall South
P.O. Box 95044
Lincoln, NE 68509-5044
(402) 471-2306
(402) 471-4619 fax

Nevada

State LTC Ombudsman
Compliance Investigator
340 North 11th Street, Suite 203
Las Vegas, NV 89101
(702) 486-3545
(702) 486-3572 fax

New Hampshire

State LTC Ombudsman
Division of Elderly and Adult
  Services
6 Hazen Drive
Concord, NH 03301-6505
(603) 271-4375
(603) 271-4771 fax
http://www.state.nh.us/dhhs/
  ocon.oombud

New Jersey

State LTC Ombudsman
Ombudsman Office for the Insti-
  tutionalized Elderly
Quakerbridge Plaza, Bldg 12B
P.O. Box 807
Trenton, NJ 08625-0807
(609) 588-3614
(609) 588-3365 fax

New Mexico

State LTC Ombudsman
State Agency on Aging State
LTC Ombudsman Office
228 East Palace Avenue
Santa Fe, NM 87501
(505) 827-7640
(505) 827-7649 fax
e-mail:
  ggarcia@nm-us.campus.mci.net

New York

State LTC Ombudsman
New York State Office for the
  Aging
2 Empire State Plaza
Albany, NY 12223-0001
(518) 474-0108
(518) 474-0608 fax
http://aging.state.ny.us/sofa

North Carolina

State LTC Ombudsman
Division of Aging
693 Palmer Drive
Caller Box Number 29531
Raleigh, NC 27626-0531
(919) 733-3983
(919) 733-0443 fax
http://www.dhr.state.nc.us/dhr/
  doa/home.htm

North Dakota

State LTC Ombudsman
Department of Human Services
Aging Services Division
600 S. 2nd Street
Suite 1C
Bismarck, ND 58504-5729
(701) 328-8910
(701) 328-8989 fax
e-mail: sofunh@state.nd.us.hub

Ohio

State LTC Ombudsman
Ohio Department of Aging
50 West Broad Street
9th Floor
Columbus, OH 43215-5928
(614) 466-1221
(614) 466-5741 fax
http://www. state.oh.us/age/

Oklahoma

State LTC Ombudsman
Aging Services Division
Oklahoma Department of
  Human Services
312 NE 28th Street
Oklahoma City, OK 73105
(405) 521-6734
(405) 521-2086 fax

Oregon

State LTC Ombudsman
Office of the LTC Ombudsman
3855 Wolverine NE
Building A, Suite 6
Salem, OR 97310
(503) 378-6533
(503) 373-0852 fax
e-mail: ombud@teleport.com

Pennsylvania

State LTC Ombudsman
Pennsylvania Department of
  Aging
LTC Ombudsman Program
555 Walnut Street
5th Floor
Harrisburg, PA 17101-1919
(717) 783-7247
(717) 772-3382 fax
e-mail:
  ltcomb@aging.state.pa.us

Puerto Rico

State LTC Ombudsman
Governor's Office of Elderly
  Affairs
P.O. Box 50063 Old San Juan
  Station
San Juan, PR 00902
(787) 721-8225
(787) 721-6510 fax

Rhode Island

State LTC Ombudsman
Department of Elderly Affairs
160 Pine Street
Providence, RI 02903-3708
(401) 222-2858
(401) 222-2130 fax

South Carolina

State LTC Ombudsman
Division on Aging
1801 Main Street
Columbia, SC 29202-8206
(803) 253-6177
(803) 253-4173 fax

South Dakota

State LTC Ombudsman
Office of Adult Services and
  Aging
Department of Social Services
700 Governors Drive
Pierre, SD 57501-2291
(605) 773-3656
(605) 773-6834 fax

Tennessee

Acting State LTC Ombudsman
Tennessee Commission on
  Aging
Andrew Jackson Building
9th Floor
500 Deaderick Street
Nashville, TN 37243-0860
(615) 741-2056
(615) 741-3309 fax

Texas

State LTC Ombudsman
Texas Department on Aging
  State
LTC Ombudsman Office
P.O. Box 12786
Austin, TX 78711
(512) 424-6840
(512) 424-6890 fax
e-mail: tdoa@state.tx.us
http://www.tdoa.state.tx.us

Utah

State LTC Ombudsman
Department of Human Services
Div. of Aging and Adult Services
120 North 200 West, Room 325
Salt Lake City, UT 84145
(801) 538-3924
(801) 538-4395 fax
http://www.dhs.state.ut.us

Vermont

State LTC Ombudsman
Vermont Senior Citizen Law
  Project
264 N. Winooski Avenue
P.O. Box 1367
Burlington, VT 05402
(802) 863-5620
(802) 863-7152 fax

Virginia

State LTC Ombudsman Program
Virginia Department for the
  Aging
530 East Main Street, #428
Richmond, VA 23219-2327
(804) 644-2804
(804) 644-5640 fax

Washington

State LTC Ombudsman
South King County MultiService
  Center
State LTC Ombudsman Office
1200 South 336th Street
Federal Way, WA 98003-7452
(800) 562-6028
(253) 874-7831 fax
http://www.home1.gte.net/
  skcmsc/msc.htm

West Virginia

DHHR Specialist
West Virginia Commission on
  Aging
State LTC Ombudsman Office
1900 Kanawha Boulevard East
Charleston, WV 25305-0160
(304) 558-3317
(304) 558-0004 fax

Wisconsin

State LTC Ombudsman
Board on Aging and Long-Term
  Care
214 North Hamilton Street
Madison, Wl 53703-2118
(800) 242-1060
(608) 261-6570 fax

Wyoming

State LTC Ombudsman
Wyoming Senior Citizens Inc.
756 Gilchrist
P.O. Box 94
Wheatland, WY 82201
(307) 322-5553
(307) 322-3283 fax

Chapter 40

Additional Resources for Alzheimer's Disease Patients and Caregivers

Aging Network Services
4400 East-West Highway, Suite 907
Bethesda, MD 20814
(301) 657-4329
(301) 657-3250 fax
http://www.agingnets.com

Mission. Aging Network Services is a nationwide, for-profit network of private-practice geriatric social workers who serve as care managers for older parents who live at a distance.

Services.

- The Network provides comprehensive assessment of older people in their own settings with recommendations and guidance.

- Master's-degreed social workers arrange home care services, select placements, and help older people through life transitions.

- Psychotherapy and consultation are provided for grown children dealing with an aging parent.

Publications. Brochures describe the programs and fees of Aging Network Services.

Excerpts from *Resource Directory for Older People*, National Institute on Aging, NIH Pub. No. 95-738, March 1996, updated and verified in 1998.

Alliance for Aging Research
2021 K Street NW, Suite 305
Washington, DC 20006
(202) 293-2856
(202) 785-8574 fax
http://www.agingresearch.org

Mission. The Alliance for Aging Research is the Nation's leading citizen advocacy organization for promoting scientific research in human aging and working to ensure healthy longevity for all Americans.

Services.

- The Alliance serves as a clearinghouse of information about the state of aging research in the United States and abroad and conducts educational programs to increase communication and understanding among professionals who serve older people.

- At Alliance-sponsored conferences, prominent scientists and policymakers share information about the latest findings in aging research.

- National print and broadcast media campaigns inform the public about the need for more research on human aging.

- The Alliance lobbies for additional funding for research on aging.

Publications. *Alliance Reports* are published periodically. The following are available free of charge: *Investing in Older Women's Health; Improving Health With Antioxidants; It's Time for a Heart to Heart; Everything You Wanted To Know But Were Afraid To Ask—Urinary Incontinence; Meeting the Medical Needs of the Senior Boom; Putting Aging on Hold—Delaying the Diseases of Aging; Americans' Views on Aging;* and *Report of Public Opinion on Healthcare and Medical Research*.

Alzheimer's Association
919 North Michigan Avenue, Suite 1000
Chicago, IL 60611
(800) 272-3900 Information and Referral Service
(312) 335-8700
(312) 335-1110 fax
(312) 335-8882 TTY
http://www.alz.org

Mission. The Alzheimer's Association is a voluntary organization that sponsors public education programs and offers supportive services to patients and families who are coping with Alzheimer's disease (AD).

Services.

- A 24-hour toll-free hotline provides information about Alzheimer's disease and links families with local chapters, which are familiar with community resources and can offer practical suggestions for daily living.

- The Association funds research to find a cure for Alzheimer's disease.

Publications. The *A.D. Newsletter* is distributed quarterly. Educational materials are available in both English and Spanish. A catalog is available on request.

American Association of Critical Care Nurses
101 Columbia
Aliso Viejo, CA 92656-1491
1-800-899-AACN (1-800-899-2226) Information Service
(714) 362-2050
(714) 362-2020 fax
http://www.aacn.org

Mission. The American Association of Critical Care Nurses (AACN) is a not-for-profit professional association dedicated to creating a health care system driven by the needs of patients.

Services.

- AACN offers information on critical care (intensive care), and patients' rights, including the right to execute advance directives (living will and durable power of attorney for health care).

- AACN offers a variety of audiovisual educational offerings.

- Elder groups planning programs on health promotion and maintenance or critical care topics can call AACN's speaker's bureau.

Publications. *Critical Nurse Care* is published six times a year. The *American Journal of Critical Care* is published six times a year. *AACN News*, the member newsletter, is published 12 times a year. A family brochure entitled *It's Critical That You Know* is available in Spanish and English. A catalog of materials is available on request.

American Association of Homes and Services for the Aging
901 E Street NW, Suite 500
Washington, DC 20004-2011
(202) 783-2242; (202) 783-2255
http://www.aahsa.org

Mission. The American Association of Homes and Services for the Aging (AAHSA) is the national association of not-for-profit organizations dedicated to providing quality housing, health, community, and related services to older people. AAHSA's mission is to represent and promote the common interests of its members through leadership, advocacy, education, and other services.

Services.

- To help members meet the social, health, and environmental needs of the people they serve, the AAHSA offers a number of continuing education programs.

- The AAHSA encourages community involvement in homes for the aging to ensure the highest quality of care for residents.

- The AAHSA sponsors the Continuing Care Accreditation Commission, which accredits qualified continuing care retirement communities.

Publications. *Currents*, published monthly, is distributed to AAHSA members and other groups that provide services to older people. For free information on long-term care and housing for older people, send a self-addressed, stamped envelope. A catalog of professional and consumer publications is available free of charge.

American Association of Retired Persons
601 E Street NW
Washington, DC 20049
(202) 434-2277
http://www.aarp.org

Mission. The American Association of Retired Persons (AARP) is a nonprofit organization dedicated to helping older Americans achieve lives of independence, dignity, and purpose.

Services.

- Local AARP chapters, which are listed in the telephone directory, sponsor educational programs on crime prevention, consumer protection, defensive driving, and income tax preparation.

- Members of AARP may participate in group health insurance programs; auto, life, and home insurance programs; an investment program; and an annuity program.

- The Health Care Campaign seeks to contain health care costs for older people and to make health care more responsive to consumer needs.

- Information about the special needs and concerns of older women is provided by the Women's Initiative Program.

- Through legislation and public education, the Worker Equity Program seeks to protect the rights of older workers.

- The Minority Affairs Program works to focus greater public attention on the needs of older members of minority groups.

- The AARP mail-order pharmacy service offers members discounts on brand name and generic prescription medications and a full line of drugstore products.

- AgeLine is a bibliographic database produced by AARP that provides abstracts for documents on issues related to middle age and aging, especially in social, psychological, economic, policy, and health care contexts. AgeLine can be accessed through online search services or a CD-ROM.

Publications. The *AARP Bulletin* is published monthly. *Modern Maturity* is published bimonthly. Publications are available on housing, health, exercise, retirement planning, money management, travel, leisure, and many other topics.

American Bar Association Commission on the Legal Problems of the Elderly

740 15th Street NW
Washington, DC 20005-1022
(202) 662-8690
(202) 662-8698 fax
e-mail: abaelderly@abanet.org
http://www.abanet.org/elderly

Mission. The American Bar Association's Commission on the Legal Problems of the Elderly, through the Fund for Justice and Education, works to expand the availability of legal services for the Nation's elderly. The Commission develops accessible and responsible systems of legal services for older persons by providing training and technical assistance, improving the quality of legal resources, disseminating legal materials, and enhancing public awareness of elder law-related issues.

Services.

- Serves to link the aging network with disability networks and offices of attorneys general.

- Training focuses on housing, health care decisionmaking, elder abuse, guardianship, disability, and ethical issues.

- The Commission is cosponsor of the Joint Conference on Law and Aging.

Publications. Articles are published annually in law journals and aging-policy publications. The Commission publishes *BIFOCAL*, a quarterly newsletter; the bimonthly newsletter *Bulletin to Bar Association Elder Law Committees and Sections*; a booklet jointly done with AARP and the American Medical Association entitled *Shape Your Health Care Future With Health Care Advance Directives*; *Effective Counseling of the Elderly; Where the Nation Stands*; and *Law and Aging Resource Guide*. A complete publication list is available on request.

American Federation for Aging Research

1414 Avenue of the Americas, 18th Floor
New York, NY 10019
(212) 752-2327
(212) 832-2298 fax
e-mail: amsedaging@aol.com
http://www.afar.ccom

Mission. The American Federation for Aging Research (AFAR) is a private, nonprofit, volunteer organization that supports research aimed at understanding the aging process and the diseases and conditions that affect older people.

Services.

- AFAR funds studies on the biomedical mechanisms of aging, genetics, human growth and development, environmental and lifestyle factors and their relationship to aging, and diseases that cause disability or that affect the lifespan.

- Scientific meetings offer formal and informal programs for the exchange of information and research results.

Publications. AFAR distributes a quarterly newsletter and *Putting Aging on Hold: Delaying the Diseases of Old Age*.

American Health Assistance Foundation
15825 Shady Grove Road, Suite 140
Rockville, MD 20850
1-800-437-AHAF (1-800-437-2423) Publications Service
(301) 948-3244
(301) 258-9454 fax
http://www.ahaf.org

Mission. The American Health Assistance Foundation (AHAF) funds scientific research on age-related and degenerative diseases, educates the public about these diseases, and provides financial assistance to Alzheimer's disease patients and their caregivers. AHAF is an umbrella organization that funds three research programs: Alzheimer's Disease Research, National Glaucoma Research, and National Heart Foundation. AHAF also funds a patient/caregiver program—the Alzheimer's Family Relief Program.

Services.

- AHAF supports investigations focusing on the causes of potential cures for Alzheimer's disease, glaucoma, and heart disease and stroke.

- The Alzheimer's Family Relief Program offers emergency grants of up to $500 to Alzheimer's patients and their caregivers in need.

Publications. Single copies of publications are available free. A sample of titles include *Alzheimer's: A Caregiver's Guide and Sourcebook; Through Tara's Eyes: Helping Children Cope With Alzheimer's Disease; Some Answers About Glaucoma; The Facts About Stroke: Protect*

Yourself and Your Loved Ones; and *Some Answers About Coronary Heart Disease*. Contact AHAF for a complete list of available publications.

American Health Care Association

1201 L Street NW
Washington, DC 20005
(202) 842-4444
(202) 842-3860 fax
http://www.ahca.org

Mission. The American Health Care Association (AHCA) is a professional organization that represents the interests of licensed nursing homes, assisted living, and subacute care facilities to Congress, Federal regulatory agencies, and other professional groups. AHCA also provides leadership in dealing with long-term-care issues.

Services.

- AHCA offers continuing education programs for nursing home professionals.

- The public may contact AHCA for educational and consumer materials on long-term care.

Publications. *AHCA Notes*, published monthly, is distributed to Association members, Congress, and the media. *Provider* magazine is published monthly for members. Publications on guardianship, choosing a nursing home or assisted living facility, financing long-term care, and long-term-care services are available to the public.

American Parkinson's Disease Association

1250 Hylan Boulevard, Suite 4B
Staten Island, NY 10305
(800) 223-2732 Information Hotline
(718) 981-8001
(718) 981-4399 fax
http://www.apdaparkinson.com

Mission. The American Parkinson's Disease Association is a volunteer organization that funds research to find a cure for Parkinson's disease, educates the public about the illness, and offers assistance to patients and their families.

Services.

- The toll-free hotline refers callers to local chapters and referral centers providing information about community services, doctors experienced in treating patients with Parkinson's disease, and up-to-date treatment methods.

- Patient education materials are available on Parkinson's disease, speech therapy, exercise, diet, and aids for daily living.

Publications. Publications include *Basic Information; Parkinson's Disease Handbook; Coping With Parkinson's Disease; Be Active; Be Independent; Let's Communicate; Good Nutrition*; and *How to Start a Parkinson's Disease Support Group*.

American Psychiatric Association
1400 K Street NW
Washington, DC 20005
(202) 682-6220
(202) 680-6850
e-mail: ata@psych.org
http://www.psych.org

Mission. The American Psychiatric Association (APA) is a professional society of psychiatrists, medical doctors who specialize in treating people with mental or emotional disorders.

Services.

- APA supports research to improve the diagnosis, treatment, and rehabilitation of people with mental or emotional illness, sets standards for facilities that provide psychiatric care, and offers continuing education programs for psychiatrists.

- The Council on Aging evaluates psychiatric care for older patients and offers training programs in geriatric psychiatry. Issues of particular concern include the use of medicines by older people, nursing home care, and treatment of patients with Alzheimer's disease and other dementias.

- Individuals can contact APA to locate a psychiatrist for consultation.

Publications. *The American Journal of Psychiatry* and the *Journal of Hospital and Community Psychiatry* are published monthly. *Psychiatry News* is distributed twice a month to members.

American Society on Aging
833 Market Street
Suite 511
San Francisco, CA 94103
(415) 974-9600
(415) 974-0300 fax
http://www.asa.asaging.org

Mission. The American Society on Aging (ASA) is a nonprofit, membership organization that informs the public and health professionals about issues affecting the quality of life for older people and promotes innovative approaches to meet these needs.

Services.

- The ASA sponsors professional education opportunities each year.

Publications. *Generations* is published quarterly for members and subscribers, and *Aging Today* is published bimonthly for members and subscribers.

Black Elderly Legal Assistance Support Project
National Bar Association
1225 11th Street NW
Washington, DC 20001
(202) 842-3900
(202) 289-6170 fax
http://www.nationalbar.org

Mission. This project stimulates the involvement of local chapters of the National Bar Association to establish and expand African American and other minority community care coalitions at four sites around the Nation. Outcomes are targeted to the legal assistance needs of African American and other minority elderly.

Services.

- The project uses the professional membership of the National Bar Association, statewide minority bar programs, minority law students, minority bar group alliances, and private attorneys to form linkages with community groups recognized by minority citizens as integral members of their communities and to meet the needs of low-income, vulnerable, African American, and other minority older persons.

Publications. The National Bar Association publishes an annual special issue of its magazine entitled *Elderly and the Law*. They also publish *Saving the Home* and *Defending Against Fraud and Scams*, a resource book on second mortgage frauds.

B'nai B'rith
1640 Rhode Island Avenue NW
Washington, DC 20036
(202) 857-6600
(202) 857-1099 fax
(800) 222-1188 The Caring Network
(800) 500-6533 Travel/Volunteer Programs
e-mail: seniors@bnaibrith.org
http://www.bnaibrith.org

Mission. B'nai B'rith, the world's oldest and largest Jewish service organization, engages in community service, Jewish education, and public advocacy.

Services.

- The B'nai B'rith Center for Senior Housing and Services supports expanded senior housing, advocacy on behalf of senior issues, continuing education, recreation, and travel.

- The program builds and maintains federally subsidized apartment houses for older adults and is developing programs to provide housing for seniors who require more supportive services.

- The CaringNetwork is a fee-for-service program that offers information, referrals, and advice to older persons and their families

- B'nai B'rith offers travel and travel/volunteer programs for seniors and their families.

Publications. The *International Jewish Monthly* magazine is distributed to B'nai B'rith members and subscribers. *B'nai B'rith Senior Housing Network* is a quarterly newsletter for the volunteer leadership and staff of B'nai B'rith senior housing facilities.

471

Brookdale Center on Aging
425 East 25ᵗʰ Street
New York, NY 10010
(800) 64-STAFF
(1-800-647-8233) Information Service
(212) 481-4426
(212) 481-5069 fax
http://www.hunter.cuny.edu.aging

Mission. The Brookdale Center on Aging of Hunter College offers professional training and support to those who provide services to older people.

Services.

- The Center offers up-to-date research and information on aging to policymakers and practitioners in the field of aging.

- The Center's Institute on Law and Rights of Older Adults advocates for the legal rights of older people, conducts conferences and seminars for lawyers and social workers, and publishes free and low-cost materials on elder law issues.

- The Center's National Human Resource Institute offers workshops and professional development programs, as well as videos, books, and curriculum materials.

- Technical assistance is available to local groups starting respite care services for caregivers of those with Alzheimer's disease.

Publications. The *Senior Rights Reporter* is published quarterly; the *Journal of Gerontological Social Work* is published in cooperation with Haworth Press. The *Directory of Legal Services for Older Adults* and *Benefits Checklist* are popular publications. A complete list of publications is available on request.

Catholic Charities U.S.A.
1731 King Street
Suite 200
Alexandria, VA 22314
(703) 549-1390
(703) 549-1656 fax
http://www.catholiccharitiesusa.org

Mission. Catholic Charities U.S.A. is a social service organization that offers assistance to people of all ages with a broad range of social problems and needs.

Services.

- Extensive services are provided to older people, including counseling, homemaker services, foster family programs, group homes and institutional care, public access programs, caregiver services, and emergency assistance and shelter.

- Catholic Charities U.S.A. advocates on behalf of older people in the areas of Social Security benefits, employment opportunities, and housing.

- Catholic Charities U.S.A. conducts studies of the impact of public policy on the welfare of people in need.

Publications. *Charities USA* is published quarterly. *Social Thought* is available quarterly to professionals in social ministry.

The Center for Social Gerontology, Inc.
2307 Shelby Avenue
Ann Arbor, MI 48103-3895
(734) 665-1126
(734) 665-2071 fax
http://www.tcsg.org

Mission. The Center for Social Gerontology, Inc. (TCSG) seeks to ensure that older people at all socioeconomic and health levels can use their talents and abilities to meet their needs. TCSG encourages policymakers to consider the implications of the aging population when formulating social policies. Staff conducts research, offers educational opportunities, and provides technical assistance and training. TCSG sponsors the special project—Strengthening Leadership in Legal Assistance: A Collaborative Two-Tiered Approach.

Services.

- TCSG sponsors regional and national conferences and conducts research on issues affecting older people including legal rights, guardianship and substitute decisionmaking, right to refuse treatment, elder abuse, and employment.

- TCSG conducts demonstration projects in law and aging, provides training programs on legal rights and resources to legal advocates, and offers technical assistance in developing and operating legal aid programs for older Americans.

- Strengthening Leadership in Legal Assistance: A Collaborative Two-Tiered Approach is a special project sponsored by TCSG that provides individualized technical assistance to selected States in an effort to integrate the legal assistance network with the eldercare campaign.

Publications. The Center publishes a newsletter called *Best Practice Notes, Comprehensive Guide to Delivery of Legal Assistance to Older People* and *National Study of Guardianship Systems*. Other monographs and manuals are also available.

Center for the Study of Aging of Albany
706 Madison Avenue
Albany, NY 12208-3604
(518) 465-6927
(518) 462-1339
http://membersaol.com/iapaas

Mission. The Center for the Study of Aging of Albany is a not-for-profit organization dedicated to improving the quality of life for older people through research, education, and training.

Services.

- The Center offers expert technical assistance to researchers, conducts a variety of leadership training seminars, publishes books and manuals, and sponsors national and international conferences on health, fitness, and disease prevention.

- The Center functions as a small think-tank to develop creative programs and policy papers on a variety of topics.

- Information and referral services assist professionals and lay people to locate resources nationally and locally for research and practice.

- Consulting services are available to professionals in such areas as adult day care, mental health, housing, nutrition, physical and mental fitness, disease prevention, and retirement.

Publications. Among the books published by the Center are: *Physical Activity, Aging and Sports Volumes I-IV; Safe Therapeutic Exercise for the Frail Elderly: An Introduction; The Senior Citizen School Volunteer Program: A Manual for Program Implementation; Environment and Aging (2nd Ed.)*; and *Who? Me!? Exercise? Safe Exercises for Persons Over Fifty*. Catalogs are available on request.

Children of Aging Parents
1609 Woodbourne Road
Suite 302-A
Levittown, PA 19057
(800) 227-7294 Information and Referral Service
(215) 945-6900
(215) 945-8720 fax
http://www.experts.com

Mission. Children of Aging Parents (CAPS) is a nonprofit organization that provides information and emotional support to caregivers of older people. CAPS serves as a national clearinghouse for information on resources and issues dealing with older people.

Services.

- Caregivers nationwide can contact the information and referral service to learn about local resources.

- To help the public understand the special needs of older people, CAPS provides "Instant Aging Workshops" for community groups.

- Training programs also are available for nurses and social workers in hospitals, nursing homes, and rehabilitation centers.

- CAPS produces and distributes literature for caregivers.

Publications. The newsletter *Capsule* is published bimonthly for members. Material is available on starting a self-help group. Brochures and factsheets also are available. For information on membership and publications, send $1.00 for printing and handling and a self-addressed, stamped envelope.

The Dana Alliance for Brain Initiatives
1001 G Street NW
Suite 1025
Washington, DC 20001
(202) 737-9200
(202) 737-9204 fax
e-mail: danainfo@dana.org
http://www.dana.org

Mission. The Dana Alliance for Brain Initiatives was created by the Charles A. Dana Foundation to familiarize the public with the benefits of brain research and to call for public support of that research.

The Alliance seeks to educate the public about brain research and its potential to improve the quality of life. The Alliance recognizes that only widespread public understanding and appreciation will translate into the level of public support required to realize the full promise of brain research.

Services.

• The Alliance links policymakers, the press, and the public to experts and resources in the field of neuroscience.

• The Alliance hosts conferences on the brain and brain diseases.

Publications. The Alliance periodically produces and disseminates several publications that provide information about the brain, brain disorders, and brain research. Also available from the Alliance are *Brain Connections*, a source guide to information about brain diseases and disorders, and *The Brain in the News*, a monthly tabloid-size newspaper containing articles reprinted from newspapers around the country on new findings in brain research.

The Alliance can also provide free subscriptions to the Dana Foundation bimonthly newsletter, *Brain Work*, and the Harvard Mahoney Neuroscience Institute quarterly newsletter, *On the Brain*.

Eldercare Locator
Washington, DC
(800) 677-1116
(202) 296-8134 fax
http://www.aoa.dhhs.gov

476

Mission. The Eldercare Locator is a nationwide directory assistance service designed to help older persons and caregivers locate local support resources for aging Americans. The toll-free number is operated as a cooperative partnership of the Administration on Aging, the National Association of Area Agencies on Aging, and the National Association of State Units on Aging.

Services.

- Information specialists give callers the names and telephone numbers of the most appropriate local information and referral resources weekdays from 9 a.m. to 11 p.m. (e.s.t.). The specialist asks the caller for a brief description of the information desired or the problem and for the county and/or city (and ZIP code, if available) of the locale of interest. Callers can receive assistance on current needs or on long-term planning questions.

Publications. A monthly report entitled *Eldercare Locator Selected Call Statistics* is available. Requests taken by phone only.

French Foundation for Alzheimer Research
11620 Wilshire Boulevard, Suite 820
Los Angeles, CA 90025
(800) 477-2243 Information Service
(310) 445-4650
(310) 479-0516 fax

Mission. The mission of the French Foundation for Alzheimer Research is to fund scientific and medical research into the cause, cure, and prevention of Alzheimer's disease and to develop and implement educational and patient care programs.

Services.

- The Foundation, through its International Scientific Advisory Board, funds scientific projects throughout the world.

- The Foundation contributes to conferences and workshops held locally, regionally, and internationally that bring together scientists from all over the world to share research advances and to explore new theories about Alzheimer's disease.

- The Foundation sponsors various programs to foster public awareness, education, and improved patient care with regard to

Alzheimer's disease including providing educational information to families of Alzheimer victims, health professionals, and the general public; funding and coordinating an intergenerational Alzheimer educational program; and supporting patient care programs at local care facilities.

Publications. *Facts about Alzheimer's Disease: A Practitioner's Guide*, by Jeffrey L. Cummings, M.D., and D. Frank Benson, M.D., is available through the Foundation. This factbook is written for physicians, other health professionals, and caregivers to provide basic information concerning recognition and management of Alzheimer's disease.

Huntington's Disease Society of America
158 W 29th Street, 7th floor
New York, NY 10001
(800) 345-4372 hotline
(212) 242-1968
(212) 243-2443 fax
http://hdsa.mgh.harvard.edu

Mission. The Huntington's Disease Society of America (HDSA) is a volunteer organization that serves patients with Huntington's disease, a hereditary, degenerative, neurological disease.

Services.

• HDSA provides information and referral to local support groups, chapter social workers, physicians, nursing homes, and a variety of other resources via local representatives.

• HDSA provides support for research into the causes, treatment, and cure of Huntington's disease.

Publications. HDSA provides written and audiovisual materials pertaining to all aspects of Huntington's disease.

Legal Counsel for the Elderly
601 E Street NW
Washington, DC 20049
(202) 434-2120
(202) 434-6464 fax
(202) 434-6562 TTY
http://www.aarp.org

Mission. Legal Counsel for the Elderly works to expand the availability of legal services to older people and enhance the quality of existing services. It ensures that incapacitated or institutionalized older people receive quality legal care.

Services.

- The National Support Center for Law and Aging provides assistance to local legal and advocacy agencies through materials, training, workshops, and technical assistance.

- Volunteer programs recruit, train, and support volunteers to serve as long-term-care ombudsmen, monitor guardianship and conservatorship cases, and provide bill payer and representative payee assistance.

- The National Volunteer Lawyers Project matches legal cases that impact large numbers of older people with volunteer law firms.

- The Senior Lawyers Project tests ways retired lawyers can provide free legal services to needy older people.

- The National Elderlaw Studies Program provides individual home study courses in elder law as well as a paralegal certificate with the U.S. Department of Agriculture Graduate School.

Publications. Publications include *Elder Law Forum*, a bimonthly newsletter; *Planning for Incapacity: A Self Help Guide to Advance Directives; Finding Legal Help: An Older Person's Guide*; and *Effective Counseling of Older Clients*.

Legal Services for the Elderly
130 West 42nd Street, 17th Floor
New York, NY 10036
(212) 391-0120
(212) 719-1939 fax
e-mail: hn4923@handsnet.org

Mission. Legal Services for the Elderly (LSE) is an advisory center for lawyers who specialize in the legal problems of older persons.

Services.

- The LSE does not provide services directly to clients. Lawyers on the staff offer advice, memoranda of law, and briefs to other lawyers who serve older clients.

- Issues of interest to the LSE include, but are not limited to, Medicaid, Medicare, Social Security, supplemental security income, unemployment insurance, disability, voluntary and involuntary commitment, involuntary committee appointment, conservatorship, intestacy, age discrimination, pensions, elderly rent increase exemptions, rent control/housing, and nursing home care.

Publications. A variety of publications are available including *An Interview Checklist*, covering legal problems specific to the elderly; *LSE Position Paper*, dealing with the legal issues and challenges the elderly confront; *You and the Law, The Right to Work*, focusing on age discrimination in employment; and *More Years, Fewer Dollars*, discussing hotel discounts for senior citizens. A list of other publications is available on request.

National Association for Home Care

228 7ᵗʰ Street SE
Washington, DC 20003
(202) 547-7424
(202) 547-3540 fax
http://www.nahc.org

Mission. The National Association for Home Care (NAHC) is a professional organization that represents a variety of agencies providing home care services, including home health agencies, hospice programs, and homemaker/home health aid agencies.

Services.

- NAHC helps develop appropriate professional standards for agencies that provide home care services.

- Continuing education programs are offered to staff members of home health agencies.

- NAHC monitors Federal and State legislation that affects the delivery of home care services.

- Material on how to select a home care agency is available to the general public.

Publications. *Caring Magazine; Home Care News*; and *NAHC Reports* are published monthly for members. Publications on home care

are distributed by the Association. A list of these materials is available on request.

National Association of Area Agencies on Aging
1112 16th Street NW, Suite 100
Washington, DC 20036-4823
(202) 296-8130
(202) 296-8134 fax
http://www.n4a.org

Mission. The National Association of Area Agencies on Aging (NAAAA) represents the interests of Area Agencies on Aging across the country.

Services.

- Area Agencies on Aging plan, implement, coordinate, monitor, and evaluate home and community-based services such as transportation, legal aid, nutrition programs, housekeeping, senior center activities, shopping activities, employment counseling, preretirement advising, and information and referral programs.

- NAAAA provides the communication, training, and technical assistance necessary to enable the network of agencies on aging to serve and represent older people in an efficient and effective manner.

- An annual training conference and exposition conducted by NAAAA showcases innovative program developments in services to older persons.

Publications. *Network News* is published every other month. The *National Directory for Eldercare Information and Referral: Director of State and Area Agencies on Aging* is published annually.

National Association of State Units on Aging
1225 I Street NW, Suite 725
Washington, DC 20005
(800) 677-1116 Eldercare Locator
(800) 989-6537 Information Service
(202) 898-2578
(202) 898-2583 fax
e-mail: staff@nasua.org
http://nasua.org

Mission. The National Association of State Units on Aging (NASUA) is a national public interest organization that provides information, technical assistance, and professional development support to its members. NASUA works to promote social policy at the Federal and State levels responsive to the needs of older Americans. Staff assist State Units on Aging to better serve older people.

Services.

- The organizational units of NASUA include: communications and development, community services and long-term-care systems development, program management and administration, and elder rights systems development.

- State and territorial Government Units on Aging offer services to improve the social and economic well-being of older persons.

- Member services include reports on current legislative and regulatory issues and policies affecting State programs; training and technical assistance; and an annual membership meeting.

- NASUA regularly communicates with Congress and the Administration, as well as national aging organizations and other human services networks and organizations representing business, industry, and philanthropic interests.

Publications. NASUA develops and maintains publications on a wide range of program and management issues such as the Older Americans Act, State Unit program operations, home- and community-based long-term-care, older worker issues, elder abuse, State long-term-care ombudsman programs, information and referral, employee caregiving, and State leadership in minority aging and nutrition programs. A list of materials is available from NASUA on request.

National Citizens' Coalition for Nursing Home Reform
1424 16th Street NW
Suite 202
Washington, DC 20036-2211
(202) 332-2275
(202) 332-2949 fax
e-mail: nccnhr1@erols.com
http://www.nccnhr.org

Mission. The National Citizens' Coalition for Nursing Home Reform defines and achieves quality for people with long-term-care needs through informed, empowered consumers; effective citizen groups and ombudsman programs; promotion of best practices in care delivery; public policy responsive to consumers needs; and enforcement of consumer-directed health and living standards.

Services.

- Consumer/citizen action and long-term-care ombudsman groups around the country, supported by the Coalition, work on behalf of older people and people with disabilities who are institutionalized.

- The Coalition conducts advocacy training on nursing home and other long-term-care issues, holds an annual education and membership conference, and serves as a clearinghouse of current information on institutional-based, long-term care.

Publications. *Quality Care Advocate* is published bimonthly. The Coalition also distributes informational materials, including *Consumer Perspective on Quality Care: The Resident's Point of View; Community Involvement in Nursing Homes; Alternative Care Approaches to Reduce Use of Restraint (Physical and Chemical)*; and *Nursing Home Law: The Basics*. A technical assistance service keeps subscribers up-to-date on the latest national and model State activities and issues. A list of publications and their cost is available on request.

The National Council on the Aging, Inc.
409 3rd Street SW, Suite 200
Washington, DC 20024
(202) 479-1200
(202) 479-0735 fax
http://www.ncoa.org

Mission. The National Council on the Aging (NCOA)—a private, non-profit organization—serves as a resource for information, training, technical assistance, advocacy, and leadership in all aspects of aging. NCOA seeks to promote the well-being and contributions of older persons and to enhance the field of aging.

Services.

- NCOA advocates on behalf of older Americans and develops innovative methods of meeting the needs of older people.

- NCOA provides a national information and consultation center, offers conferences, conducts research, supports demonstration programs, and maintains a comprehensive library of materials on aging, with emphasis on the psychological, economic, and social aspects of aging.

- Information is available on training programs for older workers, providing services to frail older persons living in their own homes, ensuring access to health and social services, and increasing participation in artistic and cultural programs by older people.

- NCOA's special areas of interest include healthy aging and spirituality, older worker employment, lifelong learning, senior center services, adult day care, long-term care, financial issues and services for elders, senior housing, rural issues, advocacy, intergenerational programs, and volunteers in aging.

Publications. *Perspective on Aging*, NCOA's flagship quarterly magazine, offers cross-cutting issues and emerging practice models. *NCOA Networks*, a membership newspaper, concentrates on fulfilling professional needs with timely legislative and policy news, articles, and funding opportunities and resources. A number of brochures are available on topics of interest to older Americans, their families, and professionals. A catalog of resources and publications is available on request.

National Legal Support for Elderly People With Mental Disabilities
Judge David L. Bazelon Center for Mental Health Law
1101 15th Street NW
Suite 1212
Washington, DC 20005-5002
(202) 467-5730
(202) 223-0409 fax
(202) 467-4232 TTY
http://www.bazelon.org

Mission. The National Legal Support for Elderly People With Mental Disabilities project trains advocates to meet the needs of older mentally disabled people, ensuring that they can age at home with supports that strengthen their individual capabilities.

Services.

- The project writes, produces, and disseminates publications on issues facing older people with mental disabilities.

- The project trains protection and advocacy attorneys in legal aid on laws that protect older people with mental disabilities.

- The project provides technical assistance to attorneys and advocates and case consultation to attorneys.

- The project organizes workshops for the National Joint Conference on Law and Aging and a conference for the National Association of Protection and Advocacy Systems.

Publications. The project has a variety of publications on disability rights for use by elder advocates and mental health and other service providers.

National Long-Term Care Ombudsman Resource Center
National Citizens' Coalition for Nursing Home Reform
1424 16ᵗʰ Street NW, Suite 202
Washington, DC 20036
(202) 332-2275
(202) 332-2949 fax
e-mail: nccnhr1@erols.com
http://www.nccnhr.org

Mission. The National Long-Term Care Ombudsman Resource Center supports the ongoing development and operation of the 52 stateside long-term-care ombudsman programs. These programs function under a Federal mandate to investigate and try to resolve the problems experienced by the residents of long-term-care facilities. The mandate includes both individual and systemic advocacy to improve the quality of life for residents.

Services.

- The Center provides technical assistance to State and regional ombudsman programs in the area of program development, program management, and on substantive issues as they impact residents. The Center provides consultation, training, and printed resource materials. The service is housed at the National Citizens'

Coalition for Nursing Home Reform and is provided in cooperation with the National Association of State Units on Aging.

Publications. *InfoBulletin*, a newsletter published five times a year
for the network, is available on request.

National Long-Term Care Resource Center
Institute for Health Services Research
University of Minnesota School of Public Health
420 Delaware SE
Box 197 Mayo
Minneapolis, MN 55455
(612) 624-5171
(612) 624-5434 fax
e-mail: allen072@tc.umn.edu
http://www.hsr.umn.edu

Mission. The National Long-Term Care Resource Center, a collaboration between the University of Minnesota Institute for Health Services Research and the National Academy of State Health Policy,
assists the aging network to develop, administer, monitor, and refine
community-based long-term-care systems reform.

Services.

- The Center's three focal areas are ethics and decisionmaking (in
  the issues of rights, risks, and responsibilities); links between
  long-term care and acute care, rehabilitation, and health care
  reform; and assessment and case management (emphasizing
  clinical applications).

Publications. A list of publications is available on request.

National Resource and Policy Center on Housing and Long-Term Care
Andrus Gerontology Center
University of Southern California
Los Angeles, CA 90089-0191
(213) 740-1364
(213) 740-7069 fax
http://www.usc.edu/go/hmap

Mission. The Center—in partnership with the National Association of Area Agencies on Aging, Brandeis University, and the National Association of Housing and Redevelopment Officials—works to make housing an integral part of long-term care.

Services.

- The Center helps improve the aging and housing network capacities to plan and coordinate housing and services.

- The Center analyzes best practices in Government-assisted housing, assisted living, home modifications, and naturally occurring retirement communities.

- The Center conducts research and policy analysis and disseminates the results to key audiences. The Center also provides training and technical assistance.

Publications. The Center publishes technical assistance guides, policy briefs, case-study briefs and reports, issues papers on disadvantaged elders, scenarios for future actions, factsheets, and a biannual newsletter.

National Resource Center: Diversity and Long-Term Care
Heller School—Institute for Health Policy
Brandeis University
P.O. Box 9110
Waltham, MA 02254-9110
(800) 456-9966 Information Service

Mission. Brandeis University and San Diego State University jointly organize and conduct the National Resource Center: Diversity and Long-Term Care. The Center concentrates on diversity issues in four areas: resource distribution, infrastructure (systems and services), care strategies, and consumer roles and choices.

Services.

- The Center carries out research, training, technical assistance, and information dissemination.

- The Center assists Federal, State, and local policymakers and practitioners concerned with community care to recognize and respond to the increasing diversity of the frail older population and other disabled and chronically ill persons with respect to race/ethnicity, gender, age cohort and generation, community features (urban/suburban/rural), economic status, and type of disability or chronic disease.

Publications. A list of publications is available on request.

National Resource Center on Long-Term Care
National Association of State Units on Aging
1225 I Street NW, Suite 725
Washington, DC 20005
(202) 898-2578
(202) 898-4794 AgeNet Electronic Bulletin Board
(202) 898-2583 fax
e-mail: staff@nasua.org

Mission. The National Resource Center on Long-Term Care concentrates on development, improvement, and enhancement of home and community-based care (HCBC). The Center emphasizes consumer involvement in all program components.

Services.

- The Center enhances the capacity of State Units on Aging (SUA) and Area Agencies on Aging (AAA) to design, develop, and manage their community-based long-term-care infrastructures.

- The Center assists SUA and AAA in developing program and policy options in response to Federal HCBC policy changes.

- The Center collects, analyzes, and reports on State and local HCBC initiatives.

Publications. The Center provides publications on long-term care and community health services. A list of materials is available on request.

National Senior Citizens Law Center
1101 14th Street NW, Suite 400
Washington, DC 20005
(202) 289-6976
(202) 289-7224 fax
http://www.nsclc.org

Mission. The National Senior Citizens Law Center (NSCLC) provides case consultation, technical assistance, training, and legal assistance support services to local and State aging legal services networks. NSCLC seeks to enhance the capability of these service providers to plan for and deliver legal assistance to at-risk elderly.

Services.

- The Center provides a comprehensive range of litigation and consulting support services. The Center provides technical assistance with Medicare claims and Part A benefits appeals.

Publications. NSCLC produces newsletters, memoranda, an informational monthly mailing on Social Security and SSI for attorneys, training materials, and a series of nursing home manuals.

Project Ayuda
National Association for Hispanic Elderly
Asociacion Nacional Pro Personas Mayores
1452 W Temple, Suite 100
Los Angeles, CA 90026
(213) 487-1922
(213) 385-3014 fax

Mission. Project Ayuda seeks to make the aging network accessible to Hispanic elderly and their families and to broaden the base of agencies and groups involved in providing services to Hispanic elderly. It demonstrates a model of home- and community-based long-term care for Hispanic elderly by developing linkages between the formal and informal long-term-care systems.

Services.

- The Project will develop and disseminate a bilingual resource guide for training church-based volunteer caregivers and produce a 10-minute video on community care and in-home support issues for use in recruiting volunteer caregivers.

- The Project will train volunteer caregivers and conduct pilot tests at three sites. Volunteers will be linked with the formal aging network.

Publications. A 10-minute video and printed resource guide will assist volunteers. Contact the Project for publication information.

United Parkinson Foundation

833 West Washington Boulevard
Chicago, IL 60607
(312) 733-1893
(312) 733-1896 fax
e-mail: ups_itf@msn.com

Mission. The United Parkinson Foundation is a nonprofit organization that provides supportive services to patients with Parkinson's disease and their families and funds research to find a cure for this progressive, neurological condition.

Services.

- Services provided by the Foundation to people with Parkinson's disease include background literature, exercise materials, a quarterly newsletter, personal responses to written inquiries, and a physician referral service.

- Scientific seminars and patient education programs are sponsored by the Foundation.

- The Foundation funds neurological research and distributes information to the public about research in progress.

Publications. A newsletter is distributed quarterly. Other publications include *The Patient Experience; One Step at a Time*; and *The Exercise Program*. A list of materials is available on request.

Chapter 41

Further Reading for Alzheimer's Disease Patients, Caregivers, and Families

Information for AD Patients

Just For You. A booklet for people who have recently heard they have Alzheimer's disease. 1994. 14 pages.

This easy-to-read and colorful booklet is for patients who want information on what may lie ahead for them. It provides answers to common questions such as "Why do I feel this way?" and "How quickly will this get worse?". In addition, it offers suggestions for coping with memory loss, "finding your way", and talking to others.

Available from the Alzheimer Society of Canada. 1320 Yonge Street, Suite 201, Toronto, ON M4T lX2 Canada. (416) 925-3552. PRICE: $1.50.

Musings. Henderson, C.S. 1992. 7 pages.

"I think it's interesting how many places I find to lose things," writes Cary Henderson, a retired professor, in these reflections from a diary that contains his thoughts about coming to terms with Alzheimer's disease. In this often poetic essay, the author shares his views about living with some of his symptoms (his clumsiness, occasional frustrations, handling the stairs, his need to "wiggle through"

Compiled from "Alzheimer's Disease: A Caregiver and Patient Resource List," an undated document produced by the Alzheimer's Disease Education and Referral (ADEAR) Center, and selected citations from the Alzheimer's disease subfile of the Combined Health Information Database (CHID). Please contact the source listed for each item to verify current prices and availability before placing your order.

social situations, or problems feeding the dog) and other aspects of his life: love of music, career interests, and wife and family. With candor and a generous spirit, he touches on a variety of themes that people of all ages who are curious about Alzheimer's disease might want to know. In the way he talks about both the limitations and the satisfactions of his life, he places the desire to adapt ahead of the desire to conceal the many changes that go along with the illness.

Available from the Duke Family Support Program. Box 3600, Duke Medical Center, Durham, NC 27710. (919) 660-7510. PRICE: Single copy free.

My Journey into Alzheimer's Disease. Davis, R. 1989. 140 pages.

A 53-year-old minister of one of the largest Protestant congregations in Miami, Florida, writes about his "sudden unexpected journey into Alzheimer's disease." Beginning with his small-town origins, the author sketches out his struggles through bible school, college, and his early pastoral work. Tracing the course of his work, his confusing symptoms, and eventual diagnosis, the author shares with the reader the ways in which the disease affected his life, work, family, and faith.

The book includes a chapter by the author's wife on changes she noticed in her husband's memory and personality through time. Also included are suggestions people can use to aid the functioning of a patient. For example, he appreciates those who come up to him at social gatherings and tell him their names and when they met. The author often refers to his religious faith and spiritual insights as he struggles to make sense out of what is happening to him. Because his communication skills were starting to deteriorate, the author wanted to record his feelings and emotions while he was still able. His purpose was to become a voice for other people with Alzheimer's disease who are no longer able to express what they think or feel.

Available through religious bookstores or from Tyndale House, Inc. P.O. Box 80, Wheaton IL 60189. (800) 323-9400. PRICE: $7.99 plus $3.50 for shipping and handling.

Painted Diaries: A Mother and Daughter's Experience Through Alzheimer's. Zabbia, K.H. Minneapolis, MN: Fairview Press. 1996. 207 p.

This book tells the story of a mother diagnosed with AD, as told by her daughter. A former newspaper reporter, the mother kept a journal recording the changes caused by AD until she no longer could write. These diary entries show humor and courage in the face of frightening mental and emotional changes. They are woven into the daughter's account of her mother's developing illness and the family's responses. During the mother's illness, the daughter began to express her feelings in artwork. The book includes copies of several of her paintings.

Available from the Fairview Press, 2450 Riverside Avenue South, Minneapolis, MN 55454. 800-544-8207. PRICE: $24.95. ISBN: 157749007X.

Show Me the Way To Go Home. Rose, L. Forest Knolls, CA: Elder Books. 1996. 139 p.

The author presents a first-person story about his struggle with Alzheimer's disease (AD). He recounts his day-to-day experiences and frustrations in coping with the effects of the disease, provides a first-hand account of what it is like to enter a world of memory loss and confusion, and explores his own difficulties in dealing with the diagnosis. He also discusses relationships with his family and friends; use of humor; and encounters with the medical profession.

Available from: Elder Books. PO Box 490, Forest Knolls, CA 94933. (415) 488-9002. PRICE: $10.95. ISBN: 0943873088.

Information for Families and Caregivers

Alzheimer's: A Caregiver's Guide and Sourcebook. Gruetzner, H. 1992. 308 pages.

This book presents information on successful care and management techniques for caregivers. It gives both families and professionals a better understanding of the disease, of the victim's behavior, and of ways to cope effectively with the demands of caring for Alzheimer's patients. The first 10 chapters cover symptoms and stages of Alzheimer's disease, and provide an overview of what to expect as the illness progresses. A special section explores the full range of resources for Alzheimer's disease care available in the community. The book also includes guidelines on locating resources such as diagnostic services, home health services, and nursing home placements, as well as suggestions on reducing caregiver stress. The last three chapters describe current research and treatment possibilities. 271 references.

Available from American Health Assistance Foundation. 15825 Shady Grove Road, Suite 140, Rockville, MD 20850. (800) 437-2423.

493

PRICE: $9.00. Also available from John Wiley & Sons, Inc. 1 Wiley Drive, Somerset, NJ 08875-1272. (800) 225-5945. Also available through bookstores. PRICE: $14.95.

Alzheimer's: Answers to Hard Questions for Families. Nelson, J.L.; Nelson, H.L. New York, NY: Doubleday Dell Publishing Group. 1996. 224 p.

This book describes problems families of AD patients may face at different stages of the illness and gives tips for handling financial, ethical, and moral issues. The authors encourage frequent family meetings throughout the disease course to discuss concerns, assign responsibilities, and make care decisions. They recommend including early-stage patients in at least some of the family meetings and advance planning. Stories highlight the importance of family communication.

Available from the Doubleday Dell Publishing Group, Doubleday Publicity Department, 1540 Broadway, New York, NY 10036. (212) 782-9791. PRICE: $21.95. ISBN: 0385485336.

Caring for the Alzheimer Patient: A Practical Guide. 3rd ed. Dippel, R.L.; Hutton, J.T., eds. Amherst, NY: Prometheus Books. 1996. 219 p.

This book is designed for family members of AD patients and professional caregivers. The authors describe the importance of exercise and a proper diet; optimal living environments; techniques for enhancing patients' memory, orientation, and ability to communicate with others; behavioral management techniques; and nursing home selection. This book also discusses the treatment of older people with neurological impairments, family support services, and legal and ethical issues.

Available from Prometheus Books, Warehouse and Fulfillment Center, 59 John Glenn Drive, Amherst, NY 14228-2197. (800) 421-0351; (716) 691-0133 (outside the United States); (716) 691-0137 fax. PRICE: $16.95. ISBN: 1573921084.

Caring for the Caregiver: A Guide to Living with Alzheimer's Disease. Parke-Davis. 1994. 171 pages.

This practical, easy-to-read guidebook is designed for caregivers of patients with Alzheimer's disease (AD). It presents ways caregivers can help themselves through the caregiving process. Topic areas are separated by colorful index tabs and include: symptoms and stages of AD; caring for the caregiver; and combating caregiver stress. It also provides medical information about the causes of and treatments for AD, lists some guidelines for financial planning and management, and covers legal and ethical issues.

In addition, this guidebook discusses home safety and security; daily challenges of caring for an AD patient in the home; and easing caregiver burden through family and friends, support groups, family counseling services, and adult day care. It also includes a section with space for notes on a patient's daily care so that another caregiver can replace the primary caregiver periodically. 19 references.

Available from Parke-Davis. Product Information, 201 Tabor Road, Morris Plains, NJ 07950. (800) 223-0432. PRICE: Single copy free.

Family Caregiving in the U.S.: Findings from a National Survey. Final Report. Bethesda, MD: National Alliance for Caregiving. June 1997. 40 p.

This report presents the results of a nationwide telephone survey designed to summarize the experiences and attitudes of family members caring for older loved ones. Selected findings include: prevalence of care-giving in the United States; demographics of caregivers; a profile of care recipients, including age (average age: 77 years) and the presence of dementia; numbers of hours of care and activities performed; medication management; stresses of caregiving; coping mechanisms; biggest difficulty and greatest reward of caregiving; use of supportive services; unmet needs for help, information, or support; and effect of caregiving on work.

Available from the National Alliance for Caregiving, 4720 Montgomery Lane, Bethesda, MD 20814. PRICE: Free.

Home Is Where I Remember Things: A Curriculum for Home and Community Alzheimer Care. Gwyther, L.P. Raleigh, NC: North Carolina Department of Human Resources. 1997. 214 p.

This manual is designed for home and professional care providers working with AD patients. Topics include what it is like to have AD; how to talk with people who have AD; helping patients with daily activities; protecting AD patients; and issues in early-, middle-, and late-stage AD. Extensive appendices describe AD; and present guidelines for understanding the person with AD, handling challenging behaviors, administering medications, and ensuring home safety.

Available from the North Carolina Department of Human Resources, Division of Aging, CB 29531, Raleigh, NC 27626-0531. (919) 733-3983. PRICE: $13 plus $2 shipping and handling.

Home Safety for the Alzheimer's Patient. San Diego, CA: Alzheimer's Disease Center, University of California-San Diego Medical Center. 1989. 31 pages. Also available in Spanish.

This easy-to-read booklet is for people who provide in-home care for people with Alzheimer's disease or related disorders. It is organized to help caregivers make each room in their homes safer for the person for whom they are caring. It can help caregivers to cope with some of the challenges they face each day and to find creative solutions for their own and the patient's well-being.

Following a brief discussion of the nature of Alzheimer's disease, the booklet describes some of the caregiver problems associated with the disease and general safety considerations. The text then focuses on home safety on a room-by-room basis (kitchen, bedroom, bathroom, living room, laundry room, entryway, and outside approaches), home safety behavior management (wandering, rummaging/hiding things, hallucinations/delusions, and impairment of the senses), driving, and natural disaster safety.

Available from the Alzheimer's Disease Education and Referral (ADEAR) Center. P.O. Box 8250, Silver Spring, MD 20907-8250. (800) 438-4380. PRICE: $2.50.

Rush Manual for Caregivers. Revised edition. Rush Alzheimer's Disease Center. 1994. 118 pages.

This manual provides an overview of the issues that family members with relatives with Alzheimer's disease (AD) often face when they cope with dementia. Chapters describe dementia, give some information about the stages of AD, and suggest ways to bridge the communication gap that dementia creates.

This manual also outlines guidelines for providing daily care (hygiene, home safety, mobility and exercise, and nutrition) and dealing with important health and behavior problems. It addresses ways to obtain outside help, such as from community and government resources, and guidelines for selecting a nursing home or hospice care. The manual concludes with lists of selected readings for families with a member who has dementia and for professionals concerning such

496

areas as activities, public policy, and nursing home care. 30 references.

Available from the Rush Alzheimer's Disease Center. Attn: Ms. Meloney Knighton, 710 South Paulina, 8 North, Chicago, IL 60612. (312) 942-4463. PRICE: $20.00.

The 36-Hour Day: A Family Guide to Caring for Persons with Alzheimer's Disease, Related Dementing Illnesses, and Memory Loss in Later Life. Revised edition. Mace, R.L.; Rabins, P.V. 1991. 329 pages.

This reference book provides information to families about giving care to patients with Alzheimer's disease or related disorders. The book presents background information on dementia, brain disorders, and the causes of dementia. Beginning with the problem of getting medical help (both accurate diagnosis and treatment) for the impaired person, the book gives practical suggestions and advice on how families and caregivers can deal with problems arising in daily care; medical problems; problems of behavior and mood; getting outside help; financial and legal issues; nursing homes and other living arrangements; and the impact of caring for an impaired person. References in the back list health and support organizations; where to buy or rent supplies; U.S., State, and protectorate agencies; and the rights of hospital and nursing home patients. 43 references.

Available from the Johns Hopkins University Press. 701 West 40th Street, Baltimore, MD 21211. (800) 537-5487. PRICE: $11.95 plus $3.00 shipping and handling (Maryland residents add 5 percent sales tax). Also available through bookstores.

When Someone You Love Has Alzheimer's Disease: The Caregiver's Journey. Grollman, E.A.; Kosik, K.S. Boston, MA: Beacon Press. 1996. 163 p.

This book for families and friends of AD patients offers, in brief statements, insights based on personal experiences. It describes the range of emotions that families and loved ones may experience. The authors discuss spiritual and emotional issues. Their advice to caregivers is presented in short topical sections such as guilt, quiet times, crying, laughing, and accepting changes. Answers to frequently asked questions provide information about symptoms, progression, patient care, genetic factors, and safety.

Available from the Beacon Press, 25 Beacon Street, Boston, MA 02108-2892. (617) 742-2110; (617) 742-2290. PRICE: $22. ISBN: 0807027200.

Where Did Mary Go? A Loving Husband's Struggle With Alzheimer's. Wall, F.A. Amherst, NY: Prometheus Books. 1996. 148 p.

The author shares a personal account of his own and his wife's struggle with her Parkinson's disease, multi-infarct dementia, and AD. As the primary caregiver, the author candidly discusses his new-found roles and the stress- and emotion-filled time as his wife gradually got worse. This book is designed to explain some of the challenges other family caregivers may face as dementias progress, including some of the signals, symptoms, and reactions to mental confusion, incontinence, falling, wandering, and other related problems.

Available from Prometheus Books. 59 John Glenn Drive, Amherst, NY 14228-2197. (716) 691-0133; (716) 691-0137 fax. PRICE: $19.95. ISBN: 1573920703.

Index

Page numbers followed by 'n' indicate a footnote. Page numbers in *italics* indicate a table or illustration

A

A. D. Newsletter 463
AA *see* Alzheimer's Association (AA)
AACN News 463
AARP *see* Retired Persons, American Association of (AARP)
AARP Bulletin 465
Abbott Laboratories, Drug Discovery Groups 428
acetaminophin 250
acetylcholine (ACh)
  Alzheimer's disease 29, 34–35, 248
  brain cells 11, 187–88, 223
  defined 369
  see also neurotransmitters
ACh *see* acetylcholine (ACh)
activities of daily living (ADL)
  confusional states 176
  defined 369
  mental status testing 92
  see also instrumental activities of daily living (IADL)

Adalat (theophyllin), side effects 160
ADAP *see* Alzheimer's disease associated protein (ADAP)
ADC *see* AIDS dementia complex (ADC)
ADEAR *see* Alzheimer's Disease Education and Referral (ADEAR) Center
adenine, defined 120
ADL *see* activities of daily living (ADL)
ADRD *see* Alzheimer's disease and related dementias (ADRD)
Adult Daycare, National Institute of 410
advance directives (living wills)
  legal issues 358–60
  nursing homes 338
Advil (ibuprofen) 250
African Americans 47–65
age factor
  Huntington's disease 122–24
  mental status testing 93, 161
Aging 383
Aging, Administration on (AoA)
  Alzheimer's Disease programs 41
  Community Eldercare Awareness Campaigns 382
  community services 381

501

Index